Marine Anti-Inflammatory and Antioxidant Agents, 4th Edition

Marine Anti-Inflammatory and Antioxidant Agents, 4th Edition

Guest Editors

Donatella Degl'Innocenti
Marzia Vasarri

MDPI

Basel • Beijing • Wuhan • Barcelona • Belgrade • Novi Sad • Cluj • Manchester

Guest Editors

Donatella Degl'Innocenti
Department of Experimental and Clinical Biomedical Sciences
University of Florence
Florence
Italy

Marzia Vasarri
Department of Experimental and Clinical Biomedical Sciences
University of Florence
Florence
Italy

Editorial Office
MDPI AG
Grosspeteranlage 5
4052 Basel, Switzerland

This is a reprint of the Special Issue, published open access by the journal *Marine Drugs* (ISSN 1660-3397), freely accessible at: https://www.mdpi.com/journal/marinedrugs/special_issues/7BO7C045WT.

For citation purposes, cite each article independently as indicated on the article page online and as indicated below:

Lastname, A.A.; Lastname, B.B. Article Title. *Journal Name* **Year**, *Volume Number*, Page Range.

ISBN 978-3-7258-5311-3 (Hbk)
ISBN 978-3-7258-5312-0 (PDF)
https://doi.org/10.3390/books978-3-7258-5312-0

Cover image courtesy of Marzia Vasarri

Contents

About the Editors

Donatella Degl'Innocenti

Donatella Degl'Innocenti is Associate Professor of Biochemistry at the Department of Experimental and Clinical Biomedical Sciences "Mario Serio" at the University of Florence (Italy), where she has been a faculty member since 2001. She holds a Ph.D. in Biochemistry and has developed a strong national and international research network throughout her career. Prof. Degl'Innocenti leads an active research laboratory focused on the biochemical properties of natural and marine-derived compounds and their potential health benefits. Her work has contributed significantly to understanding the molecular mechanisms underlying oxidative stress, inflammation, and cancer progression. In particular, her recent studies have examined the health-promoting properties of natural and marine-derived compounds from marine plants in different in vitro and in vivo models. Her work also actively addresses oxidative stress in rare genetic diseases, enhancing the translational impact of her research. She is the senior author of numerous peer-reviewed publications in international journals and is a member of the Scientific Committee of the Interuniversity Center of Marine Biology and Applied Ecology (CIBM) in Livorno (Italy). Her research continues to advance the interface between marine biochemistry and human health.

Marzia Vasarri

Marzia Vasarri is a Postdoctoral Fellow at the Department of Experimental and Clinical Biomedical Sciences "Mario Serio" at the University of Florence (Italy). She holds a Ph.D. in Biomedical Sciences (2021), following her bachelor's degree in Biotechnology (2014) and master's degree in Medical and Pharmaceutical Biotechnology (2016). Her academic and research background is rooted in biochemistry and molecular biology. Dr. Vasarri's research focuses on the biochemical and functional characterization of natural bioactive compounds, particularly phytochemicals derived from marine sources. Her work explores the mechanisms of action and signaling pathways of these marine compounds involved in the modulation of key biological processes such as inflammation, oxidative stress, apoptosis, autophagy, protein glycation, and cancer cell migration. Since 2017, she has contributed to multidisciplinary research projects employing both in vitro and in vivo models. In addition to natural products research, Dr. Vasarri has developed expertise in nanotechnology-based delivery systems aimed at enhancing the bioavailability of poorly soluble compounds. She has also participated in studies on the oxidative stress of rare genetic diseases. Dr. Vasarri is the author of multiple peer-reviewed publications and is actively involved in advancing marine drug discovery and complementary medicine. Her research reflects a strong commitment to exploring marine compounds as a promising source of novel potential therapeutic agents.

Preface

The Reprint, "Marine Anti-Inflammatory and Antioxidant Agents, 4th Edition," presents a timely and comprehensive collection of recent scientific advances in the exploration of marine-derived compounds with dual antioxidant and anti-inflammatory activity. This compilation reflects the growing recognition of chronic inflammation and oxidative stress as central mechanisms driving myriad health conditions.

Marine organisms and microorganisms represent a largely untapped reservoir of bioactive metabolites. These unique compounds show immense potential to modulate key molecular pathways involved in inflammation and oxidative damage. The exploration of marine biodiversity, therefore, holds significant promise for identifying new compounds while supporting the sustainable development of marine therapeutic bioresources.

This Reprint includes original research and review articles that cover a diverse range of topics, from the isolation and structural analysis of marine natural products to their biological evaluation in different disease models. Several contributions also explore practical applications in human health, skincare, and functional foods. The multidisciplinary nature of this volume underscores the dynamic intersection of biochemistry and marine natural products.

Our aim in assembling this fourth edition was to highlight the remarkable progress in this field, while also encouraging further exploration of the marine environment as a source of safe, effective, and sustainable health solutions. This collection is addressed to researchers in marine biotechnology, natural product chemistry, pharmacology, and related biomedical disciplines. It is also relevant for graduate students, clinicians, and professionals engaged in drug discovery and development, particularly those focused on natural and environmentally friendly approaches. We hope this collection will serve as a valuable reference and stimulate further interdisciplinary collaborations aimed at unlocking the full therapeutic potential of our seas.

Donatella Degl'Innocenti and Marzia Vasarri
Guest Editors

marine drugs

MDPI

Editorial

Exploring Marine-Derived Antioxidant and Anti-Inflammatory Agents: Findings from Recent Studies

Marzia Vasarri [1,*] and Donatella Degl'Innocenti [1,2]

1 Department of Experimental and Clinical Biomedical Sciences, University of Florence, Viale Morgagni 50, 50134 Florence, Italy
2 Interuniversity Center of Marine Biology and Applied Ecology "G. Bacci" (CIBM), Viale N. Sauro 4, 57128 Leghorn, Italy; donatella.deglinnocenti@unifi.it
* Correspondence: marzia.vasarri@unifi.it

The Special Issue "Marine Anti-Inflammatory and Antioxidant Agents, 4th Edition" of *Marine Drugs* underscores the immense therapeutic potential embedded within our planet's vast marine environments. As a prolific reservoir of bioactive compounds, the seas have emerged as a vital source for discovering agents capable of targeting fundamental processes such as inflammation and oxidative stress—key contributors to numerous chronic diseases. This collection of research emphasizes a holistic approach that integrates natural marine compounds, advanced delivery systems, and diverse applications across health domains, illustrating the interconnectedness of immune modulation, antioxidative defense, and disease mitigation.

One of the themes of this Special Issue revolves around marine-derived modulators of immune activation and migration. For instance, in Contribution 1, Liu et al. (2025) demonstrate that alternariol (AOH), a secondary metabolite produced by marine fungi *Alternaria sp.*, can suppress T cell proliferation, cytokine secretion, and migration, thereby reducing lung inflammation in vivo. Such findings highlight the precision with which marine fungal metabolites can modulate immune responses, offering promising strategies for autoimmune and allergic conditions. Complementing this, Niu et al. (2024) in Contribution 2 investigate Butyrolactone-I (BTL-I), a bioactive compound from deep-sea fungus *Aspergillus* C23-3, which protects intestinal cells and mice from heat-stress-induced oxidative damage and apoptosis. This work reveals that BTL-I reduces heat stress markers (HSP70 and HSP90), diminishes oxidative stress indicators (ROS and MDA), and enhances antioxidant enzyme activity (SOD). Importantly, BTL-I attenuates apoptosis, thereby bolstering intestinal resilience under stress—an approach aligned with the sustainable management of livestock in the context of climate change.

The scope of marine bioactivities extends into natural antioxidants that can be used to promote skin health and provide systemic protection. In Contribution 3, Yang et al. (2024) provide compelling evidence that a peptide derived from seahorse (*Hippocampus abdominalis*) hydrolysate (SHP2) mitigates UVB-induced skin damage by reducing ROS levels, improving cell viability, and promoting collagen synthesis in human keratinocytes and fibroblasts. This work also demonstrates photoaging inhibition in zebrafish models, highlighting SHP2's potential in cosmetic formulations aimed at preventing skin photoaging. Furthermore, marine-derived peptides from the blue mussel Mytilus edulis are shown to exhibit promising cardiovascular benefits in Contribution 4 by Marasinghe et al., 2024; they inhibit foam cell formation and inflammation in macrophages by modulating lipid metabolism and inflammatory pathways, showcasing the translational potential of marine biochemistry in cardiovascular health.

Nutritional applications of marine resources also feature prominently. In Contribution 5, Joshi et al. (2025) develop an enzymatically stabilized squid oil enriched with omega-3 fatty acids and astaxanthin, which demonstrates enhanced oxidative stability and nutritional retention, supporting dietary strategies to combat inflammation.

Similarly, in Contribution 6, Shu et al. (2024) explore a sea cucumber polydeoxyribonucleotide from *Apostichopus japonicus* sperm (AJS-PDRN), revealing its potent free radical scavenging properties and capacity to protect macrophages from oxidative damage. Their findings suggest that AJS-PDRN can modulate immune responses, promote membrane repair, and bolster antioxidant defenses through multiple pathways.

Further exploring anti-inflammatory and antioxidant agents, in Contribution 7, Dörschmann et al. (2025) investigate a very high-molecular-weight fucoidan (FucBB04) from the brown seaweed *Laminaria hyperborea* for potential therapeutic effects in age-related macular degeneration (AMD) models in vitro. While FucBB04 reduced inflammatory cytokine secretion (IL-6 and IL-8) and modulated VEGF levels, it did not provide antioxidant protection and negatively impacted key retinal pigment epithelium (RPE) functions. These findings suggest that although high-molecular-weight fucoidans exhibit some bioactivity against AMD-related pathways, their adverse effects on RPE cell functions highlight the need for further research with smaller-molecular-weight variants. Complementary to these findings, alginate extracted from the brown seaweed *Ericaria crinita* by Lukova et al. (2024) in Contribution 8 shows promise due to its free radical scavenging and cytokine-modulating activities, notably reducing pro-inflammatory cytokines like TNF-α and IL-6 in models of systemic inflammation. These insights point toward marine polysaccharides as versatile candidates for anti-inflammatory therapies, although further mechanistic studies are necessary.

Among research on seaweeds bioactivities, Lee et al. (2025) demonstrate in Contribution 9 that a water extract of the green seaweed *Codium fragile* (WCF), rich in bioactive oleamide (9-octadecenamide), exhibits significant anti-inflammatory, antioxidant, and anti-fibrotic effects in a mouse model of allergic asthma induced by ovalbumin. WCF modulates immune responses by reducing Th2 cytokines, eosinophil infiltration, and IgE levels, while alleviating airway inflammation, mucus overproduction, and tissue fibrosis. Mechanistically, it suppresses the TLR4/NF-κB and TGF-β1/Smad signaling pathways, decreases pro-inflammatory cytokines, oxidative stress markers, and fibrosis-related proteins, and protects against apoptosis. Overall, WCF shows promise as a natural therapeutic agent for allergic respiratory diseases.

Expanding on anti-inflammatory strategies, in Contribution 10, Pruvost et al. (2024) illustrate that nanocarriers composed of chondroitin sulfate and lipids derived from salmon (*Salmo salar*) can significantly diminish inflammatory markers in human chondrocytes. This research exemplifies how marine polysaccharides and lipids synergistically attenuate joint inflammation, reinforcing the therapeutic promise of marine biochemicals.

The fourth edition of "Marine Antioxidant and Anti-Inflammatory Agents" highlights a wide variety of marine organisms that serve as sources of bioactive compounds with antioxidant and anti-inflammatory properties. The broad diversity of species and molecules listed in Table 1 emphasizes the valuable resource that the marine environment represents in the field of human health.

To harness the vast potential of marine bioresources in the search for new anti-inflammatory and antioxidant agents, we are pleased to present two in-depth reviews included in this Special Issue.

Table 1. Summary of the research collected in the Special Issue "Marine Anti-Inflammatory and Antioxidant Agents, 4th Edition".

Marine Organism	Compound	In Vitro Experimental Model	In Vivo Animal Models	Contribution
Marine fungi *Alternaria* sp.	Alternariol (AOH)	Bone marrow-derived dendritic cells (BMDCs) and macrophages (BMDMs)	C57BL/6J mice	Contribution 1 (Liu et al. (2025))
Marine fungus Aspergillus C23-3	Butyrolactone-I (BTL-I)	Intestinal porcine enterocyte (IPEC-J2) cells	C57BL/6J mice	Contribution 2 (Niu et al. (2024))
Seahorse (*Hippocampus abdominalis*)	SHP2 peptide	Human keratinocyte (HaCaT) cells; Human dermal fibroblast (HDF) cells	Zebrafish model	Contribution 3 (Yang et al. (2024))
Blue mussel (*Mytilus edulis*)	Peptides PIISVYWK (P1) and FSVVPSPK (P2)	Murine macrophage (RAW264.7) cells		Contribution 4 (Marasinghe et al. (2024))
Squid viscera	oil enriched with omega-3 fatty acids and astaxanthin			Contribution 5 (Joshi et al. (2025))
Sea Cucumber (*Apostichopus japonicus*)	Polydeoxyribonucleotide (AJS-PDRN)	Murine macrophage (RAW264.7) cells		Contribution 6 (Shu et al. (2024))
Brow seaweed (*Laminaria hyperborea)*	Fucoidan (FucBB04)	Human uveal melanoma (OMM-1) cells; primary retinal pigment epithelium (RPE) cells from pig eyes; immortalized retinal pigment epithelial (ARPE-19) cells		Contribution 7 (Dörschmann et al. (2025))
Brown seaweed (*Ericaria crinita)*	Alginate		Wistar rats	Contribution 8 (Lukova et al. (2024))
Green seaweed (*Codium fragile*)	oleamide (9-octadecenamide)		BALB/c mice	Contribution 9 (Lee et al. (2025))
Salmon (*Salmo salar*)	chondroitin sulfate and lipids	Primary human chondrocyte cells		Contribution 10 (Pruvost et al. (2024))

In order to achieve this purpose, Yang et al. (2024) present in Contribution 11 a comprehensive review of marine microorganisms, thereby demonstrating that more than 250 microbial metabolites—including polyketides, terpenoids, alkaloids, amides or peptides, and steroids—have shown promising pharmacological activities, thus enriching the pipeline for future drug development.

Furthermore, in Contribution 12, Vasarri et al. (2025) conduct a study that emphasizes the sustainable availability of seagrasses as natural sources of bioactive compounds. This review is an investigation into the antioxidant and anti-inflammatory properties of Mediterranean seagrasses, including *Posidonia oceanica*, *Cymodocea nodosa*, and *Zostera* species. It is demonstrated that the utilization of these seagrasses holds considerable potential for the mitigation of oxidative stress and chronic inflammation.

Collectively, these reviews emphasize the substantial and as yet underutilized capacity of marine ecosystems in the production of anti-inflammatory and antioxidant agents.

In conclusion, the diverse array of marine-derived bioactivities highlighted in this Special Issue underscores the profound therapeutic potential residing within marine environments. From fungal metabolites and marine peptides to polysaccharides and microbially produced compounds, these several natural products from diverse marine organisms (Figure 1) offer novel mechanisms to combat inflammation and oxidative stress—central contributors to many chronic diseases. The integration of advanced delivery systems, sustainable sourcing, and multidisciplinary research approaches further enhances their translational prospects. As our understanding of marine biochemistry deepens, the utilization of these bioresources has the potential to facilitate innovative and efficacious applications in human health, while concurrently contributing to marine ecological preservation.

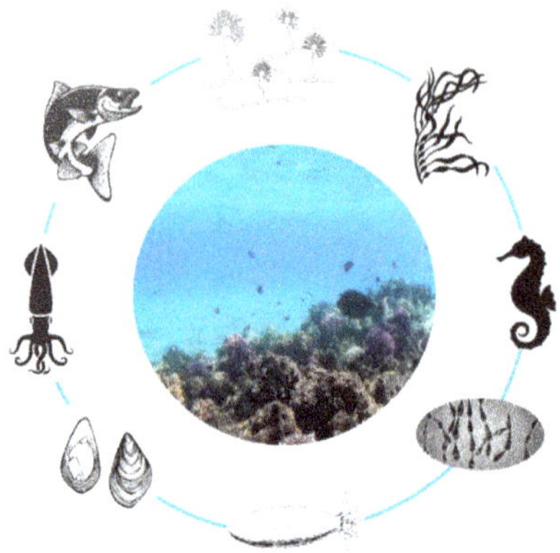

Figure 1. Scheme illustrating of the key marine organisms as sources of bioactive compounds with antioxidant and anti-inflammatory properties featured in the Special Issue "Marine Anti-Inflammatory and Antioxidant Agents, 4th Edition".

Conflicts of Interest: The authors declare no conflicts of interest.

List of Contributions:

1. Liu, C.; Gu, F.; Zou, Z.; Wang, F.; Li, D.; Song, J.; Hong, Y.; Wu, X.; Yang, X.; Liu, W.-H.; et al. Marine-Derived Alternariol Suppresses Inflammation by Regulating T Cell Activation and Migration. *Mar. Drugs* **2025**, *23*, 133. https://doi.org/10.3390/md23030133.
2. Niu, X.; Chen, S.; Wang, X.; Wen, J.; Liu, X.; Yong, Y.; Yu, Z.; Ma, X.; Abd El-Aty, A.M.; Ju, X. Butyrolactone-I from Marine Fungal Metabolites Mitigates Heat-Stress-Induced Apoptosis in IPEC-J2 Cells and Mice Through the ROS/PERK/CHOP Signaling Pathway. *Mar. Drugs* **2024**, *22*, 564. https://doi.org/10.3390/md22120564.
3. Yang, F.; Yang, Y.; Xiao, D.; Kim, P.; Lee, J.; Jeon, Y.-J.; Wang, L. Anti-Photoaging Effects of Antioxidant Peptide from Seahorse (*Hippocampus abdominalis*) in In Vivo and In Vitro Models. *Mar. Drugs* **2024**, *22*, 471. https://doi.org/10.3390/md22100471.
4. Marasinghe, C.K.; Je, J.-Y. Blue Mussel-Derived Bioactive Peptides PIISVYWK (P1) and FSVVPSPK (P2): Promising Agents for Inhibiting Foam Cell Formation and Inflammation in Cardiovascular Diseases. *Mar. Drugs* **2024**, *22*, 466. https://doi.org/10.3390/md22100466.
5. Joshi, A.; Holland, B.; Sachar, M.; Barrow, C.J. Pilot-Scale Enzymatic Conversion of Low Stability, High Free Fatty, Squid Oil to an Oxidatively Stable Astaxanthin-Rich Acylglyceride Oil Suitable for Nutritional Applications. *Mar. Drugs* **2025**, *23*, 21. https://doi.org/10.3390/md23010021.
6. Shu, Z.; Ji, Y.; Liu, F.; Jing, Y.; Jiao, C.; Li, Y.; Zhao, Y.; Wang, G.; Zhang, J. Proteomics Analysis of the Protective Effect of Polydeoxyribonucleotide Extracted from Sea Cucumber (*Apostichopus japonicus*) Sperm in a Hydrogen Peroxide-Induced RAW264.7 Cell Injury Model. *Mar. Drugs* **2024**, *22*, 325. https://doi.org/10.3390/md22070325.
7. Dörschmann, P.; Kopplin, G.; Thalenhorst, T.; Seeba, C.; Ullah, S.F.; Srivastava, V.; Roider, J.; Klettner, A. Influence of a Very High-Molecular Weight Fucoidan from *Laminaria hyperborea* on Age-Related Macular Degeneration-Relevant Pathomechanisms in Ocular Cell Models. *Mar. Drugs* **2025**, *23*, 101. https://doi.org/10.3390/md23030101.
8. Lukova, P.; Kokova, V.; Baldzhieva, A.; Murdjeva, M.; Katsarov, P.; Delattre, C.; Apostolova, E. Alginate from *Ericaria crinita* Possesses Antioxidant Activity and Attenuates Systemic Inflammation via Downregulation of Pro-Inflammatory Cytokines. *Mar. Drugs* **2024**, *22*, 482. https://doi.org/10.3390/md22110482.
9. Lee, H.L.; Ju, Y.H.; Kim, I.Y.; Choi, H.J.; Heo, Y.M.; Na, H.R.; Heo, H.J. *Codium fragile* Extract Ameliorates Respiratory Function by Controlling Allergic Inflammation in Ovalbumin-Induced Bronchial Disorders in Mice. *Mar. Drugs* **2025**, *23*, 221. https://doi.org/10.3390/md23050221.

10. Pruvost, L.; Gerlei, M.; Paris, C.; Velot, É.; Kahn, C.J.-F.; Bianchi, A.; Linder, M. Chondroitin Sulfate Nanovectorized by LC-PUFAs Nanocarriers Extracted from Salmon (*Salmo salar*) by Green Process with Decreased Inflammatory Marker Expression in Interleukin-1β-Stimulated Primary Human Chondrocytes In Vitro Culture. *Mar. Drugs* **2024**, *22*, 571. https://doi.org/10.3390/md22120571.
11. Yang, G.; Lin, M.; Kaliaperumal, K.; Lu, Y.; Qi, X.; Jiang, X.; Xu, X.; Gao, C.; Liu, Y.; Luo, X. Recent Advances in Anti-Inflammatory Compounds from Marine Microorganisms. *Mar. Drugs* **2024**, *22*, 424. https://doi.org/10.3390/md22090424.
12. Vasarri, M.; De Marchi, L.; Pretti, C.; Barletta, E.; Degl'Innocenti, D. Antioxidant and Anti-Inflammatory Properties of Four Native Mediterranean Seagrasses: A Review of Bioactive Potential and Ecological Context. *Mar. Drugs* **2025**, *23*, 206. https://doi.org/10.3390/md23050206.

marine drugs

MDPI

Article

Marine-Derived Alternariol Suppresses Inflammation by Regulating T Cell Activation and Migration

Chenfeng Liu [1,†], Fudie Gu [2,†], Zhengbiao Zou [3], Fengli Wang [1], Dashuai Li [1], Jing Song [4], Yazhen Hong [4], Xuhui Wu [5], Xianwen Yang [3], Wen-Hsien Liu [4], Guangming Liu [2,6], Yu Zhou [4,*] and Qingmei Liu [2,*]

[1] Department of Cell Biology, School of Life Science, Anhui Medical University, Hefei 230031, China; wfl19990316@163.com (F.W.); lds881008@163.com (D.L.)
[2] Xiamen Key Laboratory of Marine Functional Food, Fujian Provincial Engineering Technology Research Center of Marine Functional Food, College of Ocean Food and Biological Engineering, Jimei University, Xiamen 361021, China; 15238875906@163.com (F.G.)
[3] Hainan Academy of Medical Sciences, Hainan Medical University, Haikou 571199, China; yangxianwen@muhn.edu.cn (X.Y.)
[4] State Key Laboratory of Cellular Stress Biology, School of Life Sciences, Faculty of Medicine and Life Sciences, Xiamen University, Xiamen 361102, China
[5] School of Public Health, Xiamen University, Xiamen 361102, China
[6] Faculty of Marine Biology, Xiamen Ocean Vocational College, Xiamen 361102, China
[*] Correspondence: yu_zhou1205@163.com (Y.Z.); liuqingmei@jmu.edu.cn (Q.L.); Tel.: +86-592-6180575 (Q.L.)
[†] The authors were contributed equally to this work.

Abstract: T cells play pivotal roles in inflammation's initiation and progression. Exploring natural compounds that regulate T cell function is crucial for preventing and treating inflammation. Herein, we report that Alternariol (AOH), a marine-derived secondary metabolite, exerts an anti-inflammatory activity by targeting T cell function. Using an ovalbumin (OVA)-induced OT-II CD4$^+$ T cell activation model, we demonstrated that AOH potently suppresses T cell proliferation and cytokine secretion, mildly promotes T cell apoptosis, and spares antigen presentation processes. Mechanistically, AOH controlled early T cell activation by inhibiting the expression of activation markers (CD69, CD25, CD44) and transcription factors (T-bet, Eomes), leading to impaired Th1 cytokine production. In vivo experiments revealed that AOH attenuated OVA-induced lung injury in mice by reducing immune cell infiltration in pulmonary tissues and draining lymph nodes. Notably, AOH dramatically suppressed OVA-specific T cells migrating to the inflammatory lung while impairing T-cell-mediated other immune cell infiltration. Collectively, AOH exhibited potent anti-inflammatory effects by modulating T cell proliferation, function, and migration, offering a promising therapeutic strategy for T-cell-mediated inflammatory diseases.

Keywords: alternariol; CD4$^+$ T cells; inflammation cytokines; lung injury; cell migration

1. Introduction

The host immune system serves multiple functions in pathogen elimination, immune homeostasis and surveillance, and eliminating apoptotic and tumor cells [1,2]. However, persistent immune cell activation leads to acute and chronic inflammation, contributes to the pathogenesis of diverse diseases including autoimmune disorders, metabolic syndrome, and atherosclerosis [3], such as systemic lupus erythematosus (SLE), asthma, type 1 diabetes, and cardiovascular diseases [4]. Hence, precise immune modulation represents a critical therapeutic strategy for maintaining health. Inflammatory responses involve innate and adaptive immunity and their interaction. While lots of studies have evaluated the mechanisms of inflammation triggered by innate immune cells, particularly macrophage polarization and their proinflammatory roles [5–7], recent advances highlight the central roles of CD4$^+$ T cells in the regulation of inflammation and tumor immunity [8,9]. CD4$^+$ T cells exhibit plasticity in differentiation states (Th1/Th2/Th17/Treg), producing different cytokines (IFNγ, IL4, IL17, IL10) to activate or restrain immune responses. Consequently, therapeutic interventions targeting CD4$^+$ T cells must balance immune competence and suppression. Current immunotherapeutics have demonstrated their clinical efficacy, including cyclosporine, and are used to treat autoimmune diseases and prevent transplant rejection by inhibiting the proliferation of T cells and the release of cytokines [10]. Alemtuzumab, a CD52$^-$directed monoclonal antibody, presents the ability to deplete peripheral lymphocytes to treat relapsed or refractory lymphomas [11], and checkpoint inhibitors such as PD-1/PD-L1 antibodies enhance CD8$^+$ T cell cytotoxicity to control tumors [12]. However, these drugs also show several limitations, such as hematologic toxicities (e.g., anemia) [13], hepatorenal dysfunction [14], and high costs, which restrict their broad applicability. Thus, it is still needed to search for more drugs, compounds, or natural substances to regulate T cell function, which provides potential therapeutic strategies for T-cell-related diseases.

In contrast to the land resources that have been widely used, marine ecosystems represent a largely unexplored source of bioactive compounds with unique structural diversity and therapeutic potential [15,16]. Secondary metabolites produced by marine microorganisms were identified as diverse biological activities, such as homoseongomycin, an alphavirus inhibitor isolated from Actinomycete K3-1 [17], and macrolactins derived from *Bacillus* sp. HC001 showed anti-inflammatory ability by suppressing proinflammatory cytokines and chemokines [18]. It has been reported that the secondary metabolites of *Streptomyces* sp. induce cytotoxic activity through a variety of mechanisms, including apoptosis, necrosis, inhibition of colony formation, and cell migration [19]. Despite these discoveries, the immunomodulatory potential of marine-derived compounds in T cell-mediated diseases remains largely unexplored, which limits the provision of new immunotherapy for T-cell-related inflammatory and autoimmune diseases.

In this study, using an in vitro T cell differentiation model (Patent: CN202111226760.0), we screened marine-derived compounds to evaluate the immunomodulatory activities and found alternariol (AOH), a secondary metabolite isolated from the marine fungus *Alternaria* sp., represented a potential anti-inflammatory ability by preferring to target T cell function. Previous investigations had documented AOH had biological activities in lipopolysaccharide (LPS)-induced inflammation [20], inhibiting tumor cell viability and proliferation, and other cytotoxic effects [21]. Our previous data also found AME, a structurally analogous compound of AOH, regulated mast cell degranulation to inhibit allergy [22]. However, the role of AOH in regulating T cell function remains poorly defined. To address this question, we deeply investigated the role of AOH in regulating T cell activation, proliferation, migration, cytokine production, and potential ability to treat T-cell-mediated inflammation in the lung.

2. Results

2.1. AOH Inhibits Proinflammatory Cytokine Production of T Cell In Vitro

We established an ovalbumin (OVA)-induced CD4$^+$ T cell activation system (hereafter called the OVA-OTII system) to screen marine-derived extracts and compounds [23]. Using this system, we screened the numerous crude extracts derived from marine microorganisms; subsequently, we purified compounds from these extracts and identified alternariol (AOH), a secondary metabolite isolated from *Alternaria* sp., which represented an inhibitory effect in cytokine production from CD4$^+$ T cells (Figure 1A). AOH was purified from the *Alternaria* sp. fermented compound, and the chemical structure was confirmed via nuclear magnetic resonance (NMR) (Figures 1B and S1A–C). To delineate its immunomodulatory function, we quantified cytokine production using flow cytometry with a marked gating strategy to eliminate dead cells (Figure 1C,D). Our data revealed that greater than 50% of OVA-stimulated CD4$^+$ T cells differentiated into Th1-like cells (TNFα^+/IFNγ^+), while AOH exhibited dose-dependent inhibition of TNFα and IFNγ production (Figure 1E). Furthermore, IL2, which is central for T cell activation, proliferation, and Th1 polarization, but AOH nearly completely suppressed IL2 and IFNγ production in CD4$^+$ T cells, particularly in the Th1-polarized population (IL2$^+$IFNγ^+) (Figure 1F,G). Collecting these data, we found AOH represented an inhibitory effects for Th1-related cytokines.

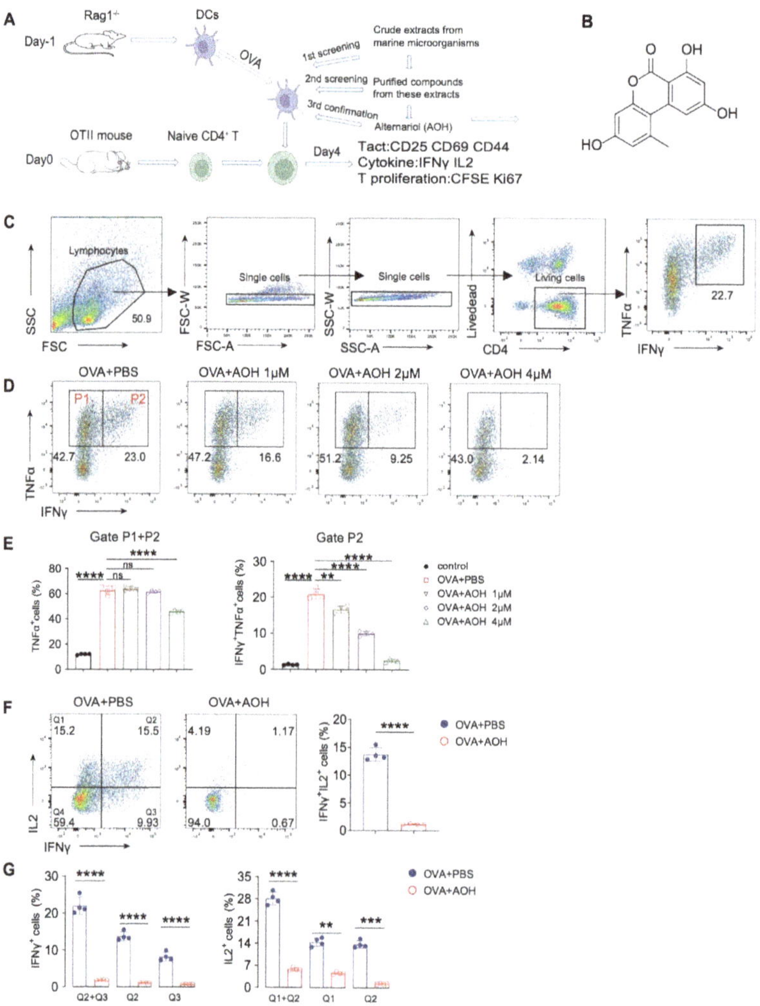

Figure 1. AOH inhibits proinflammatory cytokine production of T cells using OVA-OTII cell model. (**A**) Schematic diagram of the OT-II cell differentiation system. (**B**) Chemical structure of AOH. (**C**) Flow cytometric gating strategy for analyzing the cytokine released by T cells. (**D**) Flow cytometric analysis of IFNγ and TNFα secretion by T cells at varying concentrations of AOH. (**E**) Percentages of IFNγ and TNFα production. (**F**) Flow cytometric analysis of the inhibitory effects of AOH on IL-2 and IFNγ production. (**G**) Percentages of IFNγ and IL-2 released by T cells. Each symbol represents an independent biological replicate; the horizontal line represents the mean value (±s.e.m.). Statistical significance: **, $p < 0.01$; ***, $p < 0.001$; ****, $p < 0.0001$. ns, no significance.

2.2. AOH Affects T Cell Apoptosis and Inhibits T Cell Proliferation

T cell differentiation and cytokine production depend on multiple factors such as cell activation, proliferation, metabolic regulation, and apoptosis [24]. Flow cytometry analysis revealed that AOH treatment significantly reduced CD4$^+$ T cell numbers at days 2 and 3 after OVA stimulation (Figure 2A). Previous studies have demonstrated AOH showed an anti-tumor activity through inducing cell apoptosis [21], but little is known about the function of AOH in maintaining T cell homeostasis and survival. Using Annexin V/7AAD staining, we observed that AOH increased approximately 30% apoptotic CD4$^+$ T cells after OVA stimulation, partially contributing to the reduced cell count, but could not explain near 60% cell loss (Figure 2A–C). So, we want to ask whether AOH disturbed T cell proliferation. To address this question, we employed CFSE labeling to mark the proliferated cells with individual peaks using flow cytometry to investigate the proliferative defects by AOH. The results showed that AOH-treated cells exhibited arrested proliferation, with 80% remaining in the initiated stage (peak 1), compared to 20% P1 in control groups, with 70% proliferative cells in the P4–6 stage (Figure 2D,E). Moreover, Ki-67 expression, a marker of cellular proliferation, was also markedly downregulated by AOH (Figure 2F,G). Notably, cytokine-producing cells (IFNγ^+ or IL-2$^+$) were predominantly within the proliferating population (P6), and AOH treatment abolished both their frequency and mean fluorescence intensity (MFI) expression (Figure 2H–K). Collectively, these findings showed that AOH disrupts T cell survival, proliferation, and function.

2.3. AOH Modulates Early T Cell Activation and Transcriptional Programming

T cell activation is characterized by the upregulation of early activation markers CD69, CD25, and CD44, and the expression of differentiation-associated markers CD71 and ICOS, which are critical for T cell function. We next asked whether AOH regulated T cell activation, which caused impaired T cell proliferation and cytokine production. Activated T cells firstly enhance CD69 and CD25 expression and reduce CD62L expression, so we marked the first activated stage (P1, CD69$^+$CD62L$^+$, or CD25$^+$CD62L$^+$) and second activated stage (P2, CD69$^+$CD62L$^-$, or CD25$^+$CD62L$^-$), as shown in Figure 3A–D. Total CD69 expression (P1 + P2) was significantly reduced after AOH treatment compared to the control group at days 1 and 2, but there was no difference at day 3. Moreover, both P1 and P2 cells were decreased at days 1 and 2 after the AOH intervention, but at day 3, AOH still inhibited P1 cells but slightly enhanced the P2 percentage (Figure 3B). Notably, consideration reduced cell number after AOH treatment (Figure 2A); we also found absolutely decreased CD69$^+$ T cells at days 1–3 with AOH intervention (Figure S2). CD69 is another early activated marker, and similar results were found after AOH treatment (Figure 3C,D). In contrast to early activation markers, CD44, CD71, and ICOS represent later stages of activation and differentiation. AOH treatment resulted in a marked decrease in CD44$^+$ T cells, ICOS$^+$ T cells, and ICOS$^+$CD71$^+$ double-positive populations, accompanied by reduced expression intensity of CD71 and ICOS (Figure 3E–H). Furthermore, transcriptional regulation is essential for Th1 differentiation and function, including Eomes and T-bet. Moreover, Bcl2 and CTLA4 expression are key indicators for T cell survival and activity. We found AOH controlled T cell function in a transcriptional manner by decreasing Eomes and T-bet expression. AOH also inhibited Bcl2 and CTLA4 expression, which contribute to T cell survival and prolonged activation (Figure 3I–L). Collecting these data, AOH controls the early state of T cell activation, T cell transcription, and differentiation.

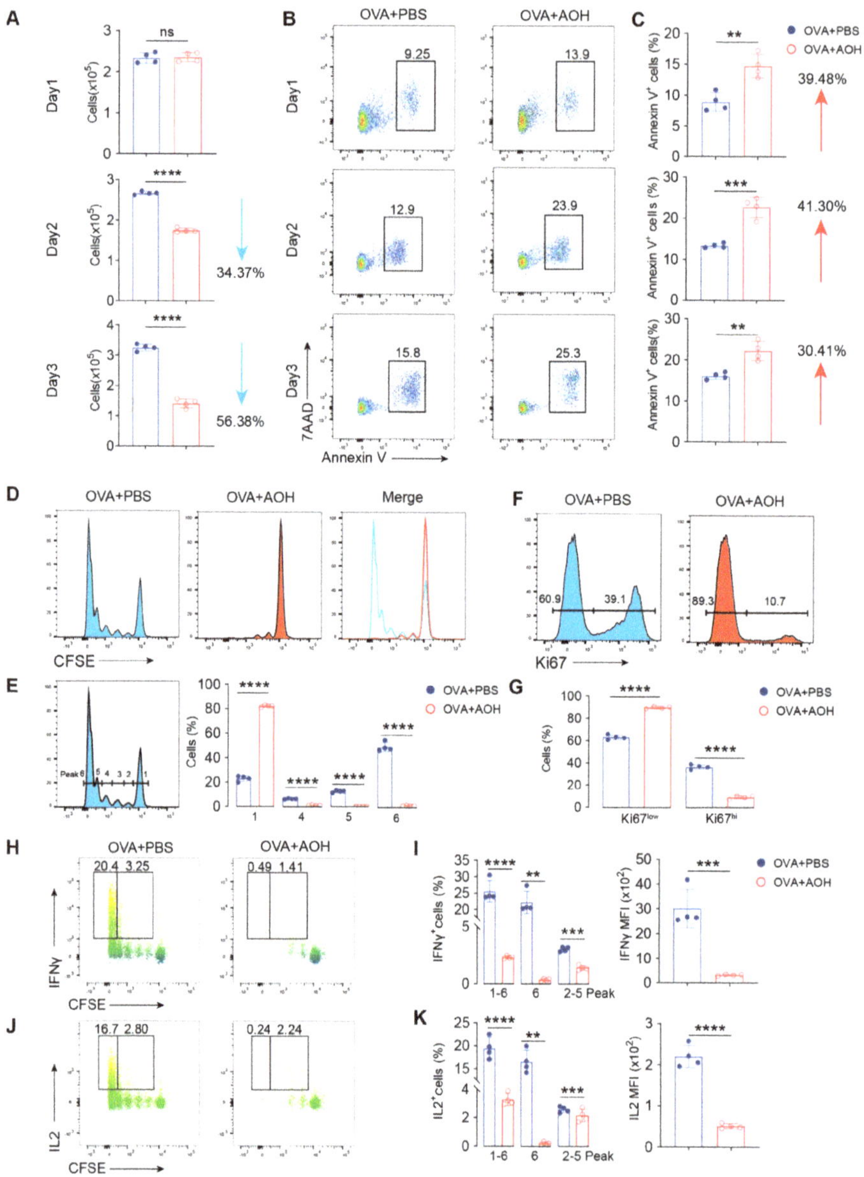

Figure 2. AOH modulates apoptosis and proliferation of T cells. (**A**) Dynamic changes in T cell counts after AOH treatment during 1–3 days. (**B**) Flow cytometric analysis of the effect of AOH on T cell apoptosis using Annexin V and 7AAD staining. (**C**) Apoptotic percentage of T cell mediated by AOH. (**D**) CFSE labeled cell proliferation in the presence of AOH. (**E**) Percentage of $CD4^+$ T cell proliferation in 1, 4–6 generations in the presence of AOH. (**F**) Ki67 expression after AOH treatment. (**G**) Percentage of Ki67 expression in the presence of AOH. (**H**) Flow cytometric analysis of CFSE marked IFNγ expression in T cells on day 4. (**I**) Percentage and immunofluorescence intensity of IFNγ released by $CD4^+$ T cells in different generations. (**J**) Flow cytometric analysis of IL-2 secretion in proliferating $CD4^+$ T cells. (**K**) Percentage and immunofluorescence intensity of IL-2 released by $CD4^+$ T cells in different generations. Each symbol represents an independent biological replicate; the horizontal line represents the mean value (±s.e.m.). Statistical significance: **, $p < 0.01$; ***, $p < 0.001$; ****, $p < 0.0001$. ns, no significance.

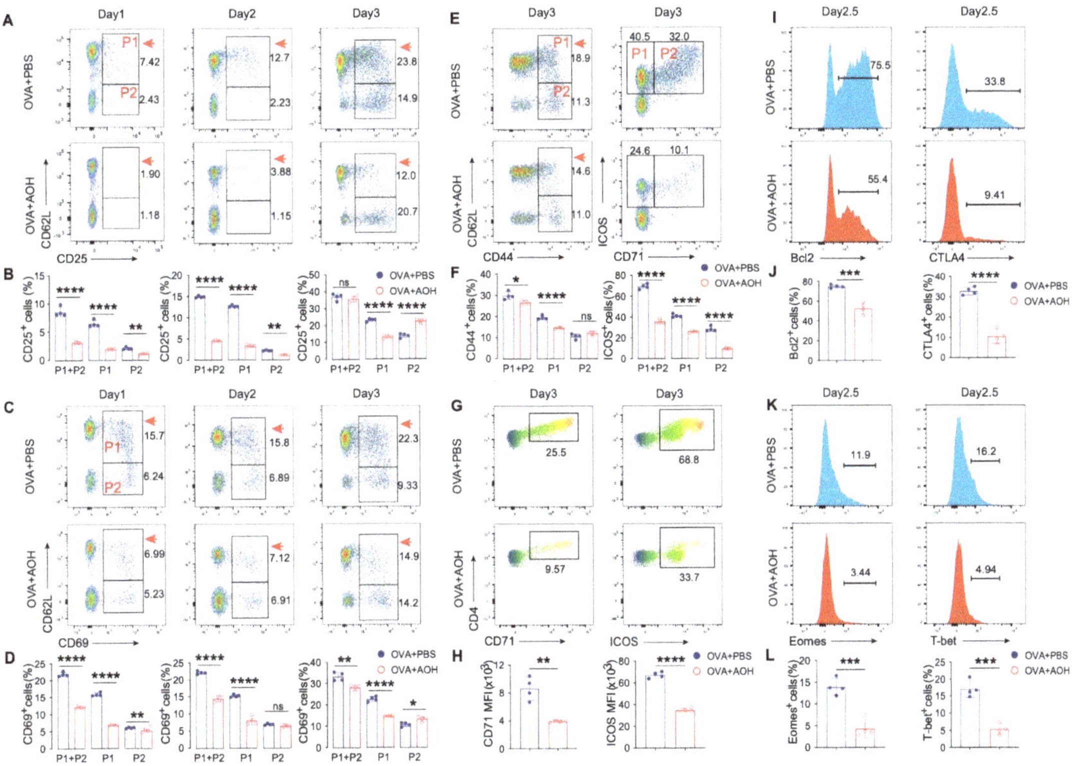

Figure 3. AOH modulates early T cell activation and related transcriptional programming. (**A**) Flow cytometric analysis of T cell activation using CD25 and CD62L expression, P1 ($CD25^+$ $CD62L^+$) and P2 ($CD25^+$ $CD62L^-$). (**B**) Proportions of CD25 expression in T cells. (**C**) Flow cytometric analysis of CD69 and CD62L expression in T cell activation, P1 ($CD69^+$ $CD62L^+$), and P2 ($CD69^+$ $CD62L^-$). (**D**) Percentages of CD69 expression in T cell subsets. (**E**) Flow cytometric analysis of T cell activation using CD44 and CD62L expression (**left**) and T cell differentiation using ICOS and CD71 expression (right), left P1 ($CD44^+$ $CD62L^+$) and left P2 ($CD44^+$ $CD62L^-$), right P1 ($ICOS^+$ $CD71^-$), right P2 ($ICOS^+$ $CD71^+$). (**F**) Proportions analysis of CD44 (**left**) and ICOS expression (**right**). (**G**) Flow cytometric detection of ICOS and CD71 expression. (**H**) Mean fluorescence intensity (MFI) of CD71 and ICOS in $CD4^+$ T cells on day 3. (**I**) Bcl-2 (**left**) and CTLA-4 (**right**) expression in $CD4^+$ T cells at day 2.5. (**J**) Quantitative analysis of Bcl-2 (**left**) and CTLA-4 (**right**) expression. (**K**) Detection of eomesodermin (Eomes) (**left**) and T-bet (**right**) expression in $CD4^+$ T cells at day 2.5. (**L**) Statistical analysis of Eomes (**left**) and T-bet (**right**) expression profiles. Each symbol represents an independent biological replicate; the horizontal line represents the mean value (±s.e.m.). Statistical significance: *, $p < 0.05$; **, $p < 0.01$; ***, $p < 0.001$; ****, $p < 0.0001$. ns, no significance.

2.4. AOH Targets Early T Cell Activation for Affecting T Cell Function Without Affecting Antigen Presentation

T cell early activation relies on antigen-presenting cells such as dendritic cells and macrophages interacting with T cells, which present peptides via MHC-II molecules to TCRs, followed by increasing CD80 and CD86 expression, thereby driving T cell entry into an activated and functional state. To determine whether AOH modulates antigen processing, we generated bone marrow-derived dendritic cells (BMDCs) and macrophages (BMDMs) and assessed MHC-II, CD80, and CD86 expression. AOH had no impact on APC maturation or antigen presentation (Figure 4A–F), indicating a dispensable role for AOH in APC maturation and antigen-presenting function. To confirm these results, in the OVA-

OTII system, we further detected the effect of AOH in DC function. AOH treatment during days 1~4 still suppressed cytokine production; however, when AOH was applied from days 1~0, which predominantly affects DC function in this time frame, cytokine production was comparable to the PBS control group (Figure 4G,H). These findings suggest that AOH preferentially targets the early T cell activation phase rather than antigen-presenting capacity by DCs.

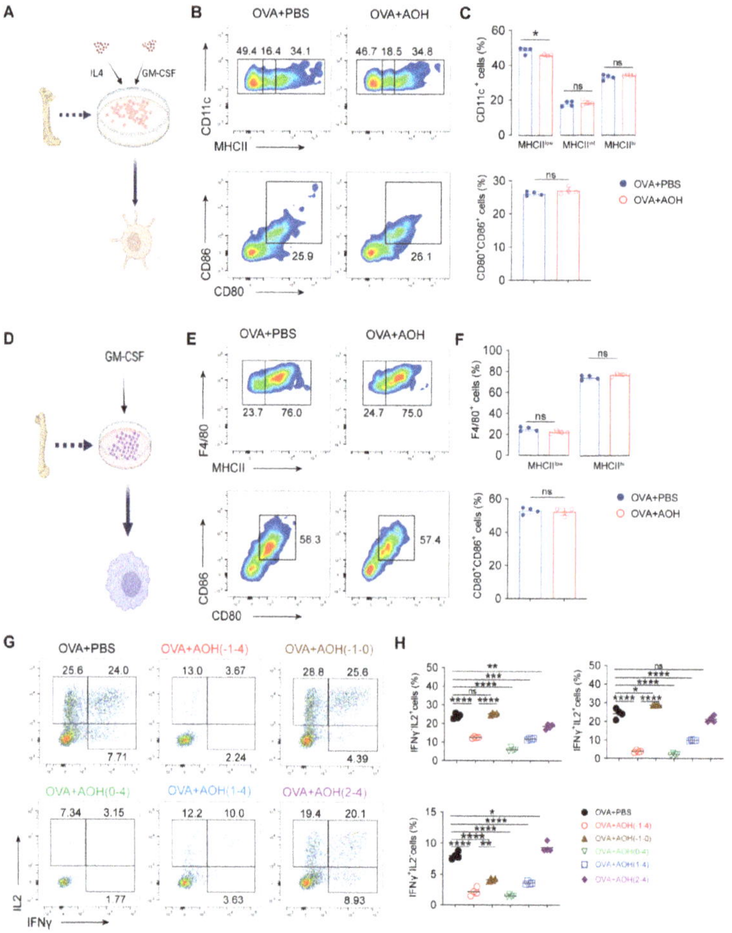

Figure 4. AOH is dispensable for the function of antigen-presenting cells. (**A**) Model of BMDC induction. (**B**) Flow cytometric analysis of AOH's effects on BMDC mature and functional markers MHCII, CD80 and CD86. (**C**) Statistical analysis of MHCII, CD80 and CD86 expression. (**D**) Model of BMDM induction. (**E**) Flow cytometric analysis of AOH's effects on BMDM mature and functional markers MHCII, CD80 and CD86. (**F**) Statistical analysis of MHCII, CD80 and CD86 expression. (**G**) Time-course analysis of AOH's effect on inflammatory cytokine (IFNγ/IL-2) release by CD4$^+$ T cells. (**H**) Percentage of IFNγ and IL-2 secreted by CD4$^+$ T cells under AOH treatment. Each symbol represents an independent biological replicate; the horizontal line represents the mean value (±s.e.m.). Statistical significance: *, $p < 0.05$; **, $p < 0.01$; ***, $p < 0.001$; ****, $p < 0.0001$. ns, no significance.

Notably, AOH treatment during days 0~4 and 1~4 significantly inhibited IFNγ and IL-2 production, consistent with our hypothesis that AOH regulated cytokine production by preferring to target T cell early activation mechanisms. To further dissect this effect, we treated AOH at day 2~4, a period that largely bypasses early T cell activation. Under these conditions, AOH exerted a marginal effect on cytokine production (Figure 4G,H). Collectively, our data show AOH selectively regulated T cell function, preferentially targeting early stages of T cell activation to inhibit cytokine production, while exerting minimal impact on antigen presentation pathways and late-stage T cell activation.

2.5. AOH Alleviates OVA-Induced Pulmonary Inflammation in Mice

Preceding data revealed that AOH suppresses T cell proliferation and cytokine production in vitro by targeting early T cell activation and transcription. Though AOH has been reported to exhibit anti-tumor activity and other biological functions in vivo, it remains unclear whether AOH regulates T cell function in vivo and its therapeutic potential in immune-related diseases. To address this issue, we employed an OVA-induced pulmonary inflammation in mice. Mice were immunized with OVA/Alum at days 0, 7, and 14, followed by intranasal OVA challenge on days 18–21. To specifically target early T cell activation, AOH was administered via gavage three times after each immunization (Figure 5A). Compared to the OVA + PBS group, AOH-treated mice exhibited improved clinical outcomes, characterized by lower weight and loss hypothermia (Figure 5B,C). OVA sensitization and re-challenge triggered aberrant T cell activation and differentiation. Pathogenic T cells migrated to the lung by OVA re-challenge and led to other immune cell infiltration in the lung, resulting in severe histopathological changes, including inflammatory solidus around the bronchioles and blood vessels, bronchiolar epithelial degeneration, and interstitial edema. AOH treatment significantly ameliorated pulmonary inflammation, as evidenced by reduced bronchiolar epithelial damage and interstitial edema, and decreased immune cell infiltration (Figure 5D). Collectively, these data represented that AOH acts as a potential therapeutic agent for treating T cell-mediated pulmonary inflammation in vivo.

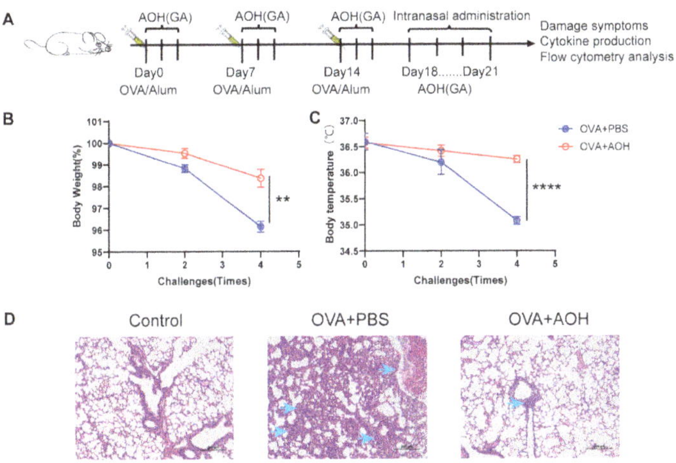

Figure 5. AOH attenuates OVA-induced pulmonary inflammation in mice. (**A**) A mouse model of pulmonary inflammation was established by immunization with OVA/Alum and nasal OVA. Mice were divided into two groups: OVA + PBS group and OVA + AOH group, with 5 mice in each group. AOH was gavaged in the OVA + AOH group, and the same volume of PBS was gavaged in OVA + PBS group. (**B**) Body weight changes of mice after nasal OVA administration. (**C**) Rectal temperature changes of mice after nasal OVA administration. (**D**) Histopathology changes in lung tissue injury between different groups. Each symbol represents an independent biological replicate; the horizontal line represents the mean value (±s.e.m.). Statistical significance: **, $p < 0.01$; ****, $p < 0.0001$.

2.6. AOH Suppresses T Cell Activation and Cytokine Production to Alleviate OVA- Induced Pulmonary Inflammation

To investigate whether AOH alleviated OVA-induced lung injury through regulating T-cell-mediated immune response in vivo, we first analyzed T cell populations, activation markers, and cytokine production in hilar lymph nodes after AOH treatment. The results indicated that although the percentages of $CD4^+$ and $CD8^+$ T cells were comparable between groups, AOH administration still resulted in a significant reduction in absolute cell numbers of $CD4^+$ and $CD8^+$ T cells (Figure 6A,B). Moreover, percentages and counts of activated $CD4^+$ T cells ($CD44^+CD62L^-$) also decreased by AOH (Figure 6C,D). In contrast to Th1-related cytokines, OVA-induced pulmonary inflammation also recruits the Th2 population for allergic response via the Th2-IgE- mast cell/eosinophil axis. AOH treatment disrupted Th2 polarization, evidenced by reduced IL-4 secretion from $CD4^+$ T cells (Figure 6 E,F). Additionally, cytokine-producing ($TNF\alpha^+CD4^+$ T or $IFN\gamma^+CD4^+$ T) cells were markedly diminished, especially the dual-positive DP ($TNF\alpha^+IFN\gamma^+CD4^+$ T) subset, which is known to promote tissue inflammation and immune cell recruitment, exhibiting the pronounced reduction (Figure 6G–I). Furthermore, AOH modulated $CD8^+$ T cell activation ($CD44^+CD62L^-$) and IFNγ production (Figure 6J–M), suggesting a broader impact on adaptive immune responses.

To investigate the immunomodulatory effects of AOH on lung inflammation, we quantified immune cell infiltration in the lung after AOH treatment. AOH administration represented a significant reduction in total immune cells in the lung (Figure 7A) and a marked attenuation of innate immune populations (size of innate immune cells is larger than adaptive immune cells, as shown in Figure 7B,C), including eosinophils, macrophages, and neutrophils (Figure 7D,E). Notably, while the relative percentage of neutrophils was slightly elevated, their absolute counts remained significantly lower in the AOH-treated group compared to PBS controls. Dramatically decreased innate immune cells disturbed the immune landscape in the lung, resulting in increased $CD4^+$ and $CD8^+$ T cell frequencies; however, the absolute numbers of these adaptive immune cells were concurrently diminished, consistent with suppression of IFNγ and IL-4 production by $CD4^+$ T cells in the lung after AOH administration (Figure 7F–J). Collectively, these data demonstrate AOH suppressed pathogenic immune responses in pulmonary inflammation.

Previous studies reported AOH-induced cell toxicity via mitochondrial damage and enhanced an embryotoxic and immunotoxin risk in vivo. Consideration of the concerns, whether AOH dampened immune organ homeostasis, immune cell development, and survival in vivo, needs to be explored in detail. AOH was administrated to WT mice without any other stimulation for 14 days, then the spleen, lymph nodes, and thymus were analyzed, and no difference was found in PBS or AOH treatment, with similar results of cell numbers of thymocytes, splenocytes, lymph node cells, and normal T cell development, B cell development, and cytokines produced by $CD4^+$T and $CD8^+$T cells (Figure S3). Taken together, AOH inhibited T cell activation and cytokine production and showed an expected immuno-safety in vivo.

We previously indicated that AOH selectively targets the early phase of T cell activation to suppress proliferation and cytokine production, accompanied by fewer inhibitory effects on T cell function with AOH treatment at a later stage (Figure 4G,H). To confirm the mechanisms in vivo, as shown in Figure S4A, we treated AOH in the late stage after OVA/Alum immunization and then detected the inhibitory effect on T cell function in LNs and lung; the results showed no significant difference in T cell numbers and cytokine production in LNs and lungs (Figure S4). These results confirmed again that AOH regulated the early stage of T cell activation to inhibit T cell function in vivo and in vitro.

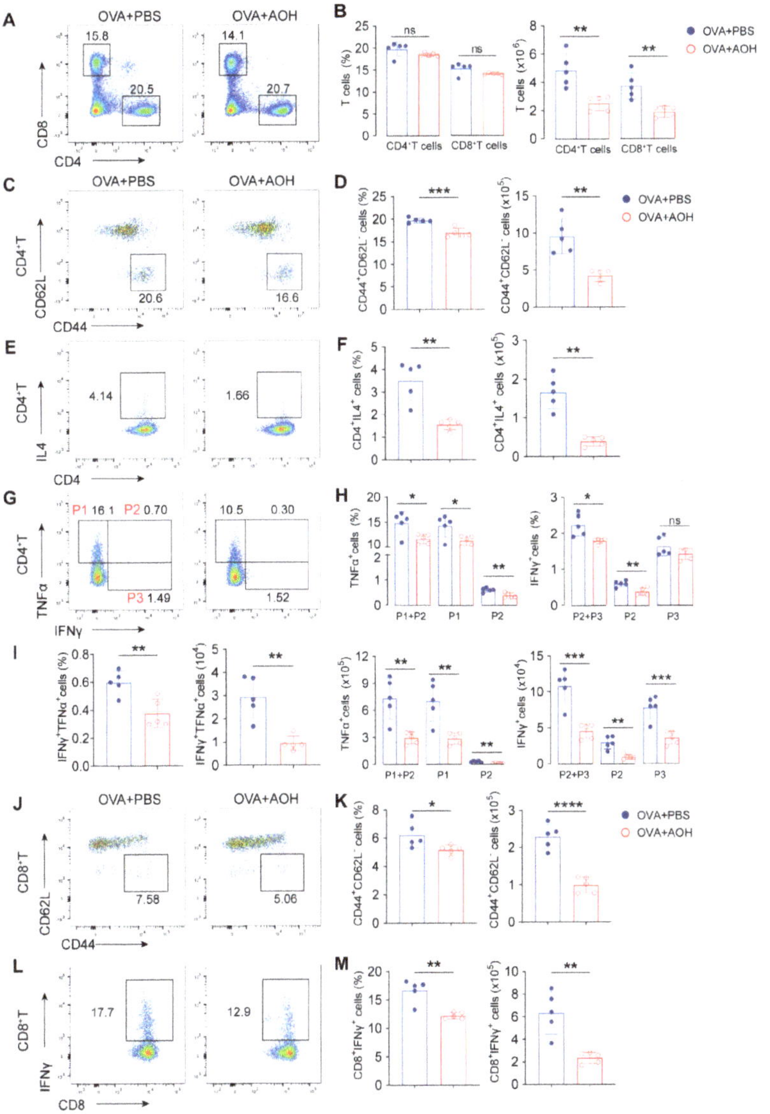

Figure 6. AOH controls T cell activation and cytokine production in hilar lymph nodes after lung injury. (**A**) Flow cytometric analysis of $CD4^+$ T and $CD8^+$ T cells in LNs. (**B**) Statistical analysis of proportions and absolute counts of $CD4^+$ T and $CD8^+$ T cell in LNs. (**C**) Flow cytometric analysis of $CD4^+$ T cell activation by $CD44^+CD62L^-$ expression. (**D**) Statistical analysis of the proportion and counts of activated $CD4^+$ T cells. (**E**) Flow cytometry analysis of IL4 production by $CD4^+$ T cells. (**F**) Statistical analysis of the proportion and counts of IL-4^+ $CD4^+$ T cells in the LNs. (**G**) Flow cytometric analysis of IFNγ and TNFα expression by $CD4^+$ T cells. (**H**) Statistical analysis of IFNγ and TNFα produced by $CD4^+$ T cells. (**I**) Proportion and counts of IFNγ and TNFα released by $CD4^+$ T cells. (**J**) Flow cytometric analysis of $CD8^+$ T cell activation. (**K**) Statistical analysis of the percentage and counts of activated $CD8^+$ T cells. (**L**) Cytokine of IFNγ expression produced by $CD8^+$ T cells. (**M**) Statistical analysis of the proportion and counts of IFNγ released by $CD8^+$ T cells. Each symbol represents an independent biological replicate; the horizontal line represents the mean value (±s.e.m.). Statistical significance: *, $p < 0.05$; **, $p < 0.01$; ***, $p < 0.001$; ****, $p < 0.0001$. ns, no significance.

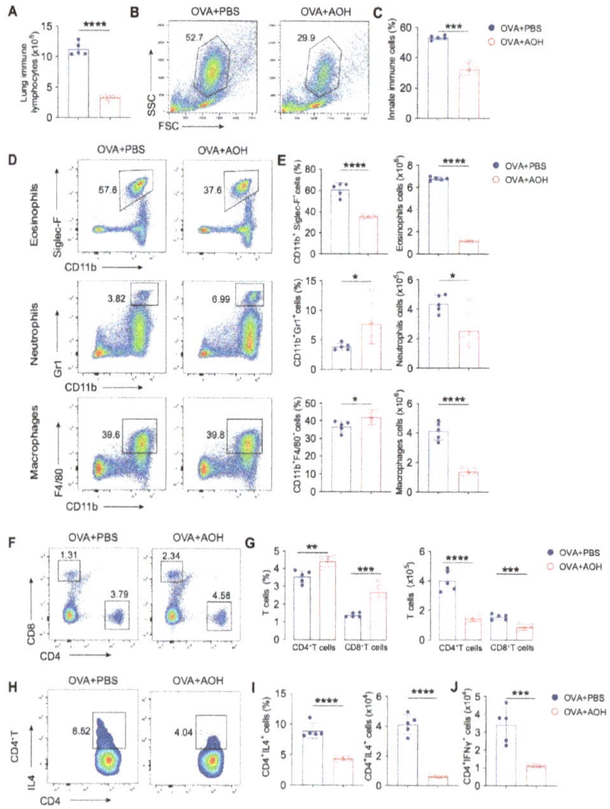

Figure 7. AOH inhibits immune cell infiltration and function to alleviate pulmonary inflammation. (**A**) Total immune cell counts in lung tissues. (**B**) Flow diagram for gating innate immune cell subsets (eosinophils, neutrophils, macrophages) in lung. (**C**) Statistics of absolute counts of innate immune cells in the lung. (**D**) Flow cytometric analysis of eosinophil, neutrophil, and macrophage proportions of CD45$^+$ cells in lung. (**E**) Statistical analysis of the proportion and absolute counts of eosinophils, neutrophils and macrophages in lung. (**F**) Flow cytometric detection of CD4$^+$ T and CD8$^+$ T cell proportions. (**G**) Statistical analysis of the proportion and absolute counts of CD4$^+$ T and CD8$^+$ T cells in lung. (**H**) Flow cytometric analysis of IL4-secreting CD4$^+$ T cells in lung. (**I**) Statistical analysis of the proportion and absolute counts of IL4 released by CD4$^+$ T cells. (**J**) Statistical analysis of absolute counts of IFNγ released by CD4$^+$ T cells. Each symbol represents an independent biological replicate; the horizontal line represents the mean value (±s.e.m.). Statistical significance: *, $p < 0.05$; **, $p < 0.01$; ***, $p < 0.001$; ****, $p < 0.0001$.

2.7. AOH Inhibits T Cell Migration to the Lung

In the OVA-induced pulmonary inflammation, dramatically decreased immune cell infiltration in the lung led us to hypothesize that AOH may regulate T cell trafficking to the lung. To test this question, we isolated activated OTII CD4$^+$ T cells (CD90.1 background) with or without AOH pretreatment in vitro under OVA stimulation, adoptively transferred these cells into WT mice (CD90.2 background), and intranasally challenged the recipients with OVA. LNs, infiltrated immune cells in the lung and bronchoalveolar lavage fluid (BALF) were analyzed at days 1 and 2 after OVA sensitization by flow cytometry (Figure 8A). Though CD90.1$^+$CD4$^+$ T cells were a normal frequency in LNs at day 1, the proportion and numbers were significantly diminished by day 2 in AOH-treated mice (Figure 8B,C). Consistent with previous results, IFNγ and IL-2 production by OTII CD4$^+$ T cells was also reduced following AOH administration (Figure 8D,E). Strikingly, the infiltrated numbers of OTII CD90.1$^+$CD4$^+$ T cells in the lung were profoundly decreased at both day 1 and day 2 under pre-treatment by AOH (Figure 8F,G), with a corresponding reduction of OTII CD90.1$^+$CD4$^+$ T cells in BALF at day 2 (Figure 8H,I). These data indicated that AOH affected CD4$^+$ T cell homeostasis and migration to the lung, and the combined results contributed to inhibiting T cell function. Furthermore, the decrease in total lung immune cells, including macrophages, neutrophils, and eosinophils (Figure 8J), supporting AOH, inhibited the pulmonary inflammation by regulating T cell activation, cytokine production, and migration. Collectively, these results demonstrated that AOH exerted its therapeutic effects by selectively targeting the early stages of T cell activation and migration, thereby reducing T cell function and pulmonary inflammation.

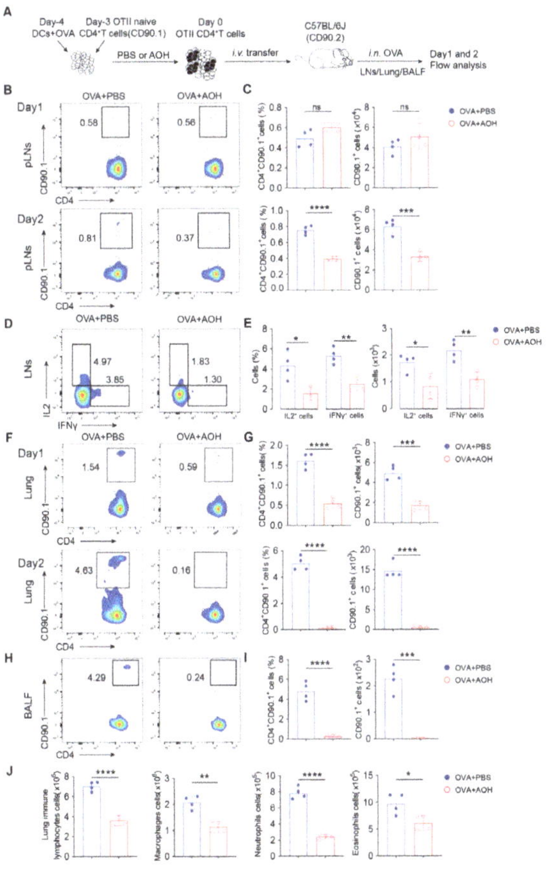

Figure 8. AOH regulates CD4$^+$ T cell migration in vivo. (**A**) Experimental model diagram. (**B**) Quantitative analysis of CD4$^+$ CD90.1$^+$ T cells in peripheral lymph nodes(pLNs) on day 1 and 2. (**C**) Proportion and absolute counts of CD4$^+$ CD90.1$^+$ T cells in pLNs at day 1 and 2. (**D**) IFNγ and IL-2 release by CD4$^+$ CD90.1$^+$ T cells in LNs. (**E**) Proportions and absolute counts of IFNγ and IL-2 in pLNs. (**F**) Flow cytometric analysis of CD90.1$^+$CD4$^+$ T cells in lungs on days 1 and 2. (**G**) Proportions and cell numbers of CD90.1$^+$ CD4$^+$ T cell in lungs on days 1 and 2. (**H**) Flow cytometric analysis of CD4$^+$ CD90.1$^+$ cells in BALF. (**I**) Proportions and absolute counts of CD4$^+$ CD90.1$^+$ cells in BALF. (**J**) Absolute counts of total immune cell in lung, and macrophages, neutrophils, and eosinophils in lung. Each symbol represents an independent biological replicate; the horizontal line represents the mean value (±s.e.m.). Statistical significance: *, $p < 0.01$; **, $p < 0.01$; ***, $p < 0.001$; ****, $p < 0.0001$. ns, no significance.

3. Discussion

In this study, we identified AOH, a secondary metabolite derived from marine microorganisms, which potently inhibited T cell-derived inflammatory cytokines (e.g., TNFα, IFNγ) through modulating early T cell activation and migration pathways and represents a potential application for treatment of pulmonary inflammation. Currently, there is a paucity of drugs specifically targeting T cell function for treating inflammatory disorders. Cyclosporine was employed to manage autoimmune diseases and organ transplant rejection through inhibiting lymphocyte proliferation. Meanwhile, corticosteroids like dexamethasone and prednisone remained the cornerstone for controlling acute/chronic inflammation, yet long-term use of cyclosporine and corticosteroids was associated with significant adverse effects, including immunosuppression, organ toxicity (liver/kidney), and metabolic disturbances [10]. Emerging immune checkpoint inhibitors, such as pembrolizumab (Keytruda), have optimized cancer therapy through robust anti-tumor immunity but often induce extra effects like immune hepatitis or thyroiditis [25]. In contrast, AOH had shown efficacy in modulating T-cell-related inflammation while inducing tumor cell apoptosis. Combining AOH with anti-PD1 agents, which may enhance anti-tumor responses while mitigating immune-related adverse events through complementary mechanisms. Our results not only highlighted the therapeutic potential of AOH in T-cell-mediated inflammatory diseases but also underscored the value of marine microbial resources for drug discovery.

Inflammation represents a dynamic interaction and complex immune landscape between innate immune cells (e.g., macrophages, DCs) and adaptive immune cells (e.g., T cells, B cells), which is difficult to recapitulate in vitro. Relying on immortalized cell lines or simple primary cell stimulations, current in vitro models fail to capture the precise immune responses, including antigen processing, immune cell trafficking, and cytokine secretion. To address this issue, we previously reported a T cell activation and differentiation model (Patent: CN202111226760.0), represented multi-immune processes including processing and presentation by innate immune cells, as well as the activation, differentiation, and cytokine by T cells, providing a high-quality platform for screening bioactive compounds. Using the T cell differentiation model, our previous study revealed that the sulfated oligosaccharide of Gracilaria lemaneiformis (GLSO) could selectively target T cells, inhibit their activation and IFNγ production, and thereby modulate Th1 cell-mediated immunity [23]. In this study, AOH was also identified as the anti-inflammatory function by targeting T cell activation. Moreover, using this OVA-OTII system, our data revealed AOH treatment enhanced regulatory T cells (Tregs) cell differentiation in vitro and in vivo (Figure S5). Tregs are a specialized subset of CD4$^+$ T cells critical for maintaining immune homeostasis, preventing autoimmunity, and modulating immune responses [26]. These results highlighted the multi-function of our OVA-OTII system during exploring T cell differentiation. Consideration of the ocean harbors a wide range of naturally active substances with diverse structures; this model could be utilized to evaluate other natural products for their anti-inflammatory effects or immunomodulatory activities.

Restraining T cell activation controls the onset and progression of T-cell-related inflammation. Zhou et al. reported a JNK pathway-associated phosphatase controls inflammatory bowel disease by suppressing CD4$^+$ T cell activation [27]. A marine-derived compound, salinosporamide A, exhibited inhibitory activity on T cell activation, showing potential for the prevention and control of autoimmune diseases [28]. Prolonged T cell activation leads to sustained inflammation [29], tissue damage [30], and susceptibility to secondary infections [31]. Under the influence of chemokines, activated T cells migrate from lymphoid organs to the site of inflammation [32,33]. In addition to controlling T cell activation, regulating T cell migration can effectively mitigate inflammation. Yang et al. reported that a non-peptide CCR5 antagonist could regulate T cell migration to inhibit collagen-induced joint inflammation [34]. The AOH compound, screened in this study for its anti-inflammatory effect on T cells, was a type of mycotoxin. AOH had been noted for modulating inflammatory responses by altering macrophage morphology, disrupting cytokine signaling, and inhibiting LPS-induced immune reactions, which are involved in nuclear factor κB activation [20,35,36]. Our findings indicated that AOH could inhibit early T cell activation without disrupting normal antigen presentation. The early intervention of an overactive immune system is very beneficial for alleviating the pathological damage caused by viral infections or inflammation [37,38]. This study also found that early intervention with AOH in the lung injury model was able to inhibit T cell activation, differentiation, and migration, as well as reduce the recruitment of other cells to the site of inflammation, showing promise as a novel immunomodulator for inflammation-related disorders, warranting further preclinical investigation.

Therefore, our findings demonstrate that AOH exerted anti-inflammatory effects through an inhibition of early T cell activation, migration, and cytokine secretion, while our study identified limitations in the scope of disease models. Beyond verifying the anti-inflammatory efficacy of AOH in lung inflammation, we still need to focus on the pharmacological effects of AOH in more disease models, such as chronic inflammatory disorders (e.g., chronic immune enteritis), which are involved in sustained T cell differentiation and unbalance of Th17/Treg cells. Moreover, it was worth exploring whether AOH controlled immune response in tumors, while current evidence demonstrated AOH's efficacy in inducing tumor cell apoptosis [19]. In addition, although we evaluated that AOH did not influence immune homeostasis, the immunotoxicity and non-immunotoxicity of AOH still need to be further studied, such as whether AOH induced toxicity and damage to endothelial or epithelial cells and whether long-term administration or higher doses of AOH caused immune suppression, gastrointestinal reactions, and liver and kidney damage. Finally, the precise molecular mechanisms underlying AOH's inhibition of early T cell activation and migration necessitated further investigation, which will help us to provide a combination intervention of AOH with other immunomodulatory drugs to better control inflammation or with immune checkpoint inhibitors to robustly better anti-tumor effects.

4. Materials and Methods

4.1. Alternariol Extraction, Isolation, and Purification

Alternariol was obtained by culture and fermentation using *Alternaria* sp. The fungus strain (*Alternaria* sp.) was isolated from the deep-sea gammarid shrimp collected by Shanghai Rainbowfish Ocean Science and Technology at the depth of 10,870 m of the central sea of Papua New Guinea. Alternariol was obtained by culture and fermentation using *Alternaria* sp. The specimen of the fungus was preserved in the China Typical Cultures Collection Center (Wuhan, China) with the registration number of CCTCC NO: M 2022501. *Alternaria* sp. The voucher strain was preserved at the Marine Culture Collection of China, Third Institute of Oceanography, Ministry of Natural Resources, Xiamen, China, and given the accession number "Xia 20". *Alternaria* sp. Xia 20 were statically incubated in medium at 25 °C for 31 days. The fermented culture was extracted with EtOAc three times to provide a crude extract. The extract was redissolved in MeOH and extracted with petroleum ether (PE) three times. The MeOH solution was evaporated under reduced pressure to obtain a defatted extract (25 g). The EtOAc extract was then subjected to column chromatography (CC) over silica gel using gradient CH2Cl2-MeOH (100:1→10:1) to provide four fractions (Fr.1–Fr.5). Fraction Fr.5 (5.7 g) was purified by CC on Sephadex LH-20 (MeOH) to yield AOH (155.0 mg).

AOH was isolated as a yellow powder. The molecular formula C14H10O5 was determined by the negative HR-ESI-MS at [M-H]- at m/z 257.1, indicating ten degrees of unsaturation. The 1H NMR data of AOH presented the diagnostic signals of four olefinic hydrogens at δH 7.19 (1H, d, J = 1.4 Hz, H-10), 6.67 (1H, d, J = 2.3 Hz, H-2), 6.59 (1H, d, J = 2.4 Hz, H-4), and 6.33 (1H, d, J = 1.5 Hz, H-8), and one methyl group at 2.68 (3H, s, H-11). The 13C NMR spectrum showed 14 carbon resonances consisting of one methyl (δC 25.2), four methines (δC 100.8, 101.6, 104.3, 117.5), and nine quaternary carbons (δC 97.4, 108.9, 138.1, 138.3, 152.6, 158.4, 164.1, 164.7, 165.4). Comparison of NMR data with those of the compound alternariol showed their structures were similar.

4.2. In Vitro Cell Models

The OVA-OTII system was previously reported [23]. Briefly, DCs were obtained from Rag1-/- mice and added to 96-well U-plates (1×10^5 cells/well) with 5 μg/well of OVA (Sigma-Aldrich, St. Louis, MO, USA) at day 1. According to treatment with PBS or AOH, cells were divided into OVA + PBS and OVA + AOH groups. Purified naïve OTII $CD4^+$ T cells (2×10^5 cells/well) were incubated with DCs at day 0. For the iTreg differentiation, OVA-stimulated OTII $CD4^+$ T cells were cultured with IL2 (5 ng/mL) and TGFβ (1 ng/mL) at day 0. Cells were cultured in RPMI1640 containing 10% FBS at 37 °C in an incubator. After 4 days, cells were harvested for antibody staining and analyzed by flow cytometer.

For BMDC and BMDM culture, bone marrow cells were obtained from the hind leg bone of mice, primary cells were cultured in RPMI1640 containing 10% FBS for 6 days with 10 ng/mL interleukin (IL)4 and 20 ng/mL GM-CSF for BMDC induction or 20 ng/mL GM-CSF for BMDM induction. Cells were seeded into 24-well plates and divided into PBS and AOH groups. 24 h later, cells were collected for flow cytometry to examine the effect of AOH on the maturation and function of BMDCs and BMDMs.

4.3. Antibodies

The following monoclonal antibodies were used for flow cytometry: Anti-CD4 (GK1.5), anti-CD8α (53–6.7), anti-CD25 (PC61.5), anti-CD44 (IM7), anti-CD62L (MEL-14), anti-CD69 (H1.2F3), anti-CD71(RI7217.1.4), anti-ICOS(C398.4A), anti-CD11b (M1/70), anti-CD11c (N418), anti-F4/80 (BM8), anti-Gr1 (RB6-8C5), anti-Foxp3 (FJK.16s), anti-MHCII(M5/114.15.2), anti-T-bet (4B10), anti-Eomes (Dan11mag), anti-TCRβ (H57-597), anti-IFNγ (XMG1.2), anti-TNFα (MP6-XT22), anti-IL-2 (JES6-5H4), anti-CD90.1 (Thy-1.1), anti-Siglec F (1RNM44N), anti-IL4 (11B11), anti-CD80 (16-10A1a), anti-CD86 (GL1), anti-B220 (RA3-6B2), anti-IgM (11/41), anti-c-Kit (2B8), anti-Ki6/7 (16A8), anti-CTLA4 (UC10-4B9), anti-Bcl2 (10C4), PE Annexin V Apoptosis Detection Kit I (559763). All the antibodies were purchased from BD Biosciences (San Jose, CA, USA), Biolegend (San Diego, CA, USA), or eBioscience (San Diego, CA, USA).

4.4. Mouse Model

In all the in vivo experiments, we treated AOH as a dose of 8 mg/kg according to our previous report for intervention of allergy using 8 mg/kg AME, a structurally analogous compound of AOH [22]. To detect immune homeostasis in mice after AOH treatment: C57BL/6J mice (4–5 weeks old) were randomly divided into two groups: PBS group and AOH group. Mice received 200 μL of PBS or AOH (8 mg/kg) via intragastric gavage (i.g.) once daily for 14 consecutive days. On day 15, mice were euthanized to collect immune-related organs, including LN, spleen, thymus, and bone marrow; T cell and B cell development; T cell activation; cytokine production were analyzed by flow cytometry. For the mouse model of lung injury, C57BL/6J mice (6–8 weeks old) were randomly divided into two groups: OVA^+PBS group and OVA^+AOH group. The mice were immunized with OVA/Alum (100 μg OVA) on days 0, 7, and 14. During immunization, the OVA+AOH group received 200 μL of AOH (8 mg/kg) orally for three consecutive days. On day 18, mice were intranasally challenged with 20 μL of 50 mg/mL OVA solution for four consecutive days and gavaged with PBS or AOH. Mice were dissected on day 22. Lung tissues were stained with hematoxylin-eosin (H&E), and immune cells in the LN and lungs were analyzed by flow cytometry.

The OT-II mice (#004194), C57BL/6J mice (#000664), and Rag1-/- mice (#003145) used in this study were purchased from Jackson Laboratories (USA). All animals were maintained in strict accordance with the Xiamen University Guide for the Care and Use of Laboratory Animals. The culture and operation protocols of the mice were approved by the Animal Research Ethics Committee of Xiamen University (Ethics No. XMULAC20230060, approved on 14 April 2023) and complied with the international regulations on the welfare and protection of laboratory animals.

4.5. *In Vivo Cell Migration Assay*

Two groups of cells were obtained using an in vitro OT-II (CD90.1 background) T cell differentiation system, OVA+PBS and OVA+AOH. On day 1, C57BL/6J mice (expressing a CD90.2 background) were divided into two groups. Each mouse was injected with $CD4^+$ T cells (2×10^6/mouse) by intravenous injection. On day 0, the mice were intranasally stimulated with OVA. On days 1 and 2, mice were dissected and analyzed for the proportion of $CD4^+$ $CD90.1^+$ cells in bronchoalveolar lavage fluid (BALF), lymph nodes (LNs), and lung immune cells.

4.6. *Cell Acquisition*

For collecting cells from BALF, an incision in the trachea of the mouse was made, and the lagging needle was inserted into the trachea. One milliliter of saline was inhaled with a syringe; the lagging needle was attached and the saline was injected into the lungs. The suction was repeated three times, and the above operation was repeated three times. The BALF was centrifuged to obtain cells.

For obtaining infiltrated immune cells from lungs, the lungs were mechanically dissected and digested at 37 °C for 60 min in RPMI with 10% FBS, 1% penicillin/streptomycin, 1 mg/mL collagenase Type 4 (Worthington Biochemical, Lakewood, NJ, USA), and 0.1 mg/mL DNase I (Sangon Biotech, Shanghai, China). The cells obtained by Percoll (Cytiva, Uppsala, Sweden) isolation were then used for flow cytometric staining and analysis.

4.7. *Flow Cytometry*

After obtaining the single cell suspension, the cell surface antibodies were added and incubated at 4 °C for 15 min. To analyze cytokine release, cells were stimulated (37 °C, 4 h) with PMA (YEASEN, Shanghai, China), Ionomycin (YEASEN, Shanghai, China), and GolgiPlug (BD Bioscience). After surface staining, cells were fixed and permeabilized using the fixation/permeabilization buffer kit (eBioscience, Boston, MA, USA) at 4 °C for 15 min. And then intracellular protein expression was assessed by staining cells at 4 °C for 1 h. To detect intracellular expression of transcription factors, cells were stained intranuclearly using a fixation/permeabilization buffer kit after labeling with surface antibodies. To observe cell proliferation, OTII $CD4^+$ T cells (2×10^5 cells/well, 96 wells) were pre-stained with 0.5 μM CFSE for 30 min at 37 °C and co-cultured with DC cells for 3.5 days. All flow cytometry data were collected on LSR Fortessa (BD Biosciences, Franklin Lakes, NJ, USA) and analyzed using FlowJo software 10 (Treestar (BD), Ashland, OR, USA).

4.8. Statistical Analysis

Statistical values were statistically processed using GraphPad Prism software 8.0, and HE staining results and immunofluorescence staining results were graphically processed using Case Viewer software 3.0. Statistical analysis was performed using *t*-test, "*", $p < 0.05$, "**", $p < 0.001$, "****", $p < 0.0001$, ns indicates no significant differences, and the data were organized and summarized using Adobe Illustrator software v27(2023).

5. Conclusions

In conclusion, AOH isolated from marine fungi had significant anti-inflammatory activity via modulating the early activation and transcription process of T cells without targeting antigen-presenting cell function, inhibiting T cell proliferation, and reducing the release of inflammatory factors. With the inhibitory effects of inflammatory cytokine production and the regulation of T cell migration and infiltration, AOH showed an effective alleviating effect on OVA-induced lung injury and inflammation in mice. Therefore, as an active substance of marine origin, AOH is expected to provide a theoretical basis for the development of novel drugs for inflammatory and related immune diseases.

Supplementary Materials: The following supporting information can be downloaded at: https://www.mdpi.com/article/10.3390/md23030133/s1, Figure S1. NMR spectrum of AOH. Figure S2. The effect of AOH on CD4+ T cell numbers in OVA-OTII model in vitro. Figure S3. AOH does not affect immune cell development and homeostasis in steady stage. Figure S4. The impact of late-stage AOH intervention on lung-injured mice. Figure S5. AOH increases Treg differentiation in vitro and in vivo.

Author Contributions: Conceptualization, W.-H.L. and G.L.; methodology: C.L., F.G., W.-H.L. and G.L.; investigation: C.L., F.W., J.S., Y.H. and X.W.; writing—original draft: C.L. and F.G.; formal analysis: F.G., Z.Z., D.L., Y.Z., G.L. and Q.L.; data curation: Y.Z., F.G., G.L. and Z.Z.; methodology: C.L., F.G., Z.Z., F.W., D.L., J.S., Y.H., X.W., G.L. and W.-H.L.; resources: X.Y.; writing—review and editing: W.-H.L., Y.Z. and G.L.; funding acquisition: G.L., C.L. and Q.L.; supervision: Q.L.; project administration: Q.L. All authors have read and agreed to the published version of the manuscript.

Funding: This work was supported by grants from the National Natural Science Foundation of China (82202006, 32472334), Key Project of Natural Science Research of Anhui Education Department (2022AH050778), and the Xiamen Marine Development Program of China (22GYY007HJ07), the Science and Technology Program of Xiamen City (2023CXY0307).

Institutional Review Board Statement: The culture and operation protocols of the mice were approved by the Animal Research Ethics Committee of Xiamen University, Ethics No. XMULAC20230060, approved on 14 April 2023.

Data Availability Statement: The data used to support the findings of this study are included within the article. Further inquiries can be directed to the corresponding author.

Conflicts of Interest: The authors declare that they have no competing interests.

References

1. Giovanni, M.; Alessandro, M.; Alice, C.; Irene, M.; Silvia, S. Immune-mediated inflammatory diseases: Common and different pathogenic and clinical features. *Autoimmun. Rev.* **2023**, *22*, 103410.
2. Søren, R.P.; Thomas, P.; Seth, L.M.; Trine, H.M. Constitutive immune mechanisms: Mediators of host defence and immune regulation. *Nat. Rev. Immunol.* **2020**, *21*, 137–150.
3. Ruslan, M.J.N. Origin and physiological roles of inflammation. *Nature* **2008**, *454*, 428–435.
4. Alessandro, L.; Domenico, F.; Marina, F.; Alessandra, P.; Sergio, O.; Mauro, M. Bioactive lipids, inflammation and chronic diseases. *Adv. Drug Deliv. Rev.* **2020**, *159*, 133–169.
5. Li, W.S.; Zhang, Q.Q.; Li, Q.; Liu, S.Y.; Yuan, G.Q.; Pan, Y.W. Innate immune response restarts adaptive immune response in tumors. *Front. Immunol.* **2023**, *14*, 1260705. [CrossRef]
6. Katherine, A.D.; Russell, E.V. Inflammasomes and adaptive immune responses. *Nat. Immunol.* **2021**, *22*, 412–422.

7. Watanabe, S.; Alexander, M.; Misharin, A.; Budinger, G.R.S. The role of macrophages in the resolution of inflammation. *J. Clin. Investig.* **2019**, *129*, 2619–2628. [CrossRef]
8. Sun, L.; Su, Y.; Jiao, A.; Wang, X.; Zhang, B. T cells in health and disease. *Signal. Transduct. Target. Ther.* **2023**, *8*, 235.
9. Bastian, K.; Anthony, C.B.; Naveen, S.; Andreas, D.B.; Susan, G.; Kristin, K.; Joanna, P.; Johannes, P.; Paulina, D.; Miriam, M.; et al. Cd4(+) t cell-induced inflammatory cell death controls immune-evasive tumours. *Nature* **2023**, *618*, 1033–1040.
10. Asuka, T.; Kentaro, I.; Yuka, T.; Yu, S.; Marlen, D.; Hiroyuki, T.; Masahiro, O.; Hideki, O. Evaluation of T-cell immune status of reduced-dose cyclosporine and everolimus combination therapy in kidney transplant patients. *Transplant Proc.* **2023**, *55*, 797–802.
11. Tobias, R.; Sumanta, B.; Andreas, S.M.; Steffen, P.; Falk, S.; Christopher, N.; Christina, B.S.; Alice, W.; Michael, H.; Thomas, M.; et al. Alemtuzumab-induced immune phenotype and repertoire changes: Implications for secondary autoimmunity. *Brain* **2022**, *145*, 1711–1725.
12. Gou, Q.; Dong, C.; Xu, H.; Khan, B.; Jin, J.; Liu, Q.; Shi, J.; Hou, Y. PD-L1 degradation pathway and immunotherapy for cancer. *Cell. Death Dis.* **2020**, *11*, 955. [CrossRef]
13. Renée, B.; Tom, V.M.; Edwin, B. CD47-sirpα blocking-based immunotherapy: Current and prospective therapeutic strategies. *Clin. Transl. Med.* **2022**, *12*, e943.
14. Jiri, P.; Eugenie, N.; Kamil, K.; Wenda, W. Cyclosporine a: Chemistry and toxicity—A review. *Curr. Med. Chem.* **2020**, *28*, 3925–3934.
15. Khalifa, S.A.M.; Elias, N.; Farag, M.A.; Chen, L.; Saeed, A.; Hegazy, M.F.; Moustafa, M.S.; Abd El-Wahed, A.; Al-Mousawi, S.M.; Musharraf, S.G.; et al. Marine natural products: A source of novel anticancer drugs. *Mar. Drugs.* **2019**, *17*, 491. [CrossRef] [PubMed]
16. Montuori, E.; De Pascale, D.; Lauritano, C. Recent discoveries on marine organism immunomodulatory activities. *Mar. Drugs.* **2022**, *20*, 422. [CrossRef]
17. Shih-Chao, L.; Caitlin, W.L.; Allison, K.S.; Lauren, P.; Nicole, B.; Jeffrey, L.C.W.; Mikell, P.; Wendy, K.S.; Kylene, K.H. Homoseongomycin, a compound isolated from marine actinomycete bacteria k3-1, is a potent inhibitor of encephalitic alphaviruses. *Antiviral. Res.* **2021**, *191*, 105087.
18. Kim, E.N.; Gao, M.; Choi, H.; Jeong, G.S. Marine microorganism-derived macrolactins inhibit inflammatory mediator effects in LPS-induced macrophage and microglial cells by regulating bach1 and HO-1/Nrf2 signals through inhibition of tlr4 activation. *Molecules* **2020**, *25*, 656. [CrossRef]
19. Lin, H.Y.; Lin, Y.S.; Shih, S.P.; Lee, S.B.; El-Shazly, M.; Chang, K.M.; Yang, Y.S.H.; Lee, Y.L.; Lu, M.C. The anti-proliferative activity of secondary metabolite from the marine *Streptomyces* sp. against prostate cancer cells. *Life* **2021**, *11*, 1414. [CrossRef]
20. Grover, S.; Lawrence, C.B. The alternaria alternata mycotoxin alternariol suppresses lipopolysaccharide-induced inflammation. *Int. J. Mol. Sci.* **2017**, *18*, 1577. [CrossRef]
21. Karolina, K.; Dominika Ewa, H.-G.; Marta Justyna, K.; Kinga Anna, U.; Kamila, D.; Agnieszka Wanda, P.-C. Mycotoxin alternariol (AOH) affects viability and motility of mammary breast epithelial cells. *Int. J. Mol. Sci.* **2021**, *22*, 696. [CrossRef]
22. Liu, Y.; Zou, Z.B.; Gu, F.D.; Lin, Y.F.; Li, Y.; Chen, H.Y.; Liu, H.; Yang, X.W.; Liu, G.M.; Liu, Q.M. Alternariol Monomethyl Ether Alleviates Ovalbumin- Induced Food Allergy by Suppressing MAPK and NF-κB Signaling Pathways of Mast Cells. *J. Agric. Food Chem.* **2024**, *72*, 5463–5476. [CrossRef]
23. Liu, Q.; Zhou, Y.; Ma, L.; Gu, F.; Liao, K.; Liu, Y.; Zhang, Y.; Liu, H.; Hong, Y.; Cao, M.; et al. Sulfate oligosaccharide of gracilaria lemaneiformis modulates type 1 immunity by restraining t cell activation. *Carbohydr. Polym.* **2022**, *288*, 119377. [CrossRef]
24. Heikrujam Thoihen, M.; Girdhari, L. T cell receptor signaling in the differentiation and plasticity of CD4(+) t cells. *Cytokine Growth Factor Rev.* **2022**, *69*, 14–27.
25. Daniel, Y.W.; Joe-Elie, S.; Justine, V.C.; Sunandana, C.; Christian, M.; Fei, Y.; Shilin, Z.; Satya, D.; Kathryn, E.B.; Lisa, H.; et al. Fatal Toxic Effects Associated With Immune Checkpoint Inhibitors: A Systematic Review and Meta-analysis. *JAMA Oncol.* **2018**, *4*, 1721–1728.
26. Scheinecker, C.; Göschl, L.; Bonelli, M. Treg cells in health and autoimmune diseases: New insights from single cell analysis. *J. Autoimmun.* **2020**, *110*, 102376. [CrossRef]
27. Rui, Z.; Ying, C.; Jing, L.; Min, C.; Hongling, W.; Meifang, H.; Shi, L.; Xiaobing, W.; Qiu, Z. JNK pathway-associated phosphatase/dusp22 suppresses CD4(+) T-cell activation and TH1/TH17-cell differentiation and negatively correlates with clinical activity in inflammatory bowel disease. *Front. Immunol.* **2017**, *8*, 781.
28. Hyun-Su, L.; Gil-Saeng, J. Salinosporamide a, a marine-derived proteasome inhibitor, inhibits t cell activation through regulating proliferation and the cell cycle. *Molecules* **2020**, *25*, 5031. [CrossRef]
29. Raquel, G.-B.; Angela, S.; Beatriz, H.F.; Cristina, R.; Hector, S.M.; Jose, M.G.G. CD4 T-cell subsets and the pathophysiology of inflammatory bowel disease. *Int. J. Mol. Sci.* **2023**, *24*, 2696. [CrossRef]
30. Gregory, P.W.; Aubrey, M.S.; Asta, J.; Nicole, J.G.; David, G.S.; Ashley, S.H. CD4 T cells mediate brain inflammation and neurodegeneration in a mouse model of parkinson's disease. *Brain* **2021**, *144*, 2047–2059.

31. Tingxia, L.; Wei, C.; Taisheng, L. Hiv-related immune activation and inflammation: Current understanding and strategies. *Immunol Res.* **2021**, *2021*, 7316456.
32. Noor, B.; Alexander, I.M.; Tiago, Z.; Anastasia, N.R.; Evan, M.C.; Scott, A.L.; Deborah, J.F. T cell activation niches-optimizing t cell effector function in inflamed and infected tissues. *Immunol. Rev.* **2021**, *306*, 164–180.
33. Keiko, N.; Gregory, S.W.; Miranda, R.L.C.; Sara, A.G.; Christina, L.W.; Gentaro, I.; Alessandra, L.-B.; Donald, N.C.; Hideki, N. Chemokine ccl19 promotes type 2 t-cell differentiation and allergic airway inflammation. *J. Allergy Clin. Immunol.* **2023**, *153*, 487–502.
34. Yi-Fu, Y.; Takao, M.; Ping, G.; Nobuya, Y.; Shiro, O.; Hiroshi, I.; Satoshi, O.; Takeshi, I.; Takahiro, T.; Toshiyuki, H.; et al. A non-peptide ccr5 antagonist inhibits collagen-induced arthritis by modulating t cell migration without affecting anti-collagen t cell responses. *Eur. J. Immunol.* **2002**, *32*, 2124–2132.
35. Solhaug, A.; Wisbech, C.; Christoffersen, T.E.; Hult, L.O.; Lea, T.; Eriksen, G.S. Holme JAThe mycotoxin alternariol induces DNA damage and modify macrophage phenotype and inflammatory responses. *Toxicol. Lett.* **2015**, *239*, 9–21. [CrossRef]
36. Jessica, K.; Ebru, C.; Cornelia, S.; Doris, M. The mycotoxin alternariol suppresses lipopolysaccharide-induced inflammation in thp-1 derived macrophages targeting the nf-κb signalling pathway. *Arch. Toxicol.* **2018**, *92*, 3347–3358.
37. Sun, S.; Zhao, G.; Liu, C.; Fan, W.; Zhou, X.; Zeng, L.; Guo, Y.; Kou, Z.; Yu, H.; Li, J.; et al. Treatment with anti-c5a antibody improves the outcome of h7n9 virus infection in african green monkeys. *Clin. Infect Dis.* **2014**, *60*, 856–895. [CrossRef]
38. Zhou, Y.; Fu, B.; Zheng, X.; Wang, D.; Zhao, C.; Qi, Y.; Sun, R.; Tian, Z.; Xu, X.; Wei, H. Pathogenic t-cells and inflammatory monocytes incite inflammatory storms in severe COVID-19 patients. *Natl. Sci. Rev.* **2020**, *7*, 998–1002. [CrossRef]

marine drugs

Article

Butyrolactone-I from Marine Fungal Metabolites Mitigates Heat-Stress-Induced Apoptosis in IPEC-J2 Cells and Mice Through the ROS/PERK/CHOP Signaling Pathway

Xueting Niu [1,2], Shengwei Chen [1,2], Xinchen Wang [1,2], Jiaying Wen [1,2], Xiaoxi Liu [2], Yanhong Yong [2], Zhichao Yu [2], Xingbing Ma [2], A. M. Abd El-Aty [3,4] and Xianghong Ju [1,2,*]

1 Marine Medical Research and Development Centre, Shenzhen Institute of Guangdong Ocean University, Shenzhen 518120, China; nxt1208@163.com (X.N.); csw9610@163.com (S.C.); wxc1202@outlook.com (X.W.); 18718018181@139.com (J.W.)

2 College of Coastal Agricultural Sciences, Guangdong Ocean University, Zhanjiang 524088, China; liuxiaoxi_06@163.com (X.L.); yongyanhong-007@163.com (Y.Y.); yujingmary@163.com (Z.Y.); mxb1984612@126.com (X.M.)

3 Department of Pharmacology, Faculty of Veterinary Medicine, Cairo University, Giza 12211, Egypt; abdelaty44@hotmail.com

4 Department of Medical Pharmacology, Medical Faculty, Ataturk University, Erzurum 25240, Turkey

* Correspondence: juxh77@163.com; Tel.: +86-13553523590

Abstract: Heat stress poses a significant challenge to animal husbandry, contributing to oxidative stress, intestinal mucosal injury, and apoptosis, which severely impact animal health, growth, and production efficiency. The development of safe, sustainable, and naturally derived solutions to mitigate these effects is critical for advancing sustainable agricultural practices. Butyrolactone-I (BTL-I), a bioactive compound derived from deep-sea fungi (Aspergillus), shows promise as a functional feed additive to combat heat stress in animals. This study explored the protective effects of BTL-I against heat-stress-induced oxidative stress and apoptosis in IPEC-J2 cells and mice. Our findings demonstrated that BTL-I effectively inhibited the heat-stress-induced upregulation of HSP70 and HSP90, alleviating intestinal heat stress. Both in vitro and in vivo experiments revealed that heat stress increased intestinal cell apoptosis, with a significant upregulation of Bax/Bcl-2 expression, while BTL-I pretreatment significantly reduced apoptosis-related protein levels, showcasing its protective effects. Furthermore, BTL-I suppressed oxidative stress markers (ROS and MDA) while enhancing antioxidant activity (SOD levels). BTL-I also reduced the expression of p-PERK, p-eIF2α, ATF4, and CHOP, mitigating oxidative and endoplasmic reticulum stress in intestinal cells. In conclusion, BTL-I demonstrates the potential to improve animal resilience to heat stress, supporting sustainable livestock production systems. Its application as a natural, eco-friendly feed additive will contribute to the development of sustainable agricultural practices.

Keywords: Butyrolactone-I (BTL-I); heat stress; intestinal apoptosis; HSP70 and HSP90 expression; oxidative stress; endoplasmic reticulum stress

1. Introduction

As the global climate is continuously changing, high temperatures and humidity pose significant challenges to animal production. Within a suitable environmental range, heat production and heat dissipation are balanced and the physiological and metabolic conditions are good. When the ambient temperature exceeds a suitable range, the body's heat dissipation system becomes imbalanced, resulting in the accumulation of excessive heat within the body. This leads to a nonspecific physiological response called heat stress (HS). HS is a crucial factor that induces stress in tropical and subtropical regions, causing severe oxidative stress [1], damage to the intestinal mucosa [2,3], inflammatory responses [4], and apoptosis [5]. These may be among the key factors causing a reduced feed intake, decreased milk and egg production, and weight loss [6].

The intestine is an important digestive organ that absorbs nutrients and excretes metabolic waste [7]. Digested food is broken down into nutrients in the small intestine and enters the bloodstream through absorption by intestinal epithelial cells. Moreover, the intestinal barrier protects the host from harmful bacteria. Under heat stress, the intestinal blood flow is reduced, and hypoxia results in ATP depletion, decreased ion pump activity and cell activity, and cell membrane and tight junction damage; thus, many pathogenic microorganisms invade and cause disease [8]. Heat stress can cause severe cell apoptosis and tissue damage [3,9], which are important causes of heat stress pathogenesis. Research has demonstrated that heat stress (HS) can accumulate reactive oxygen species and impair mitochondrial function, thus inducing apoptosis [10]. Moreover, HS has been shown to induce mammary epithelial cell apoptosis through an ROS-independent pathway [11]. Acute HS can activate p53-mediated mitochondrial apoptosis, contributing to liver injury [12,13]. Another study reported that acute heat stress triggers the unfolded protein response (UPR), leading to endoplasmic reticulum stress and subsequent apoptosis in the liver [14,15]. These findings underscore the close relationship between apoptosis and HS.

Butyrolactone-I (BTL-I) is derived from the deep-sea fungus Aspergillus C23-3, an endophytic fungus that was isolated from Pukou coral (Porites pugorica) in Xuwen (Guangdong, China). Extensive research has highlighted its potential as a potent α-glucosidase inhibitor, offering beneficial effects in managing type 2 diabetes by modulating gut microbes [16]. Additionally, BTL-I serves as a CDK-2 kinase inhibitor, promoting the apoptosis of cancer cells while exerting a protective effect against neuronal apoptosis [17]. However, whether BTL-I has the potential to alleviate apoptosis as a heat stress therapeutic drug has not been explored.

At present, heat stress is still a prominent problem that threatens human and animal health in tropical and subtropical areas. The use of bioactive products to alleviate stress injury is highly practical. Therefore, this study aimed to establish a heat shock model using IPEC-J2 cells and a heat stress model in mice to investigate the molecular mechanism through which BTL-I intervenes in intestinal epithelial cell apoptosis.

2. Results

2.1. *Effect of BTL-I on the Expression of Related Factors in Heat-Shocked IPEC-J2 Cells*

The cytotoxicity of BTL-I on IPEC-J2 cells was evaluated via the CCK8 assay. After IPEC-J2 cells were exposed to three different concentrations of BTL-I for 24 h, the cell proliferation rate was unaffected (Figure 1A). However, as the duration of the heat shock treatment increased (1.5 h, 3.0 h, 4.5 h, and 6.0 h), there was a notable and significant decrease in the cell proliferation rate ($p < 0.01$). Since the cell proliferation rate was still greater than 80% after 1.5 h of heat shock treatment, subsequent assessments were conducted at this time point (Figure 1B).

Moreover, after pretreatment with BTL-I, the IPEC-J2 cells exhibited a dose-dependent increase in the cell proliferation rate following heat shock (Figure 1C). Additionally, Western blot analysis revealed that the expression levels of HSP70 and HSP90 significantly increased ($p < 0.01$) following heat shock treatment. Conversely, the expression levels of these proteins were significantly reduced ($p < 0.05$) after BTL-I pretreatment (Figure 1D–F).

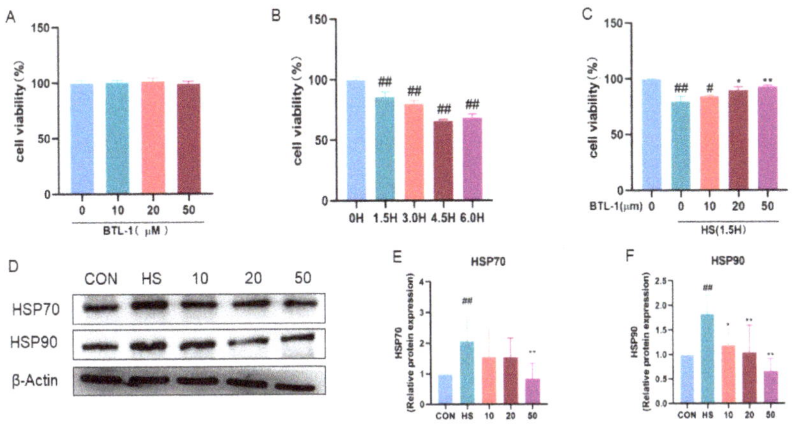

Figure 1. Effect of BTL-I on the expression of related factors in heat-shocked IPEC-J2 cells. IPEC-J2 cells were treated with different concentrations of BTL-I (10, 20, or 50 μM) for 24 h and then coincubated with the heat shock (HS) group in a 5% CO_2 incubator at 42 °C for 1.5 h. Cell viability was determined via a CCK8 assay. (**A**) Effects of BTL-I on the viability of IPEC-J2 cells; (**B**) effects of heat shock treatment on the viability of IPEC-J2 cells; (**C**) effects of BTL-I and heat shock cotreatment on IPEC-J2 cells; and (**D–F**) the expression levels of the heat shock proteins HSP70 and HSP90 were detected via Western blotting. The results are expressed as the means ± SEMs. $^{\#}$ $p < 0.05$, $^{\#\#}$ $p < 0.01$ compared with the control group; * $p < 0.05$, ** $p < 0.01$ compared with the HS group.

2.2. Effects of BTL-I on the Apoptosis of Heat-Shocked IPEC-J2 Cells

We assessed the impact of BTL-I on IPEC-J2 cell apoptosis. The findings indicated that the apoptosis rate of the IPEC-J2 cells increased following heat shock treatment compared with that in the CON group. However, after pretreatment with BTL-I, the percentage of IPEC-J2 cells that underwent apoptosis decreased (Figure 2A). Further analysis of apoptosis-related proteins revealed that the mRNA expression of *Bax* significantly increased ($p < 0.05$) after heat shock, but decreased following BTL-I pretreatment (Figure 2B). The mRNA expression of *Bcl-2* had the opposite effect ($p < 0.05$) (Figure 2C). BTL-I pretreatment led to a significant decrease in the Bax/Bcl-2 protein ratio, as determined by Western blotting ($p < 0.01$) (Figure 2D,E). Additionally, the immunofluorescence results demonstrated that the fluorescence intensity of Bcl-2 was more pronounced in the IPEC-J2 cells treated with BTL-I after heat shock, whereas the fluorescence intensity of Bax decreased upon BTL-I addition (Figure 2F,G).

2.3. Effect of BTL-I on the ROS/PERK/CHOP Signaling Pathway in IPEC-J2 Cells Subjected to Heat Shock

To investigate the mechanism underlying heat-shock-induced cell apoptosis, we examined the response of the ROS/PERK/CHOP signaling pathway, and the results are illustrated in Figure 3. Following heat shock (HS), there was a significant increase in the ROS and MDA levels in the IPEC-J2 cells ($p < 0.01$), as well as a decrease in SOD expression ($p < 0.01$) (Figure 3A–C). However, the addition of BTL-I effectively reversed the increases in ROS and MDA and the decrease in SOD ($p < 0.05$).

Furthermore, after heat shock treatment, the mRNA expression of *ATF4* and *CHOP* was significantly increased ($p < 0.05$). However, the expression of these genes was significantly downregulated after pretreatment with BTL-I ($p < 0.05$) (Figure 3D,E). Western blotting revealed significant increases in p-PERK/PERK and p-eIF2α/eIF2α expression ($p < 0.01$) after heat shock, which was consistent with the changes observed in ATF4 and CHOP expression ($p < 0.01$). However, their expression levels decreased following BTL-I pretreatment (Figure 3F–J). The immunofluorescence results indicated that the fluorescence intensity of ATF4 increased upon heat shock treatment, whereas BTL-I pretreatment led to a reduction in its expression (Figure 3K).

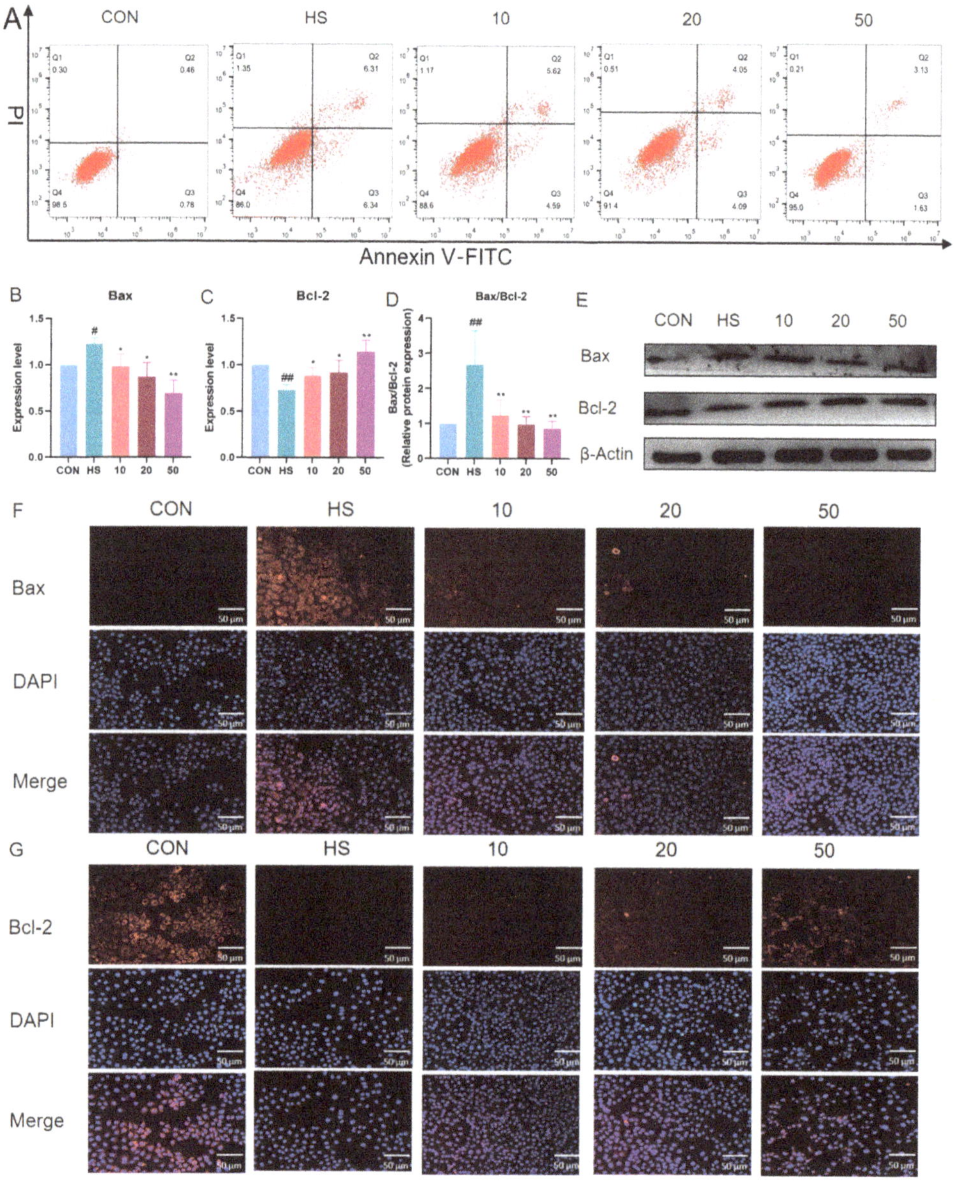

Figure 2. Effects of BTL-I on IPEC-J2 cell apoptosis after heat shock. (**A**) Flow cytometry analysis of the cell apoptosis rate; (**B**,**C**) qPCR analysis of *Bax* and *Bcl-2*; (**D**,**E**) Western blotting analysis of Bax and Bcl-2; and (**F**,**G**) IF analysis of Bax and Bcl-2; the red fluorescence represents Bcl-2 and Bax protein expression, and the blue fluorescence corresponds to the cell nuclei; the results are expressed as the means ± SEMs. # $p < 0.05$, ## $p < 0.01$ compared with the control group; * $p < 0.05$, ** $p < 0.01$ compared with the HS group.

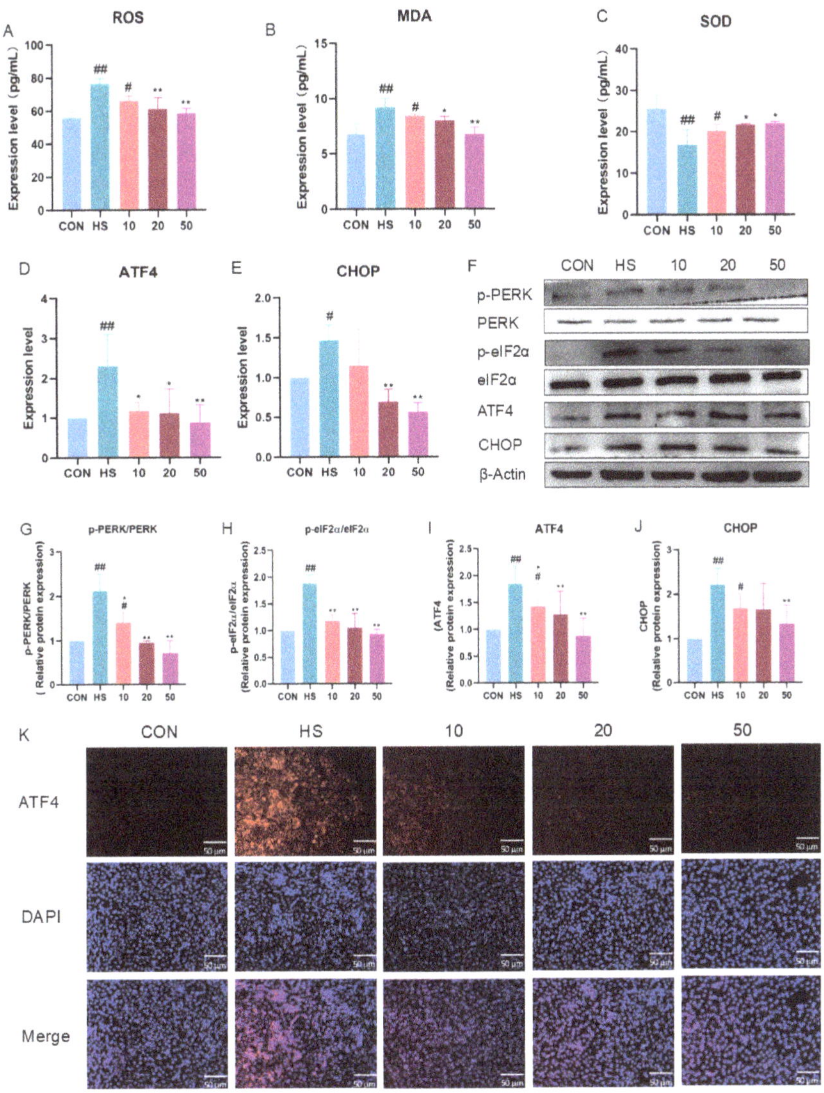

Figure 3. Effect of BTL-I on the ROS/PERK/CHOP signaling pathway in IPEC-J2 cells subjected to heat shock. (**A–C**) ELISA analysis of the levels of the oxidative markers ROS, MDA, and SOD; (**D**,**E**) qPCR analysis of the levels of the PERK/CHOP signaling pathway markers *ATF4* and *CHOP*; (**F–J**) Western blotting analysis of the levels of the PERK/CHOP signaling pathway markers p-PERK, PERK, p-eIF2α, eIF2α, ATF4, and CHOP; and (**K**) IF analysis of the levels of the PERK/CHOP signaling pathway marker ATF4. The results are expressed as the means ± SEMs. # $p < 0.05$, ## $p < 0.01$ compared with the control group; * $p < 0.05$, ** $p < 0.01$ compared with the HS group.

2.4. Effect of ROS Scavengers on the PERK/CHOP Signaling Pathway in Heat-Shocked IPEC-J2 Cells

To further investigate whether BTL-I inhibits apoptosis through endoplasmic reticulum stress (ERS), we examined the expression of PERK/CHOP-signaling-pathway-related proteins, as shown in Figure 4. The addition of the ROS scavenger NAC effectively reversed the heat-shock-induced increase in ROS accumulation ($p < 0.01$) (Figure 4A). Following heat shock treatment, the protein expressions of p-eIF2α/eIF2α, ATF4, and CHOP significantly increased ($p < 0.01$). However, the expressions of these proteins were notably inhibited after pretreatment with BTL-I or NAC ($p < 0.05$) (Figure 4B–G).

Moreover, compared with those in the CON group, the protein expression levels of Bax/Bcl-2 in the heat shock group were significantly greater ($p < 0.01$); however, pretreatment with 1 mM NAC significantly downregulated the expression of these genes ($p < 0.01$) (Figure 4H–L). These results suggest that BTL-I may exert its antiapoptotic effects through the inhibition of the ERS pathway and that the ROS scavenger NAC contributes to this protective effect.

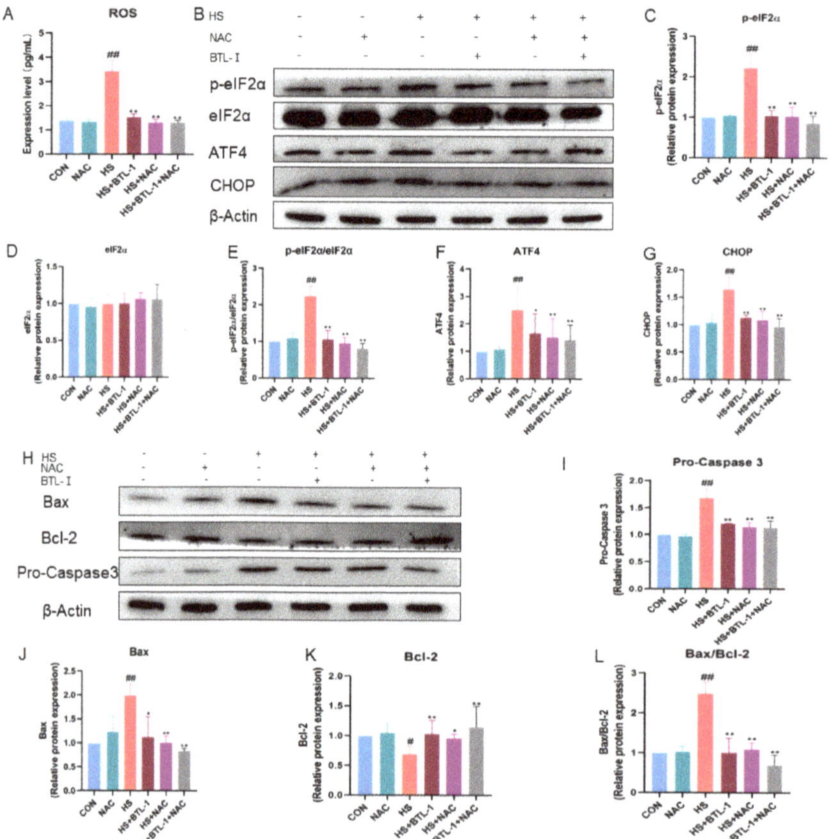

Figure 4. Effects of ROS scavengers on the PERK/CHOP signaling pathway and apoptosis in heat-shocked IPEC-J2 cells. IPEC-J2 cells were treated with BTL-I (50 μM) or NAC (1 mM) for 24 h or 3 h, respectively, and then placed together with the heat shock (HS) group in a cell incubator at 42 °C and 5% CO_2 for 1.5 h. (**A**) ELISA analysis of the oxidative marker ROS. (**B–G**) Western blot analysis of the expression of the PERK/CHOP signaling pathway markers p-PERK, PERK, p-eIF2α, eIF2α, ATF4, and CHOP. (**H–L**) Western blot analysis of the expression of the apoptosis markers Bax/Bcl-2 and procaspase 3. The results are expressed as the means ± SEMs. # $p < 0.05$, ## $p < 0.01$ compared with the control group; * $p < 0.05$, ** $p < 0.01$ compared with the HS group.

The immunofluorescence results demonstrated that, upon the addition of NAC, the fluorescence intensity of Bcl-2 was more pronounced than that in the IPEC-J2 cells treated with heat shock alone. Conversely, the fluorescence intensity of Bax decreased after the addition of NAC (Figure 5A,B).

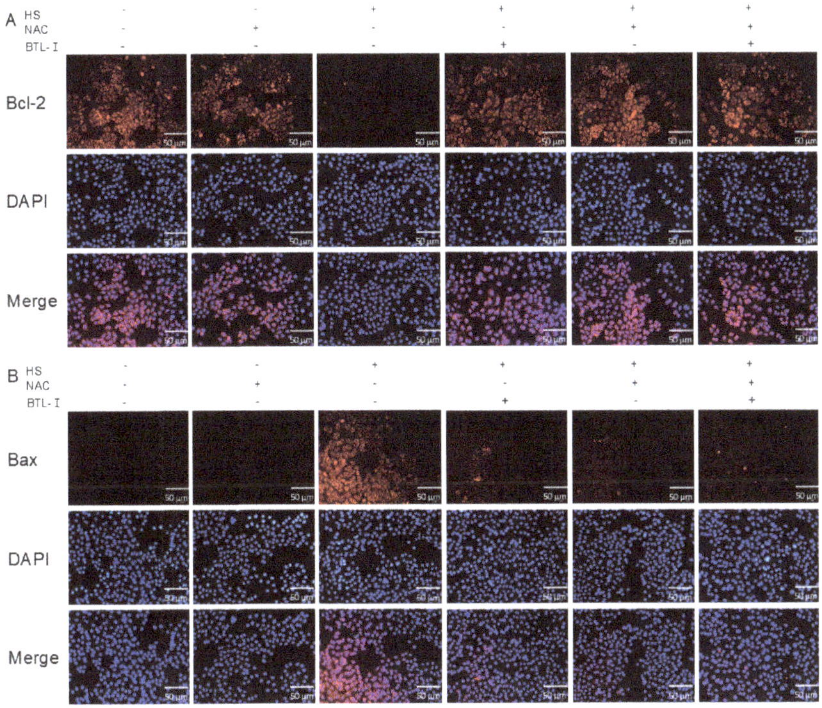

Figure 5. Effect of ROS scavengers on apoptosis in heat-shocked IPEC-J2 cells. (**A**,**B**) IF analysis of the apoptosis markers Bax and Bcl-2.

2.5. Effect of an ER Stress Inhibitor on the Apoptosis of Heat-Shocked IPEC-J2 Cells

To investigate the role of the PERK/CHOP signaling pathway, we pretreated cells with the ER stress inhibitor 4-PBA, and the results are shown in Figure 6. Compared with those in the heat shock group, the protein expression levels of p-eIF2α/eIF2α, ATF4, and CHOP were significantly lower after pretreatment with 1 mM 4-PBA ($p < 0.05$) (Figure 6A–F).

Furthermore, following pretreatment with 1 mM 4-PBA, the protein expressions of Bax/Bcl-2 and pro-caspase 3 were significantly lower than those in the HS group ($p < 0.05$) (Figure 6G–K). These findings indicate the potential involvement of the PERK/CHOP signaling pathway in these effects, and the ER stress inhibitor 4-PBA appears to play a role in mitigating apoptosis.

The immunofluorescence results revealed that, upon the addition of 4-PBA, the fluorescence intensity of Bcl-2 was more pronounced than that in the IPEC-J2 cells treated with heat shock alone. Conversely, the fluorescence intensity of Bax decreased after the addition of 4-PBA (Figure 7A,B).

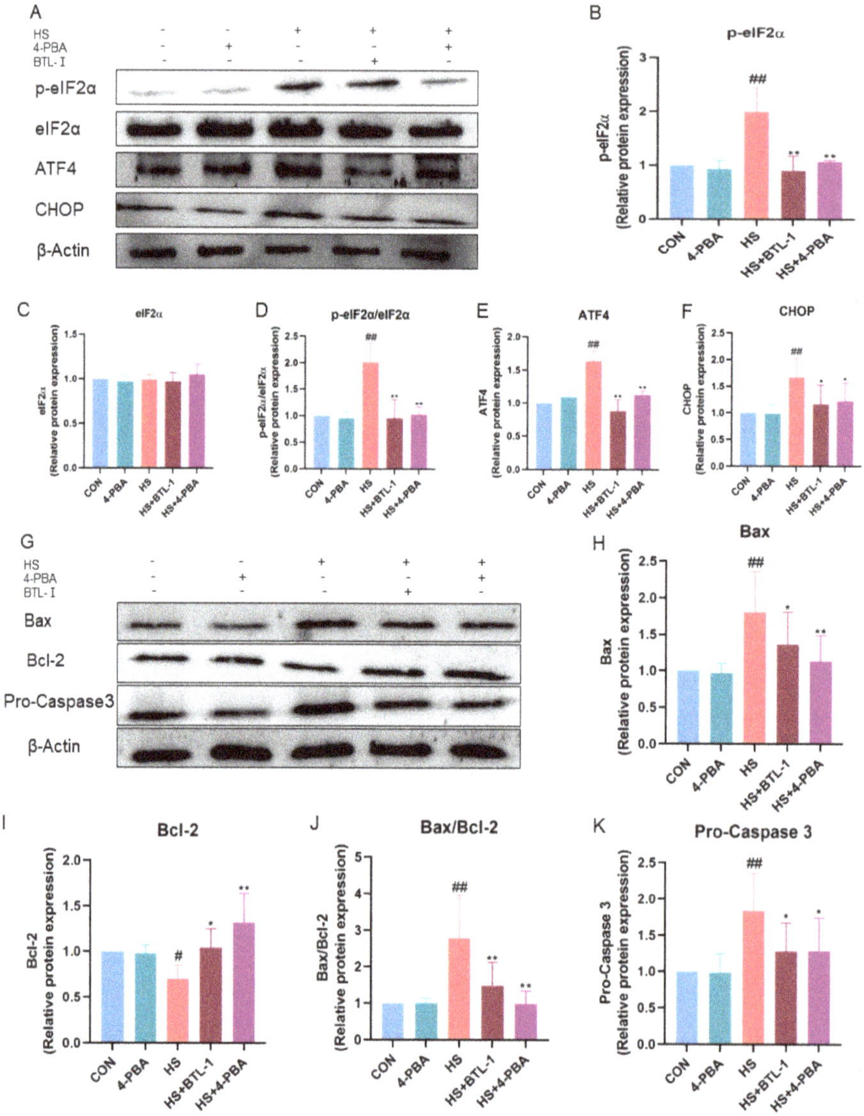

Figure 6. Effect of an ER stress inhibitor on the apoptosis of heat-shocked IPEC-J2 cells. IPEC-J2 cells were treated with BTL-I (50 μM) or 4-PBA (1 mM) for 24 h or 3 h, respectively, and then placed together with the heat shock (HS) group in a cell incubator at 42 °C and 5% CO_2 for 1.5 h. (**A–F**) Western blot analysis of the expression of the PERK/CHOP signaling pathway markers p-PERK, PERK, p-eIF2α, eIF2α, ATF4, and CHOP. (**G–K**) Western blot analysis of the expression of the apoptosis markers Bax/Bcl-2 and procaspase 3. The results are expressed as the means ± SEMs. $^{\#}$ $p < 0.05$, $^{\#\#}$ $p < 0.01$ compared with the control group; * $p < 0.05$, ** $p < 0.01$ compared with the HS group.

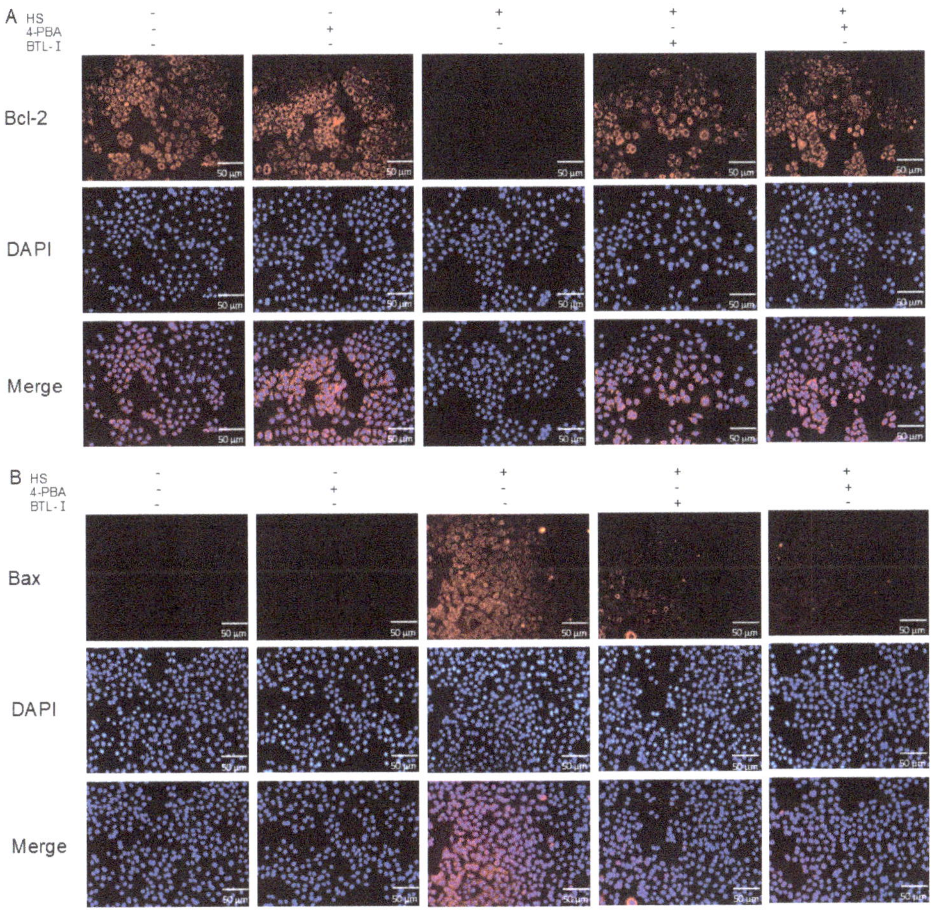

Figure 7. Effect of an endoplasmic reticulum inhibitor on the apoptosis of heat-shocked IPEC-J2 cells. (**A**,**B**) IF analysis of the apoptosis markers Bax and Bcl-2.

2.6. Protective Effect of BTL-I on Heat-Stressed Mice

We examined the impact of BTL-I on heat-stressed mice, and the results are presented in Figure 8. The expression of *HSP70* mRNA in the HS group was significantly upregulated ($p < 0.01$). Conversely, in the BTL-I group, the expression of *HSP70* mRNA was significantly downregulated ($p < 0.01$), with the most notable effect observed at a BTL-I dose of 5 mg/kg (Figure 8A). Furthermore, Western blotting revealed significant increases in the expressions of HSP70 and HSP90 after heat stress ($p < 0.05$). However, following BTL-I pretreatment, the expression levels of these genes decreased significantly ($p < 0.05$) (Figure 8B–D). As the duration of heat stress increased, the weight of the mice gradually decreased, whereas their water intake and body temperature increased (Figure 8E–G). However, after the oral administration of BTL-I, weight loss was mitigated, and water intake and body temperature gradually returned to normal levels. Additionally, the colon length of the mice decreased after heat stress, but this change was reversed after the oral administration of BTL-I (Figure 8H–I). These results suggest that BTL-I has a beneficial effect on mitigating the adverse impacts of heat stress in mice.

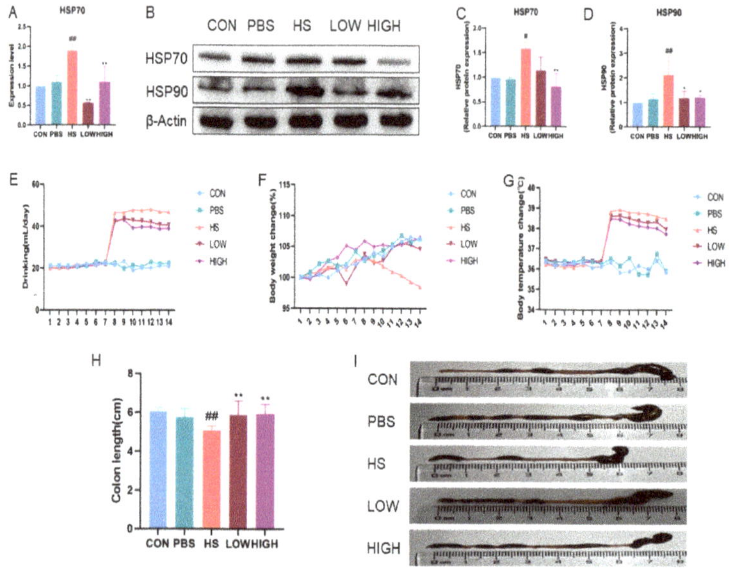

Figure 8. Protective effect of BTL-I on heat-stressed mice. The normal control group (CON) was exposed to 24 ± 1 °C and treated with PBS (0.2 mL), the heat stress group (HS) was subjected to 40 ± 1 °C for 4 h per day, the HS group had a low oral BTL-I concentration (1 mg/kg) (LOW), and the HS group had a high oral BTL-I concentration (5 mg/kg) (HIGH). Clinical changes were recorded, and colon tissues were collected. (**A–D**) qPCR and Western blotting analysis of the effects of BTL-I on HSP70 and HSP90 proteins; (**E**) water intake of the mice during the test; (**F**) body weight changes in the mice during the test; (**G**) body temperature changes; and (**H**,**I**) colon length of the mice during the test; the results are expressed as the means ± SEMs. # $p < 0.05$, ## $p < 0.01$ compared with the control group; * $p < 0.05$, ** $p < 0.01$ compared with the HS group.

2.7. Effects of BTL-I on Intestinal Cell Apoptosis in Heat-Stressed Mice

As depicted in Figure 9A, the mRNA expression level of *Bax* was significantly increased after heat stress (HS) ($p < 0.01$). However, following BTL-I administration, the mRNA level of *Bax* was significantly decreased ($p < 0.01$). Moreover, the protein expression of Bax/Bcl-2 significantly increased after heat stress ($p < 0.05$). Nonetheless, BTL-I administration notably reversed these changes ($p < 0.05$) (Figure 9B,C). Furthermore, the TUNEL results indicated that intestinal cell apoptosis was greater in the BTL-I-treated mice than in the HS-treated mice (Figure 9D). These findings suggest that BTL-I may protect against heat-stress-induced intestinal cell apoptosis.

2.8. Effect of BTL-I on the ROS/PERK/CHOP Signaling Pathway in Heat-Stressed Mice

We examined the expression of oxidative-stress-related molecules in mouse serum. The results revealed that the levels of ROS and MDA in the serum of HS mice were significantly increased ($p < 0.05$) (Figure 10A–C). However, BTL-I administration effectively inhibited the increases in the ROS and MDA levels ($p < 0.01$). Additionally, HS led to a reduction in the content of the antioxidant factor SOD in the serum ($p < 0.05$), and BTL-I administration significantly alleviated this decrease caused by HS ($p < 0.05$).

Furthermore, we explored the mechanism by which BTL-I inhibited endoplasmic reticulum stress (ERS) in HS mice by examining the key proteins of the PERK/CHOP signaling pathway. HS increased the expressions of the *ATF4* and *CHOP* mRNAs ($p < 0.05$). Additionally, the expression levels of p-PERK/PERK, p-eIF2α/eIF2α, ATF4, and CHOP were significantly increased ($p < 0.01$). However, after BTL-I administration, these changes were abolished ($p < 0.05$) (Figure 10D–J). These findings suggest that BTL-I may ameliorate ERS by modulating the PERK/CHOP signaling pathway in HS mice.

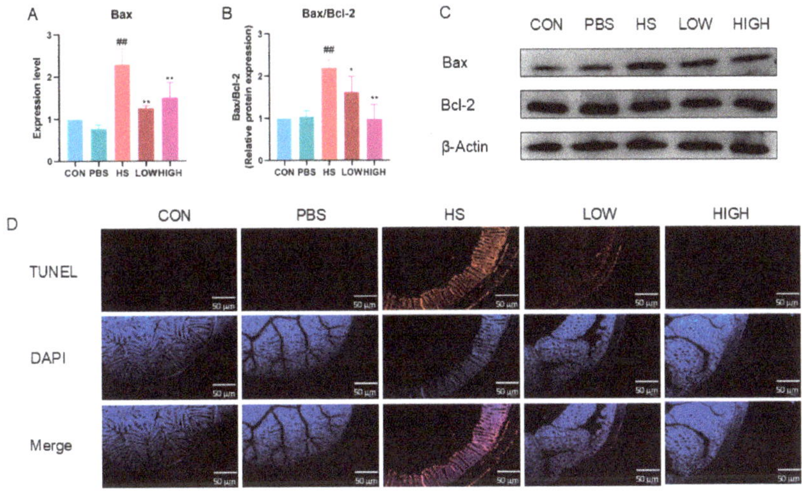

Figure 9. Effects of BTL-I on apoptosis in heat-stressed mice. (**A**) The effects of BTL-I on the expression of the apoptotic marker *Bax* were determined by qPCR. (**B–C**) The effects of BTL-I on the expression of the apoptosis markers Bax, Bcl-2, and Pro-Caspase 3 were determined by Western blotting. (**D**) Immunofluorescence staining for apoptosis was performed via the TUNEL assay. The results are expressed as the means ± SEMs. ## $p < 0.01$ compared with the control group; * $p < 0.05$, ** $p < 0.01$ compared with the HS group.

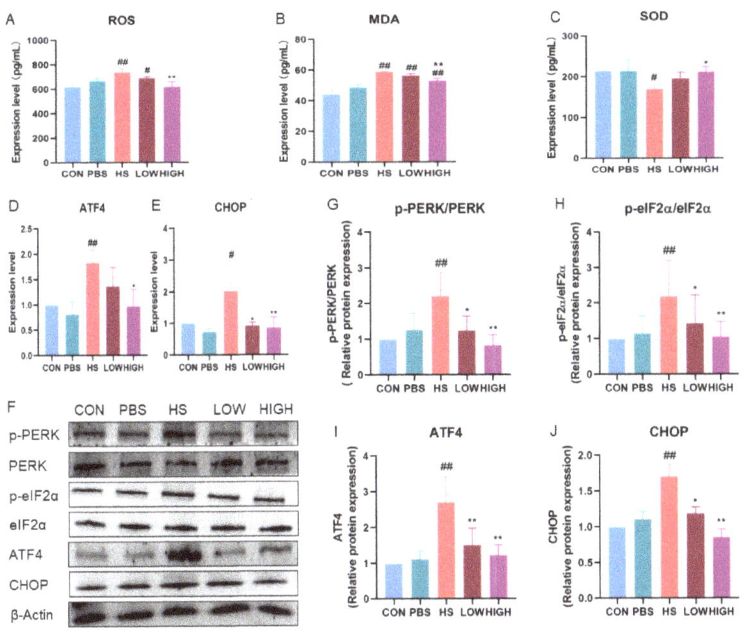

Figure 10. Effects of BTL-I on the ROS/PERK/CHOP signaling pathway in heat-stressed mice. (**A–C**) The effects of BTL-I on the expression of oxidative cytokines were determined by ELISA; (**D,E**) qPCR analysis

of the expression of the PERK/CHOP signaling pathway markers *ATF4* and *CHOP*; and (**F–J**) Western blotting analysis of the expression of the PERK/CHOP signaling pathway markers p-PERK, PERK, p-eIF2α, eIF2α, ATF4, and CHOP; the results are expressed as the means ± SEMs. $^{\#}$ $p < 0.05$, $^{\#\#}$ $p < 0.01$ compared with the control group; * $p < 0.05$, ** $p < 0.01$ compared with the HS group.

3. Discussion

Heat stress is still a prominent threat to animal husbandry in tropical and subtropical areas. Studying and developing natural active products to alleviate stress damage is highly practical. BTL-I has good anti-inflammatory, antioxidant, and intestinal balance effects, but whether BTL-I can alleviate heat stress damage and develop as a functional feed additive for livestock and poultry remains unclear. In this study, we investigated the protective mechanism of BTL-I against heat-stress-induced apoptosis in IPEC-J2 cells and intestinal cells in mice. Our results demonstrated that heat stress led to an increase in heat shock protein levels, which were effectively inhibited by BTL-I. Both in vivo and in vitro experiments revealed that heat stress increased the rate of intestinal epithelial cell apoptosis and increased the expression of apoptosis-related proteins. However, BTL-I treatment improved these effects, primarily through the regulation of the ROS/PERK/CHOP signaling pathway. These findings suggest that BTL-I has the potential to prevent heat-stress-induced intestinal cell apoptosis.

Apoptosis is a process of programmed cell death observed in pathological and specific physiological states and is characterized by active, orderly, and gene-regulated physiological changes that can alter cell shape and function [18,19]. Studies have indicated that heat stress can lead to the accumulation of ROS and mitochondrial dysfunction, triggering cell apoptosis [20]. Additionally, heat stress can induce apoptosis in mammary epithelial cells by downregulating ROS-independent pathways [21]. Acute heat stress has been associated with p53-mediated mitochondrial apoptosis in liver injury [22]. Moreover, Cui reported that acute heat stress activates the unfolded protein response (UPR), leading to endoplasmic reticulum stress (ERS) and subsequent apoptosis [23]. High temperatures can induce cell apoptosis or necrosis, and the degree of apoptosis or necrosis becomes more evident as the temperature increases [24,25].

To investigate the effects of BTL-I on intestinal cell apoptosis, the IPEC-J2 cell heat shock model and C57BL/6J mouse heat stress model were used. In our study, we observed increased apoptosis rates and upregulated expressions of Bax/Bcl-2 and Pro-Caspase 3 in IPEC-J2 cells and mice exposed to heat stress. However, pretreatment with BTL-I resulted in a reduction in the apoptosis rate and the downregulation of Bax/Bcl-2 and Pro-Caspase 3 expression. These findings highlight the potential of BTL-I as a preventive agent against heat-stress-induced intestinal cell apoptosis.

The endoplasmic reticulum (ER) plays a vital role in protein folding and maturation. ER stress, caused by unfolded or misfolded proteins, can lead to cell apoptosis. Many factors cause ER proteins to misfold or unfold, such as humidity, Ca^{2+} level disturbance, oxidative stress, nutritional deficiencies, and ischemia [26–28]. Endoplasmic reticulum stress can damage the morphological structure and physiological functions of the endoplasmic reticulum, resulting in many unfolded or misfolded proteins [29,30]. At this time, cells undergo a highly conserved stress-adaptive response (UPR), which mainly reduces the synthesis of new proteins by shutting down protein translation, inducing ER chaperones that activate protein folding, and ubiquitinating misfolded proteins/unfolded proteins, thereby relieving ER stress, protecting the ER, and reducing damage [31–33]. However, long-term stress stimulation makes the UPR insufficient to relieve endoplasmic reticulum stress and eventually leads to cell apoptosis, resulting in the occurrence of disease. For example, in the treatment of prostate cancer, resveratrol triggers ER stress by depleting ER Ca^{2+} and inducing autophagy-mediated apoptosis [34,35]. Similarly, cucurbitacin I induces cell death by activating the PERK and IRE1α signaling pathways while increasing Bax and caspase-12-dependent ER stress to induce cell apoptosis [36]. Moreover, heat stress (HS) can induce ER stress, activate the p-eIF2α/CHOP signaling pathway, trigger the apoptosis of intestinal epithelial cells, and compromise the integrity of the intestinal epithelial barrier [37]. The in vitro exposure of intestinal epithelial cells to high temperatures (41 °C) decreases cell viability, induces ER stress, and promotes cell apoptosis, ultimately disrupting barrier function [38]. Similarly, our study revealed that heat stress can induce ER stress and upregulate the PERK, eIF2α, ATF4, and CHOP proteins in IPEC-J2 and mouse cells.

Free radicals, including reactive oxygen species (ROS) and reactive nitrogen species (RNS), possess strong oxidation abilities and play significant roles in cell proliferation, differentiation, growth, and death. They are also involved in various cellular processes, such as the immune system, redox balance, and the activation of signaling pathways, including the PI3K/Akt, MAPK, eIF2α/ATF4/CHOP, and Nrf2/Keap1 pathways [39–44]. ROS, a byproduct of the electron respiratory transfer chain of mitochondria, are associated with inflammation, ER stress, and metabolic diseases due to the disruption of ROS levels [31,45–48]. MCL can induce apoptosis by targeting TrxR, triggering ROS-mediated ERS, and then inducing ICD in HCC cells [49]. Brd4 inhibition prevents FoxO4-dependent ROS production through the PI3K/AKT pathway, thereby blocking renal cell apoptosis and ERS protein expression [50]. Zinc-based ICD inducers induce mitochondrial dysfunction through ROS induction via ERS [51]. On the basis of previous reports, we hypothesized that heat-stress-induced apoptosis in IPEC-J2 and mouse intestinal epithelial cells is also regulated by the ROS/PERK/CHOP signaling pathway. To validate this hypothesis, we examined the ROS levels and observed that HS led to ROS accumulation in IPEC-J2 and mouse cells. These findings suggest that the ROS/PERK/CHOP signaling pathway mediates heat-stress-induced apoptosis.

N-acetylcysteine (NAC) scavenges reactive oxygen species (ROS) and effectively eliminates accumulated ROS [52]. In previous studies, NAC was shown to mitigate intestinal epithelial cell apoptosis by inhibiting the heat-labile enterotoxin-induced activation of the PERK/CHOP pathway [53]. Additionally, in an ischemia–reperfusion-induced acute kidney injury model, the addition of NAC effectively suppressed ROS-mediated ER stress and cell apoptosis signaling pathways [54]. In addition, TiO_2-NP-induced ER stress was significantly reduced in HT22 cells treated with NAC, as were GRP78 and caspase 12 expression [55]. In our study, the addition of NAC effectively reduced the expressions of p-PERK, p-eIF2α, ATF4, and CHOP, thereby reducing the occurrence of apoptosis. On the other hand, 4-phenyl butyric acid (4-PBA) acts as an ER stress inhibitor, clearing misfolded and unfolded proteins and inhibiting ER stress [56]. In various studies, 4-PBA has been demonstrated to inhibit ER stress and prevent acute lung injury induced by a hyperoxygen environment by upregulating Claudin 4 expression [57]. Moreover, when ER stress is inhibited, IFN-γ-mediated apoptosis is also reduced, resulting in decreased unfolded and misfolded protein responses [58]. Our study also revealed that 4-PBA effectively inhibited the expressions of p-PERK, p-eIF2α, ATF4, and CHOP and reduced the expressions of the apoptosis-related proteins Pro-Caspase 3 and Bax/Bcl-2. The results obtained with NAC and 4-PBA were consistent with those obtained with BTL-I, indicating that BTL-I mitigates heat-stress-induced apoptosis by modulating the ROS/PERK/CHOP signaling pathway. These findings further support the potential of BTL-I as a preventive measure against heat-stress-induced intestinal cell apoptosis.

The Keap1-Nrf2/ARE signaling pathway is one of the main pathways of anti-oxidative stress in vivo [59]. It can resist oxidative stress caused by various stimulating factors inside and outside the body, and improve the anti-oxidative damage and repair function of cells. It is the central defense mechanism of the system against oxidative stress. Nrf2 is a key transcription factor and the main regulator of the cellular oxidative stress response, which can induce the activation of the Nrf2-mediated expression of antioxidant enzymes, detoxification enzymes, and downstream protein molecules, such as NQO1, SOD, CAT, HO-1, and GPX [60,61]. At the same time, under environmental pressure or stimuli, ROS levels will increase dramatically, causing serious harm to cells, leading to cell function damage and even death. When a large amount of ROS accumulates in cells, Keap1 dissociates from Nrf2 and induces Nrf2 translocation to the nucleus to bind to antioxidant elements, promoting the transcription of antioxidant-related genes [62,63]. So, Nrf2 activation can effectively remove ROS accumulation and reduce oxidative stress damage. Based on the above studies, we will continue to explore whether BTL-I can alleviate apoptosis by activating Nrf2 to reduce ROS in IPEC-J2 cells in the future.

4. Materials and Methods

4.1. Chemicals and Reagents

BTL-I was purchased from Bioviotica (San Diego, CA, USA). Its chemical formula was C24H24O7. The purity of BTL-I was 99.9%. A Cell Counting Kit-8 (CCK8) was purchased from APExBIO Technology (Houston, TX, USA). Commercial-specific complete Dulbecco's modified Eagle's medium/nutrient mixture F-12 (DMEM/F12), penicillin, and streptomycin were acquired from Gibco (Carlsbad, CA, USA). An enhanced chemiluminescence (ECL) kit was obtained from Tanon (Shanghai, China). In addition, 40,6-diamidino-2-phenylindole (DAPI) was purchased from Beyotime (Shanghai, China). The primary and secondary antibodies used for Western blotting were purchased from Cell Signaling Technology (Danvers, MA, USA), Abcam (Cambridge, MA, USA) and Proteintech (Wuhan, China). Biotin-conjugated anti-rabbit IgG antibody and DyLight 594-conjugated avidin were purchased from Jackson ImmunoResearch (Cambridge, MA, USA).

4.2. Cell Culture and Viability Assay

IPEC-J2 cells obtained from Guoqiang Zhu at Yangzhou University (Yangzhou, China) and were cultured in DMEM/F12 supplemented with 10% FBS and 1% penicillin/streptomycin at 37 °C. After reaching 80% confluence, the following two sets of cells were prepared: one group was subjected to heat shock treatment, and the other group was subjected to BTL-I pretreatment. The heat shock treatment involved placing the cells in a cell incubator at 42 °C with 5% CO_2 for 1.5 h.

To assess IPEC-J2 cell viability, a CCK8 assay was performed. Initially, the cells were seeded at a density of 1×10^4 cells/mL in 96-well plates and treated with varying concentrations of BTL-I (10, 20, and 50 μM) for 24 h. The experimental concentration was set according to previously published methods [64]. Afterward, 10 μL of CCK-8 solution was added, and the cells were further incubated for 2 h. A microplate reader (BioTek, Winooski, VT, USA) was used to measure cell viability by measuring the absorbance at 450 nm.

4.3. Induction of Heat Stress in Mice

Male C57BL/6J mice aged 6–8 weeks and weighing 19–21 g were procured from a specific pathogen-free (SPF) laboratory located in Guangzhou, China. The mice were housed in a controlled environment with a temperature of 26 ± 1 °C and a 12 h light/dark cycle. All animal protocols adhered to the guidelines of the IACUC-Guangdong Ocean University and were granted ethics approval (number 2022-scuec-021). The animal experiments strictly followed the principles outlined in the National Research Council's Guide for the Care and Use of Laboratory Animals (National Institutes of Health, Bethesda, MD, USA).

Before the experiments commenced, the mice were acclimatized for one week, during which they had unrestricted access to food and water. The mice, exposed to a relative humidity (RH) of 65–85%, were randomly divided into the following five groups (n = 6): the normal control group (−HS) exposed to 24 ± 1 °C, the normal control group treated with PBS (0.2 mL), the heat stress group (+HS) subjected to 40 ± 1 °C for 4 h per day, the HS group with a low oral BTL-I concentration (1 mg/kg) (L-BTL-I), and the HS group with a high oral BTL-I concentration (5 mg/kg) (H-BTL-I). The experimental concentrations were set according to previously published methods [64]. This treatment regimen was continued for 14 days (Figure 11). The mice were subsequently euthanized, and their colons were collected for further research.

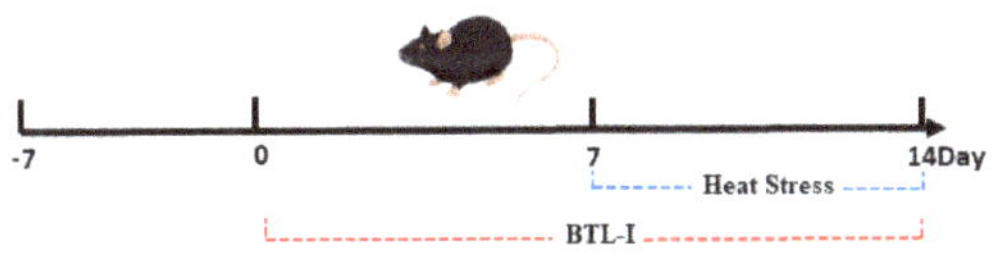

Figure 11. Mouse experiment.

4.4. Detection of Oxidative Stress Markers

To examine the inhibitory effect of BTL-I on oxidative cytokines, IPEC-J2 cells were initially seeded at a density of 5×10^6 cells/well in 6-well plates. The cells were then pretreated with different concentrations of BTL-I (10, 20, and 50 μM) for 24 h, followed by exposure to heat stress (HS) for 1.5 h. Subsequently, the cells were disrupted via an ultrasonic cell disruptor (Ningbo Shuangjia Instrument Co., Ltd., Ningbo, China) and centrifuged at 3000 rpm for 10 min. The resulting serum was collected and subjected to further centrifugation at 3000 rpm for an additional 10 min. The expression levels of ROS, MDA, and SOD (Jiangsu Meimian Industrial Co., Ltd., Nanjing, China) were detected according to the instructions of the ELISA kit according to the manufacturer's instructions.

4.5. Western Blotting Analysis

Protein levels were assessed via a BCA reagent after the homogenization of IPEC-J2 cells and colonic tissues (CWBIO, Beijing, China). To analyze the samples, sodium dodecyl sulfate–polyacrylamide gel electrophoresis (SDS–PAGE) was employed, followed by the transfer of the separated proteins to polyvinylidene fluoride (PVDF) membranes. The PVDF membranes were subsequently blocked for 30 min with QuickBlockTM Blocking Buffer (Beyotime, Shanghai, China). Following blocking, the membranes were incubated with primary antibodies at a 1:1000 dilution. The primary antibodies used were against HSP70 (Proteintech, 10995-1-AP), HSP90 (Abcam, ab59459), PERK (CST, 5683s), eIF2α (CST, 3179s), p-PERK (CST, 5324s), p-eIF2α (CST, 3398s), ATF4 (CST, 11815s), CHOP (Abcam, ab11419), Bax (Proteintech, 60267-1-lg), Bcl-2 (Proteintech, 60267-1-lg), and β-actin (TransGen Biotech, Lot# R10602). For the next step, secondary antibodies, namely, goat anti-rabbit and anti-mouse IgG conjugated with horseradish peroxidase (HRP), were used at a 1:1000 dilution.

The Western blot normalization method is shown below. The first step was to quantify the target protein and housekeeping protein in each lane. Next, the reference lane on the blot was selected. The reference lane was the CON group lane. Then, the normalization factor was determined by dividing the signal of the reference channel by the signals of the other channels, the normalization factor of each channel was obtained, and the signal of the target protein was multiplied by the normalization factor.

4.6. Total RNA Extraction and qPCR

RNA extraction was performed via TRIzol, and the isolated RNA was subsequently reverse-transcribed into cDNA. To assess the gene expression levels, SYBR fluorescence quantitative PCR was used, and the obtained data were normalized via the $2^{-\Delta\Delta CT}$ method, with β-actin serving as the reference gene. The specific primer sequences utilized in the PCR analysis can be found in Table 1.

Table 1. Mouse primer sequences.

Gene Name	Sequence (5′-3′)
m-ATF4	F: TCTGCCTTCTCCAGGTGGTTCC R: GCTGCTGTCTTGTTTTGCTCCATC
m-CHOP	F: CTACTCTTGACCCTGCGTCCCTAG R: TCTTCCTTGCTCTTCCTCCTCTTCC
m-HSP70	F: GGTGCTGACGAAGATGAAGGAGATC R: CTGCCGCTGAGAGTCGTTGAAG

Table 1. *Cont.*

Gene Name	Sequence (5′-3′)
m-Bcl-2	F: GATGACTTCTCTCGTCGCTAC R: GAACTCAAAGAAGGCCACAATC
m-Bax	F: TTGCCCTCTTCTACTTTGCTAG R: CCATGATGGTTCTGATCAGCTC
m-β-actin	F: CTACCTCATGAAGATCCTGACC R: CACAGCTTCTCTTTGATGTCAC
p-ATF4	F: GATCCTCCTGGAGAGAAGGTGGTAG R: CCGAGTGGCTGCTGTCTTGTTC
P-CHOP	F: TCTGGCTTGGCTGACTGAGGAG R: TTTCCGTTTCCTGGGTCTTCTTTGG
p-HSP70	F: CAACAAGATCACCATCACCAAC R: ACCCTTAAGGAGCTTATTGAGG
p-Bcl-2	F: TCGCCCTGTGGATGACTGAGTAC R: CCTTCAGAGACAGCCAGGAGAAATC
p-Bax	F: GCTTCAGGGTTTCATCCAGGATCG R: ACTCGCTCAACTTCTTGGTAGATGC
p-β-actin	F: CTACCTCATGAAGATCCTGACC R: CACAGCTTCTCTTTGATGTCAC

4.7. *Immunofluorescence*

IPEC-J2 cells at 50% confluency were treated with BTL-I in a 24-well plate. The cells were subsequently gently washed, fixed, and blocked. Next, the cells were incubated with anti-Bcl-2 (1:100; Abcam, Cambridge, MA, USA), anti-ATF4, and anti-Bax antibodies (1:100; Cell Signaling Technology, Danvers, MA, USA) overnight in the dark at 4 °C. After thorough washing with PBS, the cells were incubated with the appropriate secondary antibody conjugated with DyLight 594 fluorescent probes in the dark for 2 h. Subsequently, the cells were washed again with PBS and stained with a fluorescently labeled protein (DyLight 594-conjugated avidin) for 1 h. Finally, the cells were observed under a fluorescence microscope (Olympus, Tokyo, Japan) with DAPI-stained nuclei.

4.8. *Flow Cytometry*

The apoptosis analysis was conducted via the Annexin V-FITC/PI Apoptosis Detection Kit from Yeasen Biotechnology (Shanghai, China) following the provided instructions. Cell samples were collected and subjected to flow cytometry to determine the percentage of apoptotic cells. The percentage of apoptotic cells was calculated as the sum of the percentages in the first and fourth quadrants of a two-dimensional scatter plot.

4.9. *H&E Staining*

Colon tissue obtained from the mice was preserved in 4% phosphate-buffered paraformaldehyde. Afterward, the tissues were embedded in paraffin, and thin sections were prepared. These sections were then stained with hematoxylin–eosin (H&E), after which, pathological changes were observed via optical microscopy (Olympus, Tokyo, Japan).

4.10. *Terminal Deoxynucleotidyl Transferase-Mediated dUTP-Biotin Nick End Labeling (TUNEL) Assay*

Following the guidelines of Yeasen Biotechnology (Shanghai, China), the paraffin sections were dewaxed. Proteinase K treatment was conducted for 20 min, followed by incubation with equilibration buffer for 10 min. The sections were then subjected to TdT solution and incubated for 30 min at 37 °C. Finally, DAPI was added to the sealing solution, which enabled observation and imaging under a fluorescence microscope (Olympus, Tokyo, Japan).

4.11. Statistical Analyses

One-way analysis of variance, followed by Tukey's multiple comparisons test (LSD), was performed via IBM SPSS 19.0 (SPSS, Chicago, IL, USA). The results are expressed as the mean ± SEM. $p < 0.05$ was considered to indicate statistical significance. Graphs were created via GraphPad Prism 8.0 software (San Diego, CA, USA).

5. Conclusions

In conclusion, our study demonstrated that BTL-I exerts a beneficial effect on heat-stress-induced apoptosis by regulating the ROS-mediated PERK/CHOP signaling pathway, effectively inhibiting apoptosis. The positive effects of BTL-I in the heat stress model suggest its potential as a novel marine drug for preventing heat stress. These findings provide a solid theoretical basis for the defense against and treatment of heat stress, opening up new possibilities for managing this condition. Owing to the complex preparation process and high cost of BTL-I, it is not suitable for livestock breeding at present. With continuous optimization of the preparation process, BTL-I is expected to be used as a feed additive in pig production.

Author Contributions: X.J. and Y.Y.: funding acquisition. X.N.: methodology and writing—original draft. X.N., S.C., X.W. and J.W.: validation. X.N. and X.J.: formal analysis. X.N.: investigation and data curation. X.N., X.J., Y.Y., X.L., Z.Y. and X.M.: conceptualization. X.J. and X.L.: resources. A.M.A.E.-A. and X.J.: supervision; formal analysis; validation; writing—review and editing. All authors have read and agreed to the published version of the manuscript.

Funding: This study was supported by the National Natural Science Foundation of China [grant number 32273077]; the Natural Science Foundation of Guangdong Province, China [grant number 2019A1515011142]; the Innovation Team Project of Guangdong Provincial Department of Education [grant number 2022KCXTD014]; the Guangdong Postgraduate Education Innovation Project [grant number 040510052201]; the National Natural Science Foundation of Shenzhen [grant number JCYJ20220530162008018]; and the Program for Scientific Research Start-Fund of Guangdong Ocean University [grant number 101402/R17088].

Institutional Review Board Statement: All animal protocols were performed at IACUC-Guangdong Ocean University. The ethics approval number was 2022-scuec-021 (approved 10 June 2022). The animals were housed at Guangdong Ocean University Animal Hospital in Zhanjiang, China. Furthermore, all the animal experiments were conducted in accordance with the guidelines provided by the National Research Council's Guide for the Care and Use of Laboratory Animals.

Data Availability Statement: The data will be made available upon request.

Conflicts of Interest: The authors declare that the research was conducted without any commercial or financial relationships construed as potential conflicts of interest.

References

1. Varasteh, S.; Fink-Gremmels, J.; Garssen, J.; Braber, S. α-Lipoic acid prevents the intestinal epithelial monolayer damage under heat stress conditions: Model experiments in Caco-2 cells. *Eur. J. Nutr.* **2018**, *57*, 1577–1589. [CrossRef] [PubMed]
2. Pearce, S.C.; Mani, V.; Weber, T.E.; Rhoads, R.P.; Patience, J.F.; Baumgard, L.H.; Gabler, N.K. Heat stress and reduced plane of nutrition decreases intestinal integrity and function in pigs. *J. Anim. Sci.* **2013**, *91*, 5183–5193. [CrossRef]
3. Li, H.; Zhang, G.; Liu, Y.; Gao, F.; Ye, X.; Lin, R.; Wen, M. Hypoxia-inducible factor 1α inhibits heat stress-induced pig intestinal epithelial cell apoptosis through eif2α/ATF4/CHOP signaling. *Sci. Total Environ.* **2024**, *924*, 171649. [CrossRef]
4. Zheng, Y.; Zhao, Y.; He, W.; Wang, Y.; Cao, Z.; Yang, H.; Wang, W.; Li, S. Novel organic selenium source hydroxy-selenomethionine counteracts the blood-milk barrier disruption and inflammatory response of mice under heat stress. *Front. Immunol.* **2022**, *13*, 1054128. [CrossRef] [PubMed]
5. Jolly, C.; Morimoto, R.I. Role of the heat shock response and molecular chaperones in oncogenesis and cell death. *J. Natl. Cancer Inst.* **2000**, *92*, 1564–1572. [CrossRef]
6. Vandana, G.D.; Sejian, V.; Lees, A.M.; Pragna, P.; Silpa, M.V.; Maloney, S.K. Heat stress and poultry production: Impact and amelioration. *Int. J. Biometeorol.* **2021**, *65*, 163–179. [CrossRef] [PubMed]
7. Garrett, W.S.; Gordon, J.I.; Glimcher, L.H. Homeostasis and inflammation in the intestine. *Cell* **2010**, *140*, 859–870. [CrossRef]
8. Lambert, G.P. Stress-induced gastrointestinal barrier dysfunction and its inflammatory effects. *J. Anim. Sci.* **2009**, *87*, E101–E108. [CrossRef] [PubMed]

9. Lee, S.; Kang, H.-G.; Jeong, P.-S.; Kim, M.J.; Park, S.-H.; Song, B.-S.; Sim, B.-W.; Kim, S.-U. Heat stress impairs oocyte maturation through ceramide-mediated apoptosis in pigs. *Sci. Total Environ.* **2021**, *755 Pt 1*, 144144. [CrossRef]
10. Jing, J.; Zeng, H.; Shao, Q.; Tang, J.; Wang, L.; Jia, G.; Liu, G.; Chen, X.; Tian, G.; Cai, J.; et al. Selenomethionine alleviates environmental heat stress induced hepatic lipid accumulation and glycogen infiltration of broilers via maintaining mitochondrial and endoplasmic reticulum homeostasis. *Redox Biol.* **2023**, *67*, 102912. [CrossRef] [PubMed]
11. Li, L.; Su, Z.; Zou, Z.; Tan, H.; Cai, D.; Su, L.; Gu, Z. Ser46 phosphorylation of p53 is an essential event in prolyl-isomerase Pin1-mediated p53-independent apoptosis in response to heat stress. *Cell Death Dis.* **2019**, *10*, 96. [CrossRef] [PubMed]
12. Lin, Z.; Cai, Z.; Li, L.; Wei, Y.; Ling, Q. c-Jun N-terminal kinase 1/P53 signaling mediates intrinsic apoptosis of largemouth bass (Micropterus salmoides) hepatocytes under heat stress. *Sci. Total Environ.* **2024**, *947*, 174664. [CrossRef]
13. Choi, S.; Chen, M.; Cryns, V.L.; Anderson, R.A. A nuclear phosphoinositide kinase complex regulates p53. *Nat. Cell Biol.* **2019**, *21*, 462–475. [CrossRef]
14. Samanta, S.; Yang, S.; Debnath, B.; Xue, D.; Kuang, Y.; Ramkumar, K.; Lee, A.S.; Ljungman, M.; Neamati, N. The Hydroxyquinoline Analogue YUM70 Inhibits GRP78 to Induce ER Stress-Mediated Apoptosis in Pancreatic Cancer. *Cancer Res.* **2021**, *81*, 1883–1895. [CrossRef]
15. López, I.; Tournillon, A.-S.; Prado Martins, R.; Karakostis, K.; Malbert-Colas, L.; Nylander, K.; Fåhraeus, R. p53-mediated suppression of BiP triggers BIK-induced apoptosis during prolonged endoplasmic reticulum stress. *Cell Death Differ.* **2017**, *24*, 1717–1729. [CrossRef]
16. Wu, W.; Liu, L.; Zhu, H.; Sun, Y.; Wu, Y.; Liao, H.; Gui, Y.; Li, L.; Liu, L.; Sun, F.; et al. Butyrolactone-I, an efficient α-glucosidase inhibitor, improves type 2 diabetes with potent TNF-α-lowering properties through modulating gut microbiota in db/db mice. *FASEB J.* **2019**, *33*, 12616–12629. [CrossRef]
17. Nishio, K.; Ishida, T.; Arioka, H.; Kurokawa, H.; Fukuoka, K.; Nomoto, T.; Fukumoto, H.; Yokote, H.; Saijo, N. Antitumor effects of butyrolactone I, a selective cdc2 kinase inhibitor, on human lung cancer cell lines. *Anticancer Res.* **1996**, *16*, 3387–3395. [PubMed]
18. Pritchard, D.M.; Watson, A.J. Apoptosis and gastrointestinal pharmacology. *Pharmacol. Ther.* **1996**, *72*, 149–169. [CrossRef]
19. Stewart, B.W. Mechanisms of apoptosis: Integration of genetic, biochemical, and cellular indicators. *J. Natl. Cancer Inst.* **1994**, *86*, 1286–1296. [CrossRef] [PubMed]
20. Chi, J.; Li, Z.; Hong, X.; Zhao, T.; Bie, Y.; Zhang, W.; Yang, J.; Feng, Z.; Yu, Z.; Xu, Q.; et al. Inhalation of Hydrogen Attenuates Progression of Chronic Heart Failure via Suppression of Oxidative Stress and P53 Related to Apoptosis Pathway in Rats. *Front. Physiol.* **2018**, *9*, 1026. [CrossRef]
21. Wang, H.-L.; Xing, G.-D.; Qian, Y.; Sun, X.-F.; Zhong, J.-F.; Chen, K.-L. Dihydromyricetin attenuates heat stress-induced apoptosis in dairy cow mammary epithelial cells through suppressing mitochondrial dysfunction. *Ecotoxicol. Environ. Saf.* **2021**, *214*, 112078. [CrossRef]
22. Huang, W.; Xie, W.; Zhong, H.; Cai, S.; Huang, Q.; Liu, Y.; Zeng, Z.; Liu, Y. Cytosolic p53 Inhibits Parkin-Mediated Mitophagy and Promotes Acute Liver Injury Induced by Heat Stroke. *Front. Immunol.* **2022**, *13*, 859231. [CrossRef] [PubMed]
23. Cui, Y.; Zhou, X.; Chen, L.; Tang, Z.; Mo, F.; Li, X.C.; Mao, H.; Wei, X.; Wang, C.; Wang, H. Crosstalk between Endoplasmic Reticulum Stress and Oxidative Stress in Heat Exposure-Induced Apoptosis Is Dependent on the ATF4-CHOP-CHAC1 Signal Pathway in IPEC-J2 Cells. *J. Agric. Food Chem.* **2021**, *69*, 15495–15511. [CrossRef]
24. Alsharif, I. Comprehensive exploration of the molecular response, clinical signs, and histological aspects of heat stress in animals. *J. Therm. Biol.* **2022**, *110*, 103346. [CrossRef]
25. Baechler, B.L.; Bloemberg, D.; Quadrilatero, J. Mitophagy regulates mitochondrial network signaling, oxidative stress, and apoptosis during myoblast differentiation. *Autophagy* **2019**, *15*, 1606–1619. [CrossRef]
26. Salaroglio, I.C.; Panada, E.; Moiso, E.; Buondonno, I.; Provero, P.; Rubinstein, M.; Kopecka, J.; Riganti, C. PERK induces resistance to cell death elicited by endoplasmic reticulum stress and chemotherapy. *Mol. Cancer* **2017**, *16*, 91. [CrossRef]
27. Liu, Y.; Ma, Y.; Xu, J.; Zhang, G.; Zhao, X.; He, Z.; Wang, L.; Yin, N.; Peng, M. VMP1 prevents Ca^{2+} overload in endoplasmic reticulum and maintains naive T cell survival. *J. Exp. Med.* **2023**, *220*, e20221068. [CrossRef] [PubMed]
28. Esmaeili, Y.; Yarjanli, Z.; Pakniya, F.; Bidram, E.; Łos, M.J.; Eshraghi, M.; Klionsky, D.J.; Ghavami, S.; Zarrabi, A. Targeting autophagy, oxidative stress, and ER stress for neurodegenerative disease treatment. *J. Control Release* **2022**, *345*, 147–175. [CrossRef] [PubMed]
29. Tapella, L.; Dematteis, G.; Moro, M.; Pistolato, B.; Tonelli, E.; Vanella, V.V.; Giustina, D.; La Forgia, A.; Restelli, E.; Barberis, E.; et al. Protein synthesis inhibition and loss of homeostatic functions in astrocytes from an Alzheimer's disease mouse model: A role for ER-mitochondria interaction. *Cell Death Dis.* **2022**, *13*, 878. [CrossRef]
30. Jeschke, M.G.; Finnerty, C.C.; Herndon, D.N.; Song, J.; Boehning, D.; Tompkins, R.G.; Baker, H.V.; Gauglitz, G.G. Severe injury is associated with insulin resistance, endoplasmic reticulum stress response, and unfolded protein response. *Ann. Surg.* **2012**, *255*, 370–378. [CrossRef] [PubMed]
31. Ming, S.; Tian, J.; Ma, K.; Pei, C.; Li, L.; Wang, Z.; Fang, Z.; Liu, M.; Dong, H.; Li, W.; et al. Oxalate-induced apoptosis through ERS-ROS-NF-κB signalling pathway in renal tubular epithelial cell. *Mol. Med.* **2022**, *28*, 88. [CrossRef]
32. Ong, G.; Ragetli, R.; Mnich, K.; Doble, B.W.; Kammouni, W.; Logue, S.E. IRE1 signaling increases PERK expression during chronic ER stress. *Cell Death Dis.* **2024**, *15*, 276. [CrossRef]
33. Loi, M.; Raimondi, A.; Morone, D.; Molinari, M. ESCRT-III-driven piecemeal micro-ER-phagy remodels the ER during recovery from ER stress. *Nat. Commun.* **2019**, *10*, 5058. [CrossRef]

34. Richter, M.; Vidovic, N.; Honrath, B.; Mahavadi, P.; Dodel, R.; Dolga, A.M.; Culmsee, C. Activation of SK2 channels preserves ER Ca^{2+} homeostasis and protects against ER stress-induced cell death. *Cell Death Differ.* **2016**, *23*, 814–827. [CrossRef] [PubMed]
35. Lin, Y.F.; Lee, Y.F.; Liang, P.H. Targeting β-tubulin:CCT-β complexes incurs Hsp90- and VCP-related protein degradation and induces ER stress-associated apoptosis by triggering capacitative Ca^{2+} entry, mitochondrial perturbation and caspase overactivation. *Cell Death Dis.* **2012**, *3*, e434. [CrossRef] [PubMed]
36. Li, H.; Chen, H.; Li, R.; Xin, J.; Wu, S.; Lan, J.; Xue, K.; Li, X.; Zuo, C.; Jiang, W.; et al. Cucurbitacin I induces cancer cell death through the endoplasmic reticulum stress pathway. *J. Cell Biochem.* **2019**, *120*, 2391–2403. [CrossRef]
37. Cui, Y.-J.; Chen, L.-Y.; Zhou, X.; Tang, Z.-N.; Wang, C.; Wang, H.-F. Heat stress induced IPEC-J2 cells barrier dysfunction through endoplasmic reticulum stress mediated apoptosis by p-eif2α/CHOP pathway. *J. Cell Physiol.* **2022**, *237*, 1389–1405. [CrossRef] [PubMed]
38. Zhou, J.-Y.; Huang, D.-G.; Zhu, M.; Gao, C.-Q.; Yan, H.-C.; Li, X.-G.; Wang, X.-Q. Wnt/β-catenin-mediated heat exposure inhibits intestinal epithelial cell proliferation and stem cell expansion through endoplasmic reticulum stress. *J. Cell Physiol.* **2020**, *235*, 5613–5627. [CrossRef]
39. Yu, L.; Wei, J.; Liu, P. Attacking the PI3K/Akt/mTOR signaling pathway for targeted therapeutic treatment in human cancer. *Semin. Cancer Biol.* **2022**, *85*, 69–94. [CrossRef]
40. Slomovitz, B.M.; Coleman, R.L. The PI3K/AKT/mTOR pathway as a therapeutic target in endometrial cancer. *Clin. Cancer Res.* **2012**, *18*, 5856–5864. [CrossRef] [PubMed]
41. Pereira, L.; Igea, A.; Canovas, B.; Dolado, I.; Nebreda, A.R. Inhibition of p38 MAPK sensitizes tumour cells to cisplatin-induced apoptosis mediated by reactive oxygen species and JNK. *EMBO Mol. Med.* **2013**, *5*, 1759–1774. [CrossRef] [PubMed]
42. Kim, M.-H.; Aydemir, T.B.; Kim, J.; Cousins, R.J. Hepatic ZIP14-mediated zinc transport is required for adaptation to endoplasmic reticulum stress. *Proc. Natl. Acad. Sci. USA* **2017**, *114*, E5805–E5814. [CrossRef]
43. Ma, Y.; Zhang, M.; Yu, H.; Lu, J.; Cheng, K.K.Y.; Zhou, J.; Chen, H.; Jia, W. Activation of G0/G1 switch gene 2 by endoplasmic reticulum stress enhances hepatic steatosis. *Metabolism* **2019**, *99*, 32–44. [CrossRef]
44. Ichimura, Y.; Waguri, S.; Sou, Y.-S.; Kageyama, S.; Hasegawa, J.; Ishimura, R.; Saito, T.; Yang, Y.; Kouno, T.; Fukutomi, T.; et al. Phosphorylation of p62 activates the Keap1-Nrf2 pathway during selective autophagy. *Mol. Cell* **2013**, *51*, 618–631. [CrossRef] [PubMed]
45. Zorov, D.B.; Juhaszova, M.; Sollott, S.J. Mitochondrial reactive oxygen species (ROS) and ROS-induced ROS release. *Physiol. Rev.* **2014**, *94*, 909–950. [CrossRef]
46. He, J.; Ma, M.; Li, D.; Wang, K.; Wang, Q.; Li, Q.; He, H.; Zhou, Y.; Li, Q.; Hou, X.; et al. Sulfiredoxin-1 attenuates injury and inflammation in acute pancreatitis through the ROS/ER stress/Cathepsin B axis. *Cell Death Dis.* **2021**, *12*, 626. [CrossRef]
47. Kokubo, K.; Hirahara, K.; Kiuchi, M.; Tsuji, K.; Shimada, Y.; Sonobe, Y.; Shinmi, R.; Hishiya, T.; Iwamura, C.; Onodera, A.; et al. Thioredoxin-interacting protein is essential for memory T cell formation via the regulation of the redox metabolism. *Proc. Natl. Acad. Sci. USA* **2023**, *120*, e2218345120. [CrossRef]
48. Raimundo, N.; Song, L.; Shutt, T.E.; McKay, S.E.; Cotney, J.; Guan, M.-X.; Gilliland, T.C.; Hohuan, D.; Santos-Sacchi, J.; Shadel, G.S. Mitochondrial stress engages E2F1 apoptotic signaling to cause deafness. *Cell* **2012**, *148*, 716–726. [CrossRef] [PubMed]
49. Xu, Z.; Xu, J.; Sun, S.; Lin, W.; Li, Y.; Lu, Q.; Li, F.; Yang, Z.; Lu, Y.; Liu, W. Mecheliolide elicits ROS-mediated ERS driven immunogenic cell death in hepatocellular carcinoma. *Redox Biol.* **2022**, *54*, 102351. [CrossRef]
50. Liu, H.; Wang, L.; Weng, X.; Chen, H.; Du, Y.; Diao, C.; Chen, Z.; Liu, X. Inhibition of Brd4 alleviates renal ischemia/reperfusion injury-induced apoptosis and endoplasmic reticulum stress by blocking FoxO4-mediated oxidative stress. *Redox Biol.* **2019**, *24*, 101195. [CrossRef]
51. Liao, L.-S.; Chen, Y.; Hou, C.; Liu, Y.-H.; Su, G.-F.; Liang, H.; Chen, Z.-F. Potent Zinc(II)-Based Immunogenic Cell Death Inducer Triggered by ROS-Mediated ERS and Mitochondrial Ca^{2+} Overload. *J. Med. Chem.* **2023**, *66*, 10497–10509. [CrossRef] [PubMed]
52. Craver, B.M.; Ramanathan, G.; Hoang, S.; Chang, X.; Mendez Luque, L.F.; Brooks, S.; Lai, H.Y.; Fleischman, A.G. N-acetylcysteine inhibits thrombosis in a murine model of myeloproliferative neoplasm. *Blood Adv.* **2020**, *4*, 312–321. [CrossRef] [PubMed]
53. Lu, X.; Li, C.; Li, C.; Li, P.; Fu, E.; Xie, Y.; Jin, F. Heat-Labile Enterotoxin-Induced PERK-CHOP Pathway Activation Causes Intestinal Epithelial Cell Apoptosis. *Front. Cell Infect. Microbiol.* **2017**, *7*, 244. [CrossRef]
54. Gu, Y.; Huang, F.; Wang, Y.; Chen, C.; Wu, S.; Zhou, S.; Hei, Z.; Yuan, D. Connexin32 plays a crucial role in ROS-mediated endoplasmic reticulum stress apoptosis signaling pathway in ischemia reperfusion-induced acute kidney injury. *J. Transl. Med.* **2018**, *16*, 117. [CrossRef]
55. He, Q.; Zhou, X.; Liu, Y.; Gou, W.; Cui, J.; Li, Z.; Wu, Y.; Zuo, D. Titanium dioxide nanoparticles induce mouse hippocampal neuron apoptosis via oxidative stress- and calcium imbalance-mediated endoplasmic reticulum stress. *Environ. Toxicol. Pharmacol.* **2018**, *63*, 6–15. [CrossRef]
56. Park, H.-J.; Son, H.-J.; Sul, O.-J.; Suh, J.-H.; Choi, H.-S. 4-Phenylbutyric acid protects against lipopolysaccharide-induced bone loss by modulating autophagy in osteoclasts. *Biochem. Pharmacol.* **2018**, *151*, 9–17. [CrossRef] [PubMed]
57. Pao, H.-P.; Liao, W.-I.; Tang, S.-E.; Wu, S.-Y.; Huang, K.-L.; Chu, S.-J. Suppression of Endoplasmic Reticulum Stress by 4-PBA Protects Against Hyperoxia-Induced Acute Lung Injury via Up-Regulating Claudin-4 Expression. *Front. Immunol.* **2021**, *12*, 674316. [CrossRef] [PubMed]
58. Fang, C.; Weng, T.; Hu, S.; Yuan, Z.; Xiong, H.; Huang, B.; Cai, Y.; Li, L.; Fu, X. IFN-γ-induced ER stress impairs autophagy and triggers apoptosis in lung cancer cells. *Oncoimmunology* **2021**, *10*, 1962591. [CrossRef]

59. Hybertson, B.M.; Gao, B.; Bose, S.K.; McCord, J.M. Oxidative stress in health and disease: The therapeutic potential of Nrf2 activation. *Mol. Asp. Med.* **2011**, *32*, 234–246. [CrossRef]
60. Zenkov, N.K.; Menshchikova, E.B.; Tkachev, V.O. Keap1/Nrf2/ARE redox-sensitive signaling system as a pharmacological target. *Biochemistry* **2013**, *78*, 19–36. [CrossRef]
61. Guan, T.; Li, N.; Xu, X.; Xiong, D.; Wang, B.; Xiao, L.; Yang, W.; Chu, G.; Yusuf, A.; Zhang, J.; et al. Involvement of the Keap1-Nrf2-ARE pathway in the antioxidant activity of sinomenine. *Arch. Biochem. Biophys.* **2024**, *753*, 109928. [CrossRef]
62. Liu, C.; Rokavec, M.; Huang, Z.; Hermeking, H. Curcumin activates a ROS/KEAP1/NRF2/miR-34a/b/c cascade to suppress colorectal cancer metastasis. *Cell Death Differ.* **2023**, *30*, 1771–1785. [CrossRef] [PubMed]
63. Chi, F.; Cheng, C.; Zhang, M.; Su, B.; Hou, Y.; Bai, G. Resveratrol targeting NRF2 disrupts the binding between KEAP1 and NRF2-DLG motif to ameliorate oxidative stress damage in mice pulmonary infection. *J. Ethnopharmacol.* **2024**, *332*, 118353. [CrossRef] [PubMed]
64. Chen, S.; Zhang, Y.; Niu, X.; Mohyuddin, S.G.; Wen, J.; Bao, M.; Yu, T.; Wu, L.; Hu, C.; Yong, Y.; et al. Coral-Derived Endophytic Fungal Product, Butyrolactone-I, Alleviates Lps Induced Intestinal Epithelial Cell Inflammatory Response Through TLR4/NF-κB and MAPK Signaling Pathways: An in vitro and in vivo Studies. *Front. Nutr.* **2021**, *8*, 748118. [CrossRef]

marine drugs

MDPI

Article

Anti-Photoaging Effects of Antioxidant Peptide from Seahorse (*Hippocampus abdominalis*) in In Vivo and In Vitro Models

Fengqi Yang [1], Yang Yang [2], Dandan Xiao [1], Poongho Kim [3], Jihee Lee [3], You-Jin Jeon [1,*] and Lei Wang [2,4,*]

1 Department of Marine Life Sciences, Jeju National University, Jeju 63243, Republic of Korea; yfq426@naver.com (F.Y.); dandanxiao98@gmail.com (D.X.)
2 State Key Laboratory of Marine Food Processing & Safety Control, College of Food Science and Engineering, Ocean University of China, Qingdao 266404, China; yangy72000@163.com
3 South Sea Fisheries Research Institute, National Institute of Fisheries Science, Yeosu 59780, Republic of Korea; phkim1@korea.kr (P.K.); easyhee2@korea.kr (J.L.)
4 Sanya Oceanographic Institution, Ocean University of China, Sanya 572024, China
* Correspondence: youjin2014@gmail.com (Y.-J.J.); leiwang2021@ouc.edu.cn (L.W.); Tel.: +82-64-754-3475 (Y.-J.J.)

Abstract: Overexposure to ultraviolet (UV) radiation can lead to photoaging, which contributes to skin damage. The objective of this study was to evaluate the effects of an antioxidant peptide (SHP2) purified from seahorse (*Hippocampus abdominalis*) alcalase hydrolysate on UVB-irradiated skin damage in human keratinocyte (HaCaT) and human dermal fibroblast (HDF) cells and a zebrafish model. The data revealed that SHP2 significantly enhanced cell viability by attenuating apoptosis through the reduction of intracellular reactive oxygen species (ROS) levels in UVB-stimulated HaCaT cells. Moreover, SHP2 effectively inhibited ROS, improved collagen synthesis, and suppressed the secretion of matrix metalloproteinases (MMPs) in UVB-irradiated HDF cells. SHP2 restored the protein levels of HO-1, Nrf2, and SOD, while decreasing Keap1 expression in UVB-treated HDF, indicating stimulation of the Keap1/Nrf2/HO-1 signaling pathway. Furthermore, an in vivo study conducted in zebrafish confirmed that SHP2 inhibited photoaging by reducing cell death through the suppression of ROS generation and lipid peroxidation. Particularly, 200 μg/mL of SHP2 exerted a remarkable anti-photoaging effect on both in vitro and in vivo models. These results demonstrate that SHP2 possesses antioxidant properties and regulates skin photoaging activities, suggesting that SHP2 may have the potential for use in the development of cosmetic products.

Keywords: *Hippocampus abdominalis*; UVB irradiation; antioxidant peptide; photoprotective

1. Introduction

UVB radiation is a well-known environmental factor that causes skin aging. Exposure to UVB radiation induces DNA damage, cell apoptosis, and oxidative stress, resulting in the upregulation of metalloproteinases (MMPs) and degradation of the extracellular matrix (ECM) [1,2]. UVB radiation can cause skin photoaging by inducing the generation of ROS and disrupting the balance of ECM formation and degradation, leading to collagen degradation, which is characterized by wrinkle formation, sagging, and pigmentation [3,4]. Therefore, studying the interactions between UVB radiation, MMPs, and ECM degradation, as well as maintaining the ROS balance, is crucial for discovering protective ingredients against photoaging and maintaining skin health.

Marine bioresources encompass various organisms living in the ocean, including algae, shellfish, fish, mollusks, and marine microorganisms [5]. In recent years, marine bioresources have received significant attention owing to their rich bioactive compound content, such as bioactive peptides. These peptides have attracted considerable interest due to their diverse biological activities, including antioxidant, anti-inflammatory, anticancer, and antimicrobial properties [6]. They hold immense potential for application in cosmetics, functional foods, pharmaceuticals, and other fields. Marine-derived bioactive peptides are known for their superior safety profiles, intestinal bioavailability, and homology with human collagen [7]. Their unique structural features and bioavailability make them attractive candidates for incorporation into cosmetics and development as functional ingredients.

Seahorses have been used in traditional medicine due to their antioxidant, anti-arthritis, and anti-fatigue properties [8,9]. Among the various seahorse species, *H. abdominalis*, commonly known as the big-belly seahorse, is renowned for its large size, capable of growing up to 35 cm in length, as well as its unique characteristics, such as pale coloration and smooth skin [10,11]. Additionally, *H. abdominalis* is notable for its rich protein content, featuring a high ratio of essential amino acids, including aromatic and heterocyclic amino acids, as well as acidic amino acids [12]. Peptides extracted from seahorse tissues have attracted the interest of researchers because of their biological properties and potential therapeutic effects. These peptides have long been studied for their pharmacological effects and are valuable resources for biomedical research and drug development. A previous study identified *H. abdominalis* peptide sequences and investigated their alkyl radical scavenging activity [13]. Additionally, the *H. abdominalis* peptide demonstrated significant protective effects against AAPH-induced oxidative damage in Vero cells and zebrafish in a previous study [10]. To further explore the bioactivity of SHP2, we evaluated its potential antioxidant and anti-photoaging effects in vitro using HaCaT and HDF cells, as well as in vivo in zebrafish. This study aimed to elucidate the potential of SHP2 in mitigating UVB-induced skin damage and to investigate its possible applications in cosmetic product development.

2. Results

2.1. Protective Effect of SHP2 against UVB-Irradiated HaCaT Cell Skin Damage

UV exposure induces oxidative damage and generates intracellular ROS, leading to cell death. Previous studies have demonstrated that *H. abdominalis* peptides effectively scavenge alkyl radicals and have an antioxidant effect [13,14]. In the present study, we investigated the effects of SHP2 on UVB-induced oxidative stress and apoptosis in HaCaT cells. We analyzed the effects of different concentrations of SHP2 on the viability of HaCaT cells. As depicted in Figure 1A, concentrations of SHP2 ranging from 12.5 to 200 μg/mL did not significantly affect HaCaT cell viability, indicating that SHP2 is not toxic to the cells. Next, we evaluated the effect of UVB radiation on intracellular ROS levels and determined whether SHP2 inhibited the increase in ROS levels induced by UVB radiation. As shown in Figure 1B, UVB radiation significantly increased intracellular ROS levels in HaCaT cells, whereas SHP2 reduced the amount of UVB-induced ROS in a concentration-dependent manner, indicating its antioxidant properties. Furthermore, as illustrated in Figure 1C, UVB radiation significantly decreased the viability of UVB-irradiated HaCaT cells, whereas SHP2 increased it in a dose-dependent manner. Additionally, as shown in Figure 2, the cells exhibited significant damage due to UVB radiation, with an increased intensity and clustering of blue spots, suggesting cell stress or death. In contrast, SHP2 significantly inhibits apoptosis, particularly at high concentrations. These results suggest that SHP2 provides a substantial protection against UVB-induced damage. Overall, SHP2 protects HaCaT cells against UVB-induced photoaging by inhibiting intracellular ROS and apoptosis.

2.2. Protective Effect of SHP2 against UVB-Induced HDF Cell Model

UV irradiation can stimulate the expression of MMPs, inducing oxidative damage to cells and ECM degradation. Collagen, a major component of the ECM, is highly susceptible to degradation when the level of MMP collagenases increases, which is a key cause of skin aging [15]. To further demonstrate the protective benefits of SHP2 against UVB-induced skin damage, we evaluated its photoprotective effects on HDF cells by assessing the ROS levels, collagen synthesis, and MMP expression. As shown in Figure 3A, SHP2 showed no toxicity on HDF cells at concentrations ranging from 12.5 to 200 μg/mL. In Figure 3B, intracellular ROS levels sharply increased following UVB radiation, but SHP2 treatment groups ranging from 50 to 200 μg/mL showed significantly lower values compared to that in the model group. Concurrently, cell viability in the SHP2 treatment groups steadily increased, indicating protection against UVB-triggered damage in HDF (Figure 3C).

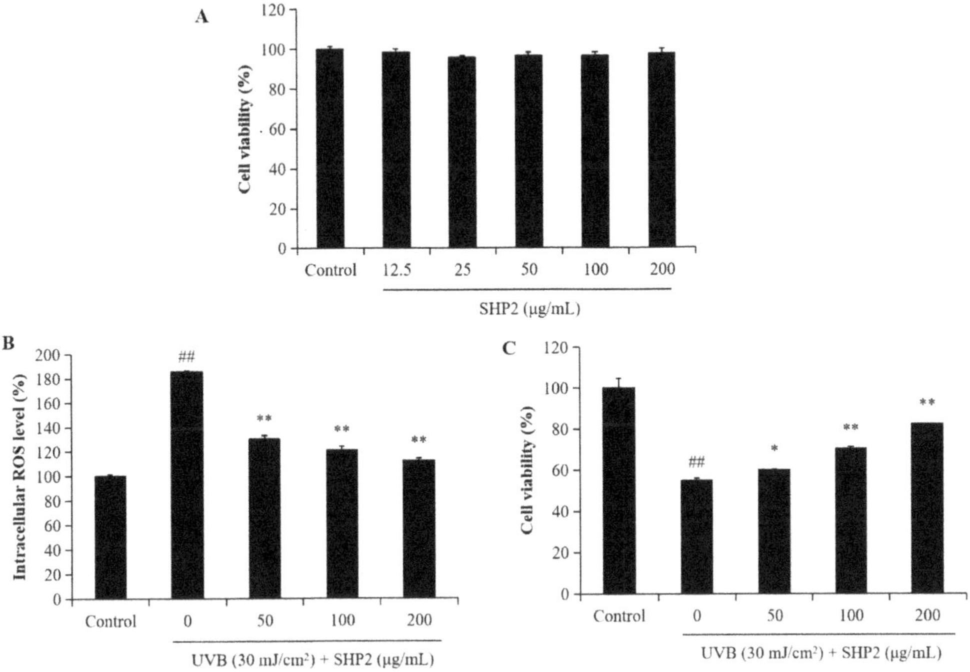

Figure 1. SHP2 protects HaCaT cells against UVB-induced photodamage. (**A**) Cytotoxicity of SHP2 on HaCaT cells; (**B**) intracellular ROS scavenging effect of SHP2 in UVB-irradiated HaCaT cells; (**C**) protective effect of SHP2 against UVB-induced cell death in HaCaT cells. The experiments were conducted in triplicate and the data are expressed as the mean ± SE. * $p < 0.05$, ** $p < 0.01$ as compared to the UVB-irradiated group and ## $p < 0.01$ as compared to the control group.

As shown in Figure 4A, collagen levels decreased following UVB irradiation. However, co-treatment with SHP2 at concentrations ranging from 50 to 200 μg/mL significantly restored the collagen synthesis level. This result indicated that treatment with SHP2 enhanced collagen production, contributing to its anti-wrinkle effect. Additionally, Figure 4B–F shows the high MMP levels in UVB-irradiated HDF. However, SHP2 significantly reduced the expression levels of MMP-1,2,8,9, and 13. In particular, the reduction in MMP-8 and MMP-13 stimulated by UVB exposure was restrained in a concentration-dependent manner when HDF cells were incubated with SHP2. SHP2-treated groups exhibited a downward trend in MMPs' expression, indicating a reduction in MMPs' activity, which may be beneficial for maintaining ECM integrity. These results demonstrate that SHP2 can inhibit the generation of MMPs in the HDF cells induced by UVB radiation and stimulate the synthesis of collagen proteins, providing evidence for SHP2 as a potential cosmetic ingredient.

To evaluate the protective effects of SHP2 against UVB-induced photoaging in HDF cells, we analyzed the expression levels of Keap1, Nrf2, HO-1, and SOD. As shown in Figure 5, UVB treatment significantly decreased the protein levels of HO-1, Nrf2, and SOD, which are the key proteins involved in cellular defense against oxidative stress, while increasing Keap1 expression compared to the control group. Supplementation with 50 μg/mL to 200 μg/mL of SHP2 significantly restored the levels of HO-1, Nrf2, and SOD. Additionally, Keap1 expression significantly decreased following SHP2 treatment. These results further support the hypothesis that SHP2 exerts protective effects against UVB-induced oxidative damage and photoaging in HDF cells by modulating the Keap1/Nrf2/HO-1 signaling pathway.

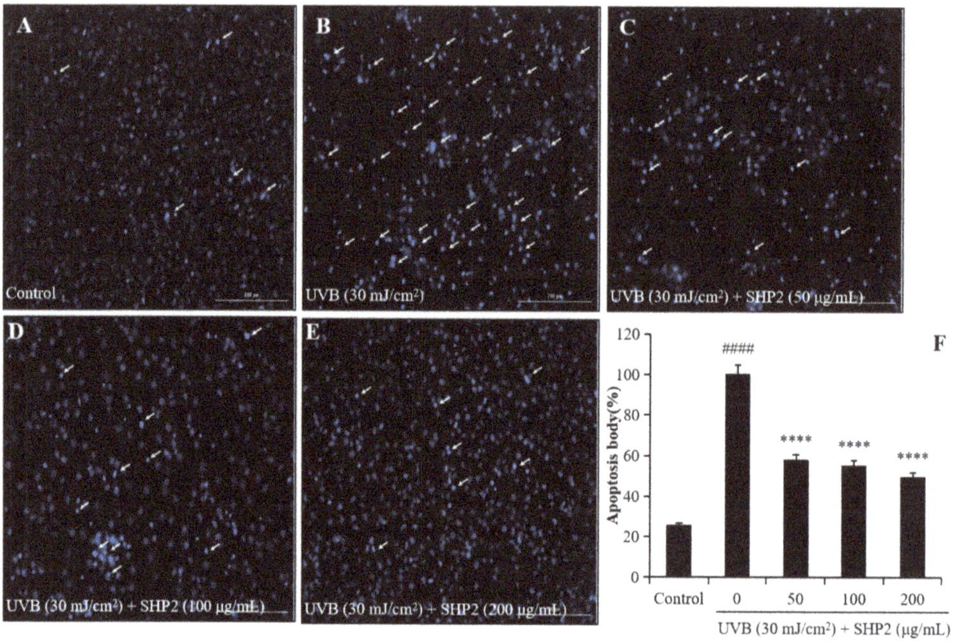

Figure 2. SHP2 protects HaCaT cells against UVB-induced apoptosis. (**A**) Morphology of the normal cells; (**B**) morphology of the cells irradiated by UVB; (**C**) morphology of the cells treated with 50 µg/mL SHP2 and irradiated by UVB; (**D**) morphology of the cells treated with 100 µg/mL SHP2 and irradiated by UVB; (**E**) morphology of the cells treated with 200 µg/mL SHP2 and irradiated by UVB; (**F**) quantification of apoptotic cells. The apoptotic body formation was evaluated by Hoechst 33342 staining assay. White arrows indicate apoptotic bodies. **** $p < 0.0001$ as compared to the UVB-irradiated group and #### $p < 0.0001$ as compared to the control group.

2.3. *Protective Effect of SHP2 in UVB-Irradiated Zebrafish Model*

Previous studies have suggested that because of the genetic and organ system similarities of zebrafish to humans, ease of cultivation, high throughput, and low cost, zebrafish can be used as an in vivo model to measure UVB irradiation-induced cell death, intracellular ROS levels, and lipid peroxidation to evaluate the photoprotective activities of active substances [3,16,17]. In this study, we explored the in vivo photoprotective activity of SHP2 in UVB-irradiated zebrafish. As shown in Figure 6, after UVB exposure, there was a significant increase in ROS generation, cell death, and lipid peroxidation, leading to elevated oxidative stress, cytotoxicity, and oxidative damage caused to the cell membrane. However, SHP2 significantly inhibited ROS production, cell death, and lipid peroxidation in UVB-exposed zebrafish across all the SHP2 treatment groups. These results imply that SHP2 prevents photoaging in vivo in zebrafish.

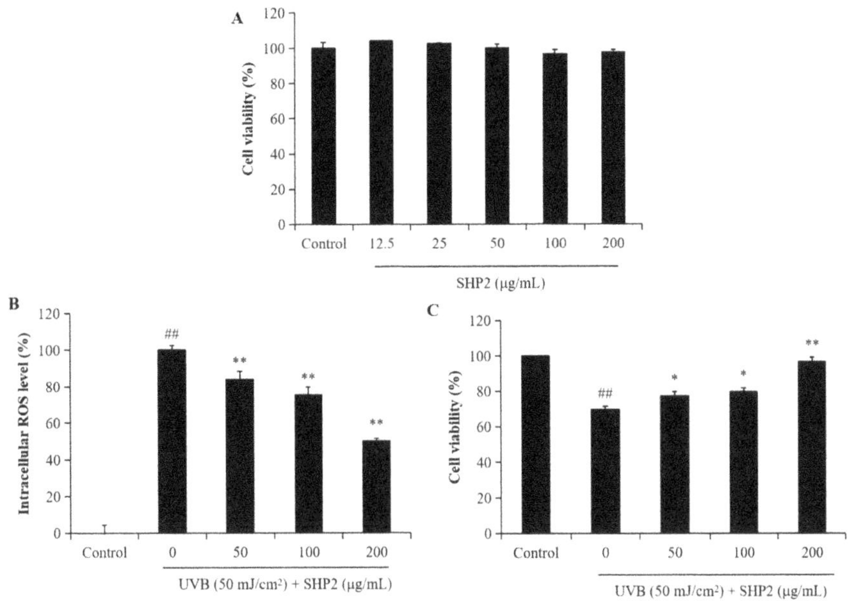

Figure 3. SHP2 protects HDF cells against UVB-induced damage. (**A**) Cytotoxicity of SHP2 on HDF cells; (**B**) intracellular ROS scavenging effect of SHP2 in UVB-irradiated HDF cells; (**C**) protective effect of SHP2 against UVB-induced cell death in HDF cells. The experiments were conducted in triplicate and the data are expressed as the mean ± SE. * $p < 0.05$, ** $p < 0.01$ as compared to the UVB-irradiated group and ## $p < 0.01$ as compared to the control group.

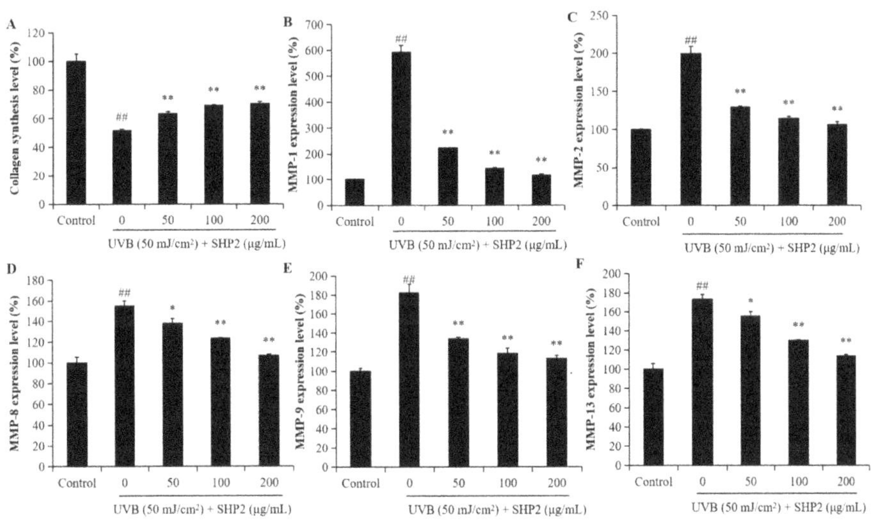

Figure 4. SHP2 improves collagen synthesis and inhibits MMPs' expression in UVB-irradiated HDF cells. (**A**) Collagen contents in UVB-irradiated HDF cells; (**B**) MMP-1 expression levels in UVB-irradiated HDF cells; (**C**) MMP-2 expression levels in UVB-irradiated HDF cells; (**D**) MMP-8 expression levels in UVB-irradiated HDF cells; (**E**) MMP-9 expression levels in UVB-irradiated HDF cells; (**F**) MMP-13 expression levels in UVB-irradiated HDF cells. The experiments were conducted in triplicate and the data are expressed as the mean ± SE. * $p < 0.05$, ** $p < 0.01$ as compared to the UVB-irradiated group and ## $p < 0.01$ as compared to the control group.

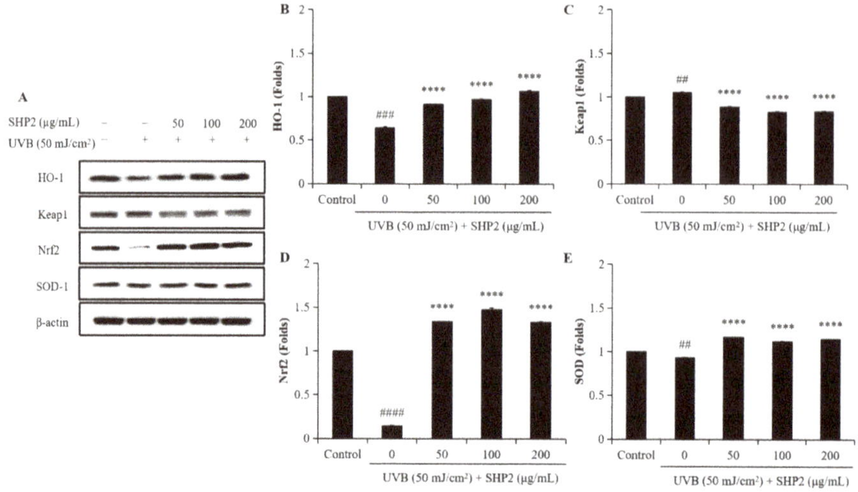

Figure 5. Protective effects of SHP2 on Keap1/Nrf2/HO-1 signaling pathway in UVB-irradiated HDF cells. (**A**) Western blot bands; (**B**) HO-1 protein expression; (**C**) Keap1 protein expression; (**D**) Nrf2 protein expression; (**E**) SOD protein expression. The experiments were conducted in triplicate and the data are expressed as the mean ± SE. **** $p < 0.0001$ as compared to the UVB-irradiated group and ## $p < 0.01$, ### $p < 0.001$, #### $p < 0.0001$ as compared to the control group.

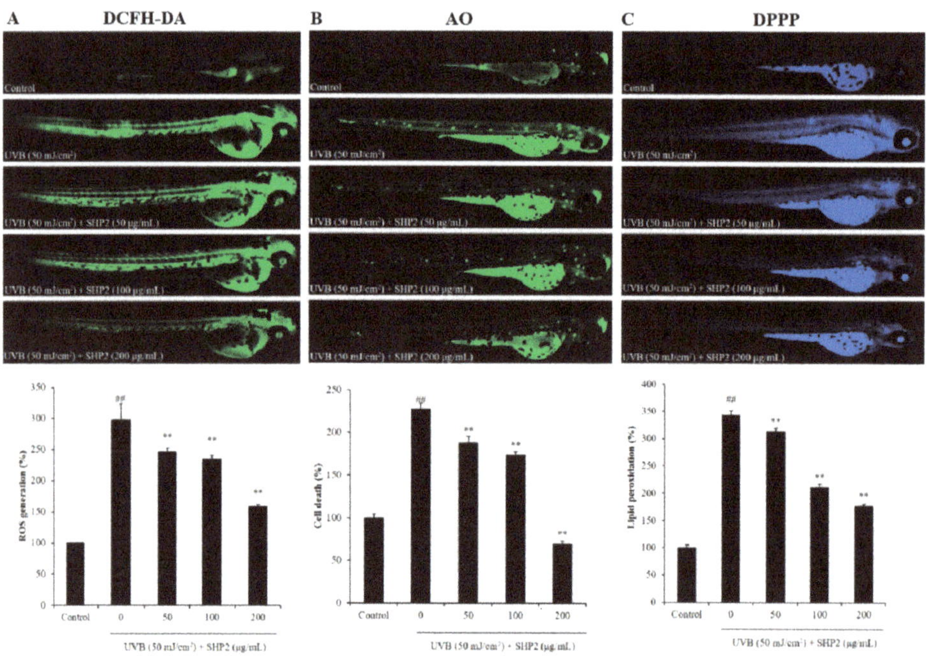

Figure 6. SHP2 protects zebrafish against UVB-induced oxidative stress in the zebrafish. (**A**) ROS generation in zebrafish; (**B**) cell death level in zebrafish; (**C**) lipid peroxidation level in zebrafish. ROS, cell death, and lipid peroxidation levels were measured by Image J software (v.1.8.0). The data are expressed as means ± SE. ** $p < 0.01$ as compared to the UVB-treated group and ## $p < 0.01$ as compared to the control group.

3. Discussion

Under normal circumstances, the human body maintains a balance between the antioxidant and oxidative defenses. However, when endogenous factors, such as inflammation and metabolism, or exogenous factors, such as ultraviolet (UV) radiation, lead to the excessive production of ROS, this balance is disrupted. UV radiation can decrease cellular antioxidant levels and stimulate the production of intracellular ROS, leading to cell death, and is considered a primary environmental factor contributing to skin aging. The skin aging induced by UV radiation is commonly referred to as photoaging [18,19].

Antioxidant peptides have wide applications in various fields such as cosmetics, food, and pharmaceuticals. Because of their rich bioactivity, many researchers have focused on the extraction of new peptides from plants, terrestrial organisms, and marine animals. Marine peptides exhibit an extensive range of biological activities, including antioxidant, anti-aging, anti-hypertensive, anti-fatigue, immunomodulatory, and other functions [20,21]. The seahorse is a precious marine animal belonging to the Syngnathidae family. Reports suggest that the peptides extracted from *H. abdominalis* possess anti-fatigue, antihypertensive, and antioxidant effects [8,22,23]. However, the photoprotective role of *H. abdominalis* antioxidant peptides still needs to be evaluated. Traditional in vitro experiments such as free-radical scavenging and metal ion chelation assays cannot easily simulate the natural physiological environment of the human body. Therefore, we conducted the experiments using two types of skin cells in vitro and a zebrafish model in vivo to verify the cosmeceutical effects of SHP2 from multiple perspectives, including its antioxidant, anti-apoptotic, and anti-photoaging effects.

UVB radiation can induce the excessive production of free radicals in the human body, and an overabundance of ROS can lead to skin aging, resulting in dullness, wrinkles, and dysfunction by triggering cell apoptosis [24]. Antioxidant peptides possess the ability to scavenge free radicals, rapidly absorb them, exhibit excellent stability, and effectively delay skin aging. SHP2 significantly reduced ROS levels in a dose-dependent manner and inhibited UVB-induced apoptosis in HaCaT and HDF cells, thereby demonstrating photoprotective effects. The antioxidant activity of protein hydrolysates is highly dependent on the sequence, molecular weight, and composition of peptides. SHP2 is a low-molecular-weight peptide (913 Da) containing proline and tryptophan at the carboxyl terminus [13], which contributes to its bioactivity and anti-photoaging effects.

UVB radiation can cause wrinkles and skin damage by stimulating MMP expression and inducing the excessive production of intracellular ROS. Increased skin enzyme activity results in protein hydrolysis in the ECM [25]. Furthermore, UVB stimulation leads to the overexpression of MMP-1, resulting in the degradation of the type I and III collagen as well as the upregulation of MMP-2 and MMP-9, contributing to ECM degradation. Prolonged exposure to UV radiation accelerates the loss of collagen, reducing the synthesis of elastic fiber proteins, which are the major causes of wrinkling and skin aging [26,27]. SHP2 significantly reduced cell apoptosis, enhanced collagen synthesis, and inhibited MMP 1, 2, 8, 9, and 13 expression in a dose-dependent manner. Therefore, SHP2 demonstrated strong photoprotective activity. SHP2 also exhibited an anti-skin aging effect by downregulating ROS production and preventing the UVB-induced apoptosis of HaCaT cells. Experimental evidence suggests that some antioxidant peptides can confer anti-aging effects by enhancing the type I collagen expression and reducing that of MMP-1 [28]. SHP2 inhibited MMP expression in UVB-irradiated HDF, thereby suppressing collagen degradation, indicating its ability to promote the formation of elastic fiber proteins. These data indicated that SHP2 has photoprotective activity and the potential to delay skin aging.

The Keap1/Nrf2/HO-1 signaling pathway was analyzed by Western blotting to investigate the protective effects of SHP2 against UVB-induced photoaging in HDF cells. UVB exposure disrupted this pathway, as evidenced by the downregulation of HO-1, Nrf2, and SOD, and the upregulation of Keap1 expression. Treatment with SHP2 successfully restored the protein levels of HO-1, Nrf2, and SOD while reducing Keap1 expression, thus enhancing the antioxidant defense of cells and maintaining cellular homeostasis under

UVB radiation, indicating SHP2's potential anti-photoaging effects. Nrf2 is a key transcription factor that regulates the expression of antioxidant and cytoprotective genes. Its activation induces the expression of enzymes, such as SOD and HO-1, which neutralize ROS, a major contributor to oxidative stress and photoaging [24]. Additionally, SHP2's ability to downregulate Keap1, which targets Nrf2 for degradation, facilitates its protective action against oxidative damage. As oxidative damage is the primary cause of photoaging, these findings suggest that SHP2's modulation of the Keap1/Nrf2/HO-1 pathway holds therapeutic potential for preventing or mitigating UVB-induced photoaging.

Although cell and rodent models have been widely used for activity assessment, non-rodent models, such as zebrafish, offer many advantages, e.g., low maintenance costs, small size, and short life cycle, which can effectively improve experimental efficiency [29]. Moreover, owing to their transparency, zebrafish allow the use of fluorescent probes to detect cell death, ROS generation, and lipid peroxidation, making them ideal for high-throughput drug screening [30]. In vivo results indicated that SHP2 significantly inhibits ROS generation in zebrafish, effectively reducing in vivo UVB-induced photoaging by UVB stimulation through decreasing lipid peroxidation and cell death. These results suggest that SHP2 has tremendous potential for use in the cosmetics industry and merits further exploration.

To further understand the protective role of SHP2 against UVB-induced skin damage, it is essential to focus on the mechanisms of DNA damage. Recent studies highlight the critical role of DNA damage in UVB-induced skin injury, which, if unrepaired, increases skin cancer risk. For example, trigonelline prevents oxidative DNA damage by modulating the PI3K-Akt-Nrf2 signaling pathway in HDF cells and mice [31]. Similarly, asperyellone protects HDF cells from UVB-induced oxidative stress and DNA damage, reducing apoptosis and maintaining cellular integrity [32]. These findings emphasize the importance of addressing UVB-induced DNA damage to prevent the survival and proliferation of DNA-damaged cells, which may reduce the risk of developing skin cancer. Future studies will explore the potential of SHP2 in mitigating UVB-induced DNA damage to further confirm its protective effects against photoaging.

4. Materials and Methods

4.1. Materials

The dimethyl sulfoxide (DMSO), acridine orange (AO), 3-(4-5-dimethyl-2yl)-2-5-diphynyltetrasolium bromide (MTT), 2, 7-dichlorodihydroflurescin diacetate (DCFH-DA), 1,3-Bis (diphenylphosphino) propane (DPPP) phosphate-buffered saline (PBS), human matrix metalloproteinases (MMP)-1, 2, 8, 9, and 13, and Enzyme-Linked Immunosorbent Assay (ELISA) kit were purchased from Sigma Co., Ltd. (St. Louis, MO, USA). Dulbecco's modified Eagle's medium (DMEM), penicillium/streptomycin (P/S), fetal bovine serum (FBS), and trypsin-EDTA were purchased from Gibco BRL (Life Technologies, Burlington, ON, Canada). The primary antibodies, anti-heme oxygenase 1 (HO-1) (rabbit monoclonal antibody, Cat. #70081S), anti-Nrf2 (rabbit monoclonal antibody, Cat. #12721S), and anti-Keap1 (rabbit monoclonal antibody, Cat. #8047S), were purchased from Cell Signaling Technology (Beverly, MA, USA). Anti-Superoxide dismutase 1 (SOD1) (mouse monoclonal antibody, Cat. #SC-17767) and β-actin (mouse monoclonal antibody, Cat. #SC-47778) were obtained from Santa Cruz Biotechnology (Santa Cruz, CA, USA). The secondary antibodies, including the anti-rabbit IgG, HRP-linked antibody (Cat. #7074S) and anti-mouse IgG, HRP-linked antibody (Cat. #7076S), were obtained from Cell Signaling Technology (Beverly, MA, USA).

4.2. Purification of Bioactive Peptides from H. abdominalis

The extraction and purification of peptides from *H. abdominalis* alcalase hydrolysate (HA) were performed according to previously reported methodologies [13]. To isolate the antioxidant peptides, a process combining ultrafiltration and Sephadex purification was employed, followed by enzyme-assisted hydrolysis. This process resulted in the separation of three distinct molecular weight fractions: HA-I (>10 kDa), HA-II (5–10 kDa), and HA-III (<5 kDa). Among these fractions, HA-III, which exhibited the strongest bioactivity, was selected for further purification of the antioxidant peptides using a Sephadex G10 column. Finally, three peptides were identified: GIIGPSGSP (Glycine–Isoleucine–Isoleucine–Glycine–Proline–Serine–Glycine–Serine–Proline: SHP1), IGTGIPGIW (Isoleucine–Glycine–Threonine–Glycine–Isoleucine–Proline–Glycine–Isoleucine–Tryptophan: SHP2), and QIGFIW (Glutamine–Isoleucine–Glycine–Phenylalanine–Isoleucine–Tryptophan: SHP3). Previous studies have shown that IGTGIPGIW possesses strong free radical scavenging properties in both in vivo and in vitro models [10]. Additionally, Kim [11] showed that among the peptides extracted from seahorses, IGTGIPGIW had a relatively stronger alkyl radical scavenging capability compared to that of GIIGPSGSP and QIGFIW. Consequently, we selected SHP2 to conduct subsequent studies on UVB-caused skin damage, both in vivo and in vitro.

4.3. Cell Culture and Cell Viability Analysis

HaCaT cells were cultured in DMEM supplemented with 10% FBS and 1% streptomycin/penicillin. HDF cells were cultured in DMEM mixed with F-12 media supplemented with 10% FBS and 1% streptomycin/penicillin. The cultures were maintained at 37 °C in a humidified incubator with 5% CO_2. HaCaT and HDF cells were purchased from the Korean Cell Line Bank, subcultured, and seeded at concentrations of 1×10^5 and 5×10^4 cells/mL, respectively. The cells were subjected to treatment with concentrations ranging from 12.5 to 200 μg/mL, and cell viability was assessed utilizing the MTT assay.

4.4. Determination of the Anti-UVB-Induced Skin Damage Effects on HaCaT Cells

To investigate the anti-UVB-stimulated skin damage effects on HaCaT cells, the cells were exposed to SHP2 at concentrations of 50, 100, and 200 μg/mL and irradiated (30 $mJ \cdot cm^{-2}$) with UVB. After 24 h of incubation, cell viability, intracellular ROS levels, and apoptotic body formation were assessed using the MTT assay, DCFH-DA assay, and Hoechst 33342 staining, respectively [3].

4.5. Determination of the Anti-UVB-Induced Skin Damage Effects on HDF Cells

HDF cells were treated with SHP2 at concentrations of 50, 100, and 200 μg/mL and then irradiated with UVB (50 mJ/cm^2) to assess the protective effects of SHP2 against UVB-induced skin damage. Intracellular ROS levels and cell viability were evaluated using the DCFH-DA and MTT assays, respectively. To analyze collagen synthesis and MMP expression levels, SHP2-treated HDF cells were irradiated with UVB (50 mJ/cm^2) and incubated in FBS-free media for 48 h. The cell culture media were collected and used to assess MMPs expression and PIP levels, which reflect collagen synthesis. Collagen synthesis in HDF cells was evaluated using an ELISA kit (Cat. # MK101), while MMP expression levels were measured using Sigma's Sandwich ELISA kits, following the manufacturers' instructions [33].

4.6. Western Blotting

For Western blotting, cell lysates were prepared using RIPA buffer containing protease and phosphatase inhibitors. The protein concentration was measured using a BCA assay, and the sample concentrations were adjusted to ensure equal loading. Electrophoresis was performed at 80–120 V. The proteins were transferred onto nitrocellulose membranes using a transfer system at 90 V for 90 min. The membrane was then blocked with 5% skim milk in TBST and incubated with the primary antibody overnight at 4 °C, followed by incubation with an HRP-conjugated secondary antibody for 2 h. Protein bands were detected using ECL reagent, and images were captured using a Fusion Solo system (Vilber Lourmat, Collégien, France).

4.7. In Vivo Studies in Zebrafish

Adult zebrafish were maintained according to the protocols outlined in our previous study [3]. The protective effect of SHP2 against UVB was investigated using 2-day post-fertilization (2dpf) larvae by treating with SHP2 (50, 100, and 200 μg/mL). After a treatment duration of 1 h, the larvae were exposed to UVB radiation at a dose of 50 $mJ \cdot cm^{-2}$ and incubated for 6 h. ROS generation, cell death, and lipid peroxidation were assessed using DCFH-DA, acridine orange, and DPPP, respectively [34].

4.8. Statistical Analysis

All experiments were performed in triplicate. Data are presented as the mean ± standard error (SE). Statistical analysis was conducted using SPSS 20.0, employing a one-way ANOVA to compare the mean values. Significant differences between means were determined using Tukey's test.

5. Conclusions

In this study, we investigated the antioxidant and photoprotective properties of SHP2 against UVB-induced photodamage, utilizing both in vitro and in vivo models. These results indicate that SHP2 purified from *H. abdominalis* had a protective effect against UVB-induced oxidative stress in both HaCaT and HDF cells. SHP2 increased collagen synthesis by suppressing oxidative stress and inhibiting MMP expression in HDF cells, demonstrating a protective effect against UVB dermal damage. SHP2 treatment restored the expression of key antioxidant proteins such as HO-1, Nrf2, and SOD while reducing Keap1 expression in UVB-irradiated HDF cells. These results confirm the role of SHP2 in modulating the Keap1/Nrf2/HO-1 signaling pathway, contributing to its anti-photoaging activity. Furthermore, SHP2 inhibits UVB-induced damage in zebrafish by reducing cell death, lipid peroxidation, and ROS levels. Overall, this study indicates that SHP2 has anti-photoaging activity. However, a limitation of this study is the need for further exploration of SHP2's long-term effects in other in vivo and in vitro biological systems, as well as its potential mechanisms of action, to confirm its viability as a functional ingredient in cosmetics.

Author Contributions: Conceptualization, F.Y., Y.-J.J. and L.W.; methodology, F.Y., Y.Y. and D.X.; software, F.Y., Y.Y. and L.W.; validation, F.Y. and Y.-J.J.; formal analysis, Y.Y. and P.K.; investigation, P.K. and J.L.; resources, Y.-J.J.; data curation, F.Y. and D.X.; writing—original draft preparation, F.Y.; writing—review and editing, F.Y. and L.W.; supervision, Y.-J.J. and L.W.; funding acquisition, Y.-J.J. and L.W. All authors have read and agreed to the published version of the manuscript.

Funding: This research was supported by the National Institute of Fisheries Sciences, Ministry of Oceans and Fisheries, Korea (R2024057).

Institutional Review Board Statement: The study protocols were conducted in accordance with the regulations and policies after obtaining approval from the Animal Experimental Ethics Committee of Jeju National University (approval number: 2022-0005).

Data Availability Statement: Data are contained within the article.

Acknowledgments: This research was supported by the 2024 scientific promotion program funded by Jeju National University.

Conflicts of Interest: The authors declare no conflicts of interest.

References

1. Loo, Y.C.; Hu, H.-C.; Yu, S.-Y.; Tsai, Y.-H.; Korinek, M.; Wu, Y.-C.; Chang, F.-R.; Chen, Y.-J. Development on potential skin anti-aging agents of Cosmos caudatus Kunth via inhibition of collagenase, MMP-1 and MMP-3 activities. *Phytomedicine* **2023**, *110*, 154643. [CrossRef] [PubMed]
2. Lee, H.R.; Yang, J.H.; Lee, J.H.; Kim, K.M.; Cho, S.S.; Baek, J.S.; Kim, J.M.; Choi, M.-H.; Shin, H.-J.; Ki, S.H. Protective Effect of Castanopsis sieboldii Extract against UVB-Induced Photodamage in Keratinocytes. *Molecules* **2023**, *28*, 2842. [CrossRef] [PubMed]

3. Yang, F.; Hyun, J.; Nagahawatta, D.P.; Kim, Y.M.; Heo, M.-S.; Jeon, Y.-J. Cosmeceutical Effects of Ishige okamurae Celluclast Extract. *Antioxidants* **2022**, *11*, 2442. [CrossRef] [PubMed]
4. Tong, T.; Geng, R.; Kang, S.-G.; Li, X.; Huang, K. Revitalizing Photoaging Skin through Eugenol in UVB-Exposed Hairless Mice: Mechanistic Insights from Integrated Multi-Omics. *Antioxidants* **2024**, *13*, 168. [CrossRef] [PubMed]
5. Monteiro, J.P.; Domingues, M.R.; Calado, R. Marine Animal Co-Products—How Improving Their Use as Rich Sources of Health-Promoting Lipids Can Foster Sustainability. *Mar. Drugs* **2024**, *22*, 73. [CrossRef]
6. Abdo, A.A.A.; Al-Dalali, S.; Hou, Y.; Aleryani, H.; Shehzad, Q.; Asawmahi, O.; Al-Farga, A.; Mohammed, B.; Liu, X.; Sang, Y. Modification of Marine Bioactive Peptides: Strategy to Improve the Biological Activity, Stability, and Taste Properties. *Food Bioprocess Technol.* **2023**, *17*, 1412–1433. [CrossRef]
7. De Luca, C.; Mikhal'chik, E.V.; Suprun, M.V.; Papacharalambous, M.; Truhanov, A.I.; Korkina, L.G. Skin Antiageing and Systemic Redox Effects of Supplementation with Marine Collagen Peptides and Plant-Derived Antioxidants: A Single-Blind Case-Control Clinical Study. *Oxidative Med. Cell. Longev.* **2016**, *2016*, 4389410. [CrossRef]
8. Zhang, Y.; Ryu, B.; Cui, Y.; Li, C.; Zhou, C.; Hong, P.; Lee, B.; Qian, Z.-J. A peptide isolated from *Hippocampus abdominalis* improves exercise performance and exerts anti-fatigue effects via AMPK/PGC-1α pathway in mice. *J. Funct. Food.* **2019**, *61*, 103489. [CrossRef]
9. Li, K.; Yan, L.; Zhang, Y.; Yang, Z.; Zhang, C.; Li, Y.; Kalueff, A.V.; Li, W.; Song, C. Seahorse treatment improves depression-like behavior in mice exposed to CUMS through reducing inflammation/oxidants and restoring neurotransmitter and neurotrophin function. *J. Ethnopharmacol.* **2020**, *250*, 112487. [CrossRef]
10. Lee, H.-G.; Nagahawatta, D.P.; Yang, F.; Jayawardhana, H.H.A.C.K.; Liyanage, N.M.; Lee, D.-S.; Lee, J.M.; Yim, M.-J.; Ko, S.-C.; Kim, J.-Y.; et al. Antioxidant potential of hydrolysate-derived seahorse (*Hippocampus abdominalis*) peptide: Protective effects against AAPH-induced oxidative damage in vitro and in vivo. *Food Chem.* **2023**, *407*, 135130. [CrossRef]
11. Kodagoda, Y.K.; Liyanage, D.S.; Omeka, W.K.M.; Kim, G.; Kim, J.; Lee, J. Identification, expression profiling, and functional characterization of cystatin C from big-belly seahorse (*Hippocampus abdominalis*). *Fish Shellfish Immunol.* **2023**, *138*, 108804. [CrossRef] [PubMed]
12. Wijerathna, H.M.S.M.; Nadarajapillai, K.; Udayantha, H.M.V.; Kasthuriarachchi, T.D.W.; Shanaka, K.A.S.N.; Kwon, H.; Wan, Q.; Lee, J. Molecular delineation, expression profiling, immune response, and anti-apoptotic function of a novel clusterin homolog from big-belly seahorse (*Hippocampus abdominalis*). *Fish Shellfish Immunol.* **2022**, *124*, 289–299. [CrossRef] [PubMed]
13. Kim, H.-S.; Je, J.-G.; Ryu, B.; Kang, N.; Shanura Fernando, I.P.; Jayawardena, T.U.; Asanka Sanjeewa, K.K.; Oh, J.-Y.; Lee, T.-G.; Jeon, Y.-J. Antioxidant and angiotensin-I converting enzyme inhibitory peptides from *Hippocampus abdominalis*. *Eur. Food Res. Technol.* **2019**, *245*, 479–487. [CrossRef]
14. Kim, H.-S.; Kim, S.-Y.; Fernando, I.P.S.; Sanjeewa, K.K.A.; Wang, L.; Lee, S.-H.; Ko, S.-C.; Kang, M.C.; Jayawardena, T.U.; Jeon, Y.-J. Free radical scavenging activity of the peptide from the Alcalase hydrolysate of the edible aquacultural seahorse (*Hippocampus abdominalis*). *J. Food Biochem.* **2019**, *43*, e12833. [CrossRef] [PubMed]
15. Liu, H.; Dong, J.; Du, R.; Gao, Y.; Zhao, P. Collagen study advances for photoaging skin. *Photodermatol. Photoimmunol. Photomed.* **2024**, *40*, e12931. [CrossRef]
16. Yang, F.; Nagahawatta, D.P.; Yang, H.-W.; Ryu, B.; Lee, H.-G.; Je, J.-G.; Heo, M.-S.; Jeon, Y.-J. In vitro and in vivo immuno-enhancing effect of fucoidan isolated from non-edible brown seaweed Sargassum thunbergii. *Int. J. Biol. Macromol.* **2023**, *253*, 127212. [CrossRef]
17. Wang, L.; Jayawardena, T.U.; Hyun, J.; Wang, K.; Fu, X.; Xu, J.; Gao, X.; Park, Y.; Jeon, Y.-J. Antioxidant and anti-photoaging effects of a fucoidan isolated from Turbinaria ornata. *Int. J. Biol. Macromol.* **2023**, *225*, 1021–1027. [CrossRef]
18. Zhang, Y.; Li, Y.; Quan, Z.; Xiao, P.; Duan, J.-A. New Insights into Antioxidant Peptides: An Overview of Efficient Screening, Evaluation Models, Molecular Mechanisms, and Applications. *Antioxidants* **2024**, *13*, 303. [CrossRef]
19. Pourzand, C.; Albieri-Borges, A.; Raczek, N.N. Shedding a New Light on Skin Aging, Iron- and Redox-Homeostasis and Emerging Natural Antioxidants. *Antioxidants* **2022**, *11*, 471. [CrossRef]
20. Yang, H.; Zhang, Q.; Zhang, B.; Zhao, Y.; Wang, N. Potential Active Marine Peptides as Anti-Aging Drugs or Drug Candidates. *Mar. Drugs* **2023**, *21*, 144. [CrossRef]
21. Lu, Z.; Sun, N.; Dong, L.; Gao, Y.; Lin, S. Production of Bioactive Peptides from Sea Cucumber and Its Potential Health Benefits: A Comprehensive Review. *J. Agric. Food Chem.* **2022**, *70*, 7607–7625. [CrossRef] [PubMed]
22. Oh, Y.; Ahn, C.-B.; Je, J.-Y. Cytoprotective Role of Edible Seahorse (*Hippocampus abdominalis*)-Derived Peptides in H_2O_2-Induced Oxidative Stress in Human Umbilical Vein Endothelial Cells. *Mar. Drugs* **2021**, *19*, 86. [CrossRef] [PubMed]
23. Je, J.-G.; Kim, H.-S.; Lee, H.-G.; Oh, J.-Y.; Lu, Y.A.; Wang, L.; Rho, S.; Jeon, Y.-J. Low-molecular weight peptides isolated from seahorse (*Hippocampus abdominalis*) improve vasodilation via inhibition of angiotensin-converting enzyme in vivo and in vitro. *Process Biochem.* **2020**, *95*, 30–35. [CrossRef]
24. Kong, J.; Hu, X.-M.; Cai, W.-W.; Wang, Y.-M.; Chi, C.-F.; Wang, B. Bioactive Peptides from Skipjack Tuna Cardiac Arterial Bulbs (II): Protective Function on UVB-Irradiated HaCaT Cells through Antioxidant and Anti-Apoptotic Mechanisms. *Mar. Drugs* **2023**, *21*, 105. [CrossRef] [PubMed]
25. Zhang, C.; Lv, J.; Qin, X.; Peng, Z.; Lin, H. Novel Antioxidant Peptides from Crassostrea Hongkongensis Improve Photo-Oxidation in UV-Induced HaCaT Cells. *Mar. Drugs* **2022**, *20*, 100. [CrossRef] [PubMed]

26. Wang, L.; Lee, W.; Oh, J.Y.; Cui, Y.R.; Ryu, B.; Jeon, Y.-J. Protective Effect of Sulfated Polysaccharides from Celluclast-Assisted Extract of Hizikia fusiforme against Ultraviolet B-Induced Skin Damage by Regulating NF-κB, AP-1, and MAPKs Signaling Pathways In vitro in Human Dermal Fibroblasts. *Mar. Drugs* **2018**, *16*, 239. [CrossRef]
27. Wang, L.; Oh, J.Y.; Yang, H.-W.; Kim, H.S.; Jeon, Y.-J. Protective effect of sulfated polysaccharides from a Celluclast-assisted extract of Hizikia fusiforme against ultraviolet B-induced photoaging in vitro in human keratinocytes and in vivo in zebrafish. *Mar. Life Sci. Tech.* **2019**, *1*, 104–111. [CrossRef]
28. Lee, H.; Kim, K.; Oh, C.; Park, C.-H.; Aliya, S.; Kim, H.-S.; Bajpai, V.K.; Huh, Y.S. Antioxidant and anti-aging potential of a peptide formulation (Gal 2–Pep) conjugated with gallic acid. *RSC Adv.* **2021**, *11*, 29407–29415. [CrossRef]
29. Cao, Y.; Chen, Q.; Liu, Y.; Jin, L.; Peng, R. Research Progress on the Construction and Application of a Diabetic Zebrafish Model. *Int. J. Mol. Sci.* **2023**, *24*, 5159. [CrossRef]
30. Shimizu, N.; Shiraishi, H.; Hanada, T. Zebrafish as a Useful Model System for Human Liver Disease. *Cells* **2023**, *12*, 2246. [CrossRef]
31. Tanveer, M.A.; Rashid, H.; Nazir, L.A.; Archoo, S.; Shahid, N.H.; Ragni, G.; Umar, S.A.; Tasduq, S.A. Trigonelline, a plant derived alkaloid prevents ultraviolet-B-induced oxidative DNA damage in primary human dermal fibroblasts and BALB/c mice via modulation of phosphoinositide 3-kinase-Akt-Nrf2 signalling axis. *Exp. Gerontol.* **2023**, *171*, 112028. [CrossRef] [PubMed]
32. Santhakumaran, I.; Shanuja, S.K.; Narayanaswamy, R.; Gnanamani, A. Asperyellone prevents HDF cells from UVB irradiation damages: An elaborated study. *J. Cell. Biochem.* **2019**, *120*, 7560–7572. [CrossRef] [PubMed]
33. Wang, L.; Jayawardena, T.U.; Wang, K.; Ahn, G.; Cha, S.-H.; Jeon, Y.-J. Protective effect of the brown seaweed Padina boryana against UVB-induced photoaging in vitro in skin cells and in vivo in zebrafish. *Algal Res.* **2023**, *76*, 103316. [CrossRef]
34. Wang, L.; Kim, H.S.; Oh, J.Y.; Je, J.G.; Jeon, Y.-J.; Ryu, B. Protective effect of diphlorethohydroxycarmalol isolated from Ishige okamurae against UVB-induced damage in vitro in human dermal fibroblasts and in vivo in zebrafish. *Food Chem. Toxicol.* **2020**, *136*, 110963. [CrossRef]

marine drugs

MDPI

Article

Blue Mussel-Derived Bioactive Peptides PIISVYWK (P1) and FSVVPSPK (P2): Promising Agents for Inhibiting Foam Cell Formation and Inflammation in Cardiovascular Diseases

Chathuri Kaushalya Marasinghe [1] and Jae-Young Je [2,*]

[1] Department of Food and Nutrition, Pukyong National University, Busan 48513, Republic of Korea; chathurimarasinghe9313@gmail.com

[2] Major of Human Bioconvergence, Division of Smart Healthcare, Pukyong National University, Busan 48513, Republic of Korea

* Correspondence: jjy1915@pknu.ac.kr; Tel.: +82-51-629-4633

Abstract: Atherosclerosis is a key etiological event in the development of cardiovascular diseases (CVDs), strongly linked to the formation of foam cells. This study explored the effects of two blue mussel-derived bioactive peptides (BAPs), PIISVYWK (P1) and FSVVPSPK (P2), on inhibiting foam cell formation and mitigating inflammation in oxLDL-treated RAW264.7 macrophages. Both peptides significantly suppressed intracellular lipid accumulation and cholesterol levels while promoting cholesterol efflux by downregulating cluster of differentiation 36 (CD36) and class A1 scavenger receptors (SR-A1) and upregulating ATP binding cassette subfamily A member 1 (ABCA-1) and ATP binding cassette subfamily G member 1 (ABCG-1) expressions. The increased expression of peroxisome proliferator-activated receptor-gamma (PPAR-γ) and liver X receptor-alpha (LXR-α) further validated their role in enhancing cholesterol efflux. Additionally, P1 and P2 inhibited foam cell formation in oxLDL-treated human aortic smooth muscle cells and exerted anti-inflammatory effects by reducing pro-inflammatory cytokines, nitric oxide (NO), prostaglandin E_2 (PGE_2), inducible nitric oxide synthase (iNOS), and cyclooxygenase-2 (COX-2), primarily through inhibiting NF-κB activation. Furthermore, P1 and P2 alleviated oxidative stress by activating the Nrf2/HO-1 pathway. Our findings demonstrate that P1 and P2 have significant potential in reducing foam cell formation and inflammation, both critical factors in atherosclerosis development. These peptides may serve as promising therapeutic agents for the prevention and treatment of CVDs associated with oxidative stress and inflammation.

Keywords: blue mussel; bioactive peptides; RAW264.7 macrophages; atherosclerosis; inflammation; cholesterol flux; oxidative stress

1. Introduction

Atherosclerosis, a significant vascular pathology, has emerged as a leading cause of mortality in both Korea and Western countries [1], serving as a crucial etiological event in cardiovascular diseases (CVDs), encompassing myocardial infarction, ischemic diseases, strokes, and peripheral arterial disease [2]. The global burden of CVDs is substantial, with over 19 million reported deaths in 2019, and expected to rise to 25 million by 2030 [3]. Foam cells, a key pathological component which contribute significantly to the progression of atherosclerosis, are commonly found within atherosclerotic plaque as pathogenic cells [4]. Under normal conditions, intraplaque macrophages maintain a balanced cellular microenvironment through lipid metabolism, immune regulation and modulation, and efferocytosis. However, the recruitment of monocytes into the vascular intima and their exposure to the modified lipoproteins contribute to the formation of lipid-laden macrophage foam cells in the context of atherosclerosis [5]. These foam cells not only trigger the initial stages of atherosclerosis but also play a pivotal role in the progression of advanced plaque rupture [6].

The aggregation of altered low-density lipoproteins (LDL), particularly oxidized LDL (oxLDL), and the subsequent disruption of cholesterol metabolism are crucial factors in the ongoing presence of lipid-filled foam cells [7]. Under normal physiological circumstances, scavenger receptors facilitate lipid uptake via cholesterol influx process, while ABC transporters mediate cholesterol efflux to release excess lipid [8]. However, oxLDL disrupts these cholesterol flux processes, leading to an exacerbation of foam cell formation and its associated complications [8]. Furthermore, inflammation emerges as a fundamental contributor to the pathogenesis of atherosclerosis. Inflammatory responses are intricately involved in all stages of atherosclerosis, with oxLDL playing a major role in triggering inflammation by stimulating the generation of inflammatory factors [9]. The interplay between foam cell formation and inflammation amplifies the complexities of atherosclerosis.

Investigating natural agents with potential anti-inflammatory properties to mitigate foam cell formation presents an attractive strategy for prevention of atherosclerosis. Marine-derived organisms have garnered attention due to their perceived health benefits in preventing several chronic diseases [10]. These organisms boast a diverse array of active compounds, comprising proteins, carbohydrates, lipids, and polyphenols [11]. Of particular interest, proteins have the capacity to produce bioactive peptides (BAPs) with certain biological activities, including antioxidant, anticancer, anti-obesity, and anti-diabetes effects [12,13]. Recent studies have highlighted various BAPs with significant health benefits, particularly in the context of CVDs. For instance, BAPs derived from collagen hydrolysate of *Salmo salar* skin have been shown to reduce blood pressure and lipids [14], while pentapeptides VIAPW and IRWWW from *Miichthys miiuy* muscle exhibit hypolipidemic activities [15]. Similarly, antioxidant peptides from *Eucheuma cottonii*, a marine red alga [16], demonstrate promising cardiovascular benefits. Furthermore, antihypertensive peptides from Antarctic krill protein hydrolysates offer additional therapeutic potential [17]. The cumulative evidence suggests that these BAPs not only contribute to lowering blood pressure and lipids but also possess antioxidant and anti-inflammatory properties, making them valuable in managing heart disease and atherosclerosis.

Blue mussel (*Mytilus edulis*), a marine bivalve, is recognized as a substantial source of proteins, constituting approximately 64.5% of dry matter, along with a rich profile of amino acids [18]. Several studies, including our own, have highlighted antioxidant, hepatoprotective, anti-inflammatory, and anti-osteoporotic activities exhibited by active substances derived from blue mussel hydrolysates and isolated peptides [19–23]. Additionally, seventeen novel angiotensin-converting enzyme (ACE) inhibitory peptides have been identified from the protein hydrolysate of *Mytilus edulis*. These peptides demonstrate potential therapeutic value in the treatment of high blood pressure, atherosclerosis, and heart disease [24]. Moreover, in a preliminary investigation, blue mussel-derived hydrolysate demonstrated a promising inhibitory effect on foam cell formation [25]. Building upon these findings and acknowledging the multifunctional biological activities of BAPs [26], including our own findings related to osteogenesis effects, antioxidant properties, and anti-apoptosis effects of blue mussel-derived peptides, PIISVYWK (P1) and FSVVPSPK (P2), the present study delves into the foam cell formation inhibitory effects of these two peptides (P1 and P2) in oxLDL-treated RAW264.7 macrophages. Furthermore, the study scrutinizes the anti-inflammatory and anti-oxidative stress properties of these two peptides in oxLDL-treated RAW264.7 macrophages.

2. Results

2.1. Effects of P1 and P2 Peptides on Cell Viability and on oxLDL-Induced Macrophage Foam Cell Formation

The chemical structures of P1 and P2 peptides are depicted in Figure 1. Prior to investigating the inhibitory effects of P1 and P2 peptides on foam cell formation, the cytotoxicity of P1 and P2 peptides was measured in RAW264.7 macrophages. As illustrated in Figure 2A, there were no discernible cytotoxic effects at the concentrations tested (10~200 μM). To validate foam cell formation inhibitory activity, Oil Red O (ORO) staining assay was performed. Both P1 and P2 peptides demonstrated a dose-dependent inhibitory effect on macrophage foam cell formation induced by oxLDL exposure. Interestingly, P1 and P2 peptides showed similar intracellular lipid accumulation inhibition rates of approximately 74.0 ± 4.3% and 75.1 ± 5.2%, respectively, at 200 μM treatment (Figure 2B). Representative images further verify the inhibitory effect of P1 and P2 peptides (Figure 2C).

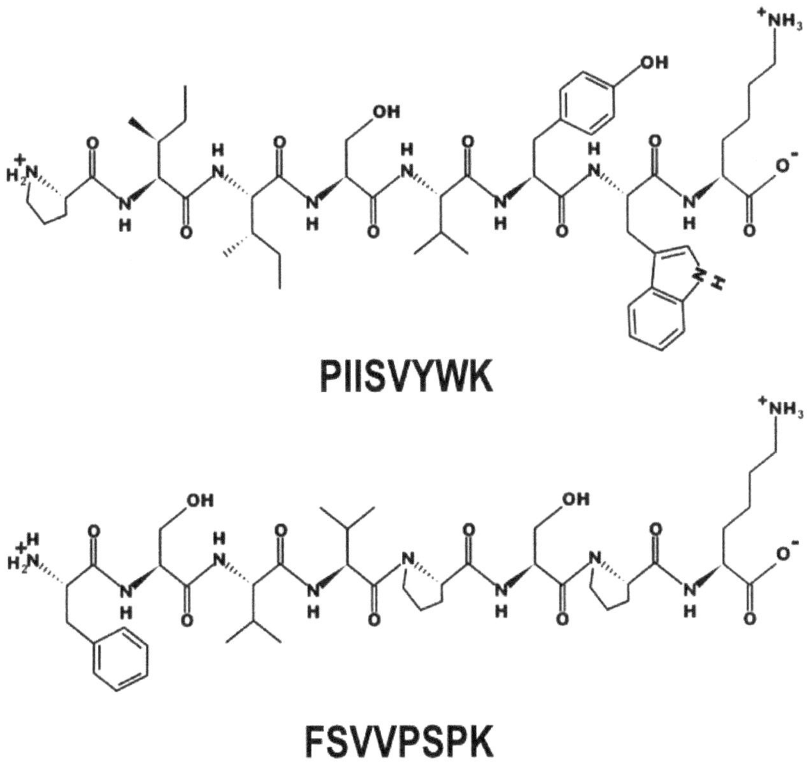

Figure 1. Chemical structures of PIISVYWK (P1) and FSVVPSPK (P2).

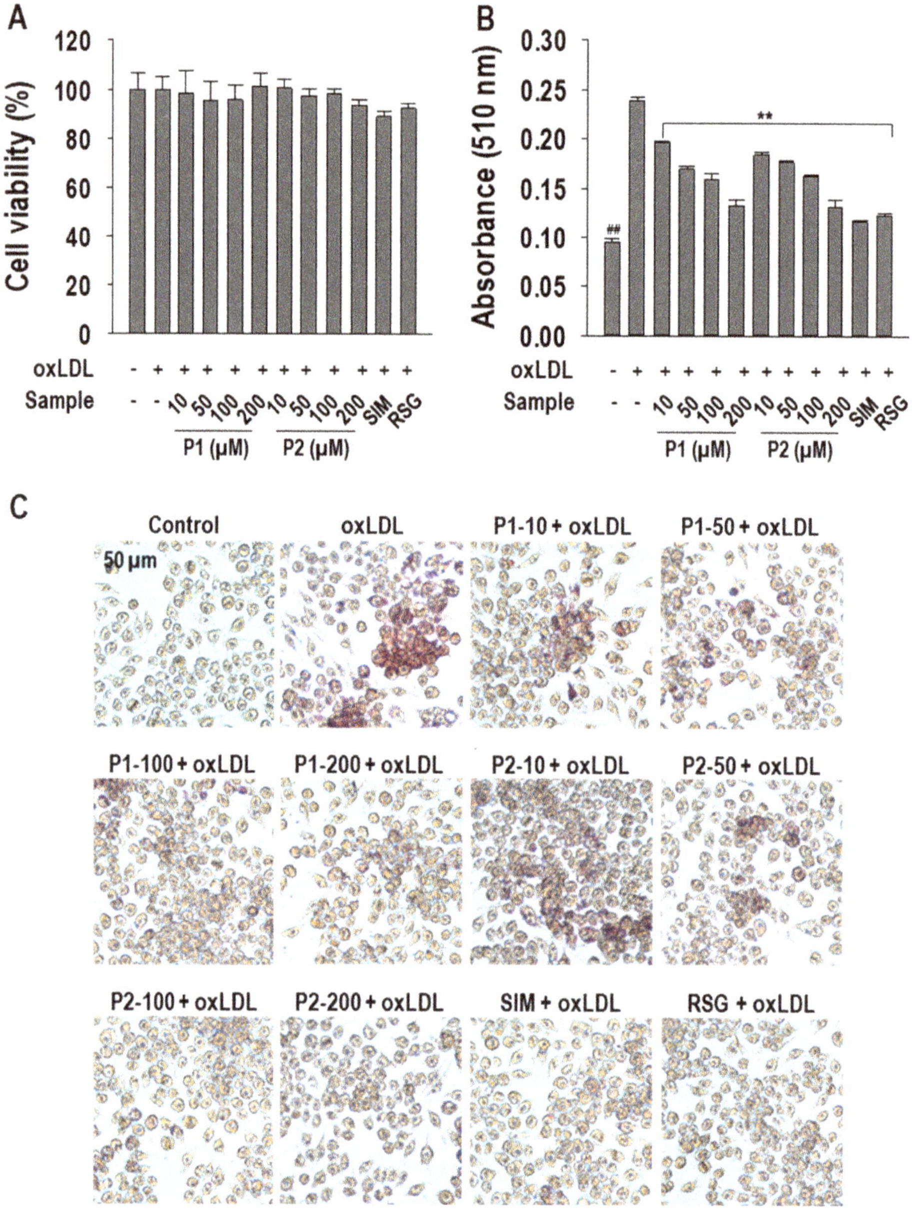

Figure 2. (**A**) Cell viability, (**B**) inhibition of intracellular lipid accumulation quantitatively, and (**C**) qualitatively (40× magnification) of PIISVYWK (P1) and FSVVPSPK (P2) peptides in oxLDL-treated RAW264.7 macrophages. The macrophages were treated with P1 and P2 peptides or positive controls (10 μM) including simvastatin (SIM) or rosiglitazone (RSG) or oxLDL (50 μg/mL) for MTT assay. For ORO staining, macrophages were treated with P1 and P2 peptides or positive controls (10 μM) including SIM or RSG for 1 h followed by oxLDL treatment for another 24 h. Experiments consisted of three independent measurements (n = 3) with ± S.D. ** $p < 0.001$ and ## $p < 0.001$, compared to the oxLDL-treated group and non-treated group, respectively. The numbers behind letters in images denote concentrations in μM.

2.2. Effects of P1 and P2 Peptides on Total Cholesterol (TC), Free Cholesterol (FC), and Cholesterol Esters (CE), and Triglyceride (TG) Levels in oxLDL-Treated Macrophages

The effects of P1 and P2 peptides on changes in TC, FC, and CE levels were analyzed in oxLDL-treated RAW264.7 macrophages. As shown in Figure 3A~D, both P1 and P2 peptides exhibited a dose-dependent suppression of TC, FC, and CE levels. However, at a concentration of 200 μM, P2 displayed a more suppressive effect on TC and FC levels compared to P1 by fully suppressing cholesterol levels. P1 treatment attenuated TC and FC by 70.7 ± 1.0% and 58.3 ± 0.8%, respectively. Additionally, both P1 and P2 peptides fully inhibited CE levels at all the tested concentrations. Moreover, P1 and P2 peptides significantly ($p < 0.05$) ameliorated TG level compared to oxLDL-treated macrophages.

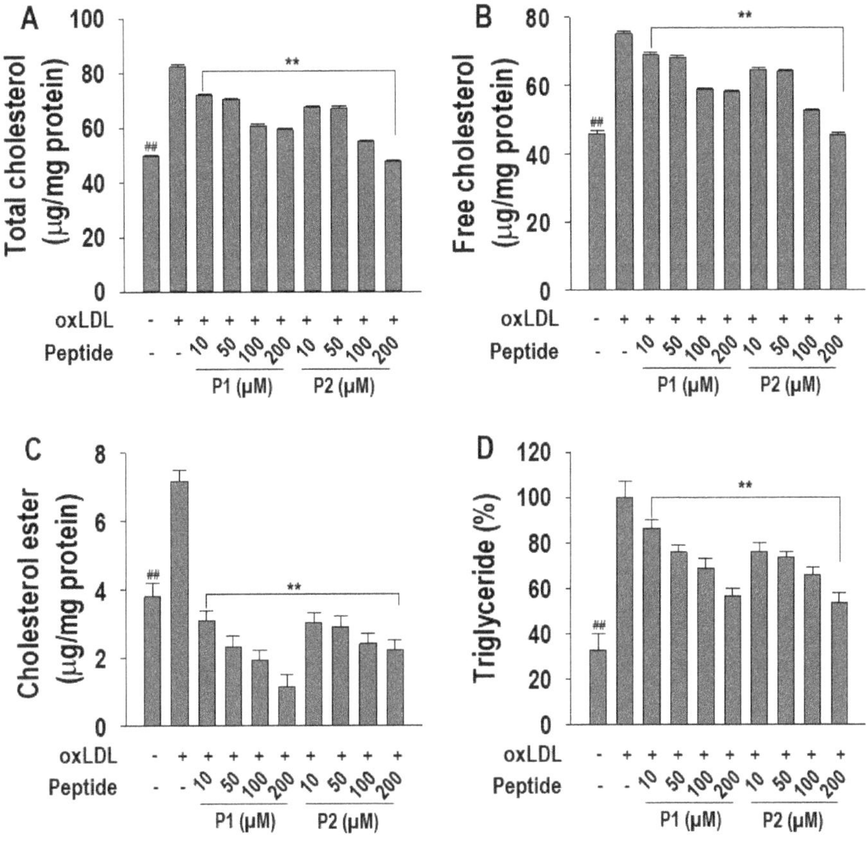

Figure 3. Effect of 10~200 μM of P1 and P2 peptides on (**A**) total cholesterol, (**B**) free cholesterol, (**C**) cholesterol ester, and (**D**) triglycerides content in oxLDL-treated RAW264.7 macrophages. The macrophages were treated with P1 and P2 peptides for 1 h followed by oxLDL treatment for 24 h. Experiments consisted of three independent measurements ($n = 3$) with ± S.D. ** $p < 0.001$ and ## $p < 0.001$, compared to the oxLDL-treated group and non-treated group, respectively.

2.3. Effects of P1 and P2 Peptides on Cellular Cholesterol Flux

To elucidate how P1 and P2 peptides affect cellular cholesterol flux, various parameters including cholesterol influx, cholesterol efflux, expression of relevant proteins, and transcription factor were examined. Since 10, 50, 100, and 200 μM of concentrations showed significant effect on above experiments, for subsequent studies, we have selected 10 μM as the lowest concentration and 200 μM as the highest concentration to further investigate the effects of these peptides. A significant increase ($p < 0.05$) in cholesterol influx rate was observed in oxLDL-treated macrophages. However, P1 and P2 peptides significantly ($p < 0.05$) reduced the rate of cholesterol influx compared to the cells with oxLDL alone. Notably, their inhibition rates were 42.2 ± 1.1% and 43.6 ± 2.2% for P1 and P2 peptides, respectively, at 200 μM treatment (Figure 4A). Simvastatin, a positive control, was shown to inhibit cholesterol influx by 61.0 ± 1.0%. Conversely, the rate of cholesterol efflux by P1 and P2 peptides significantly ($p < 0.05$) increased in a dose-dependent manner (Figure 4B). Cholesterol efflux rate was increased more than 3-fold when treated with 200 μM of P1 and P2 peptides compared to the macrophages without treatment. However, there is no change in cholesterol efflux rate in oxLDL-treated macrophages. Rosiglitazone, a positive control, showed a marked increase in cholesterol efflux rate.

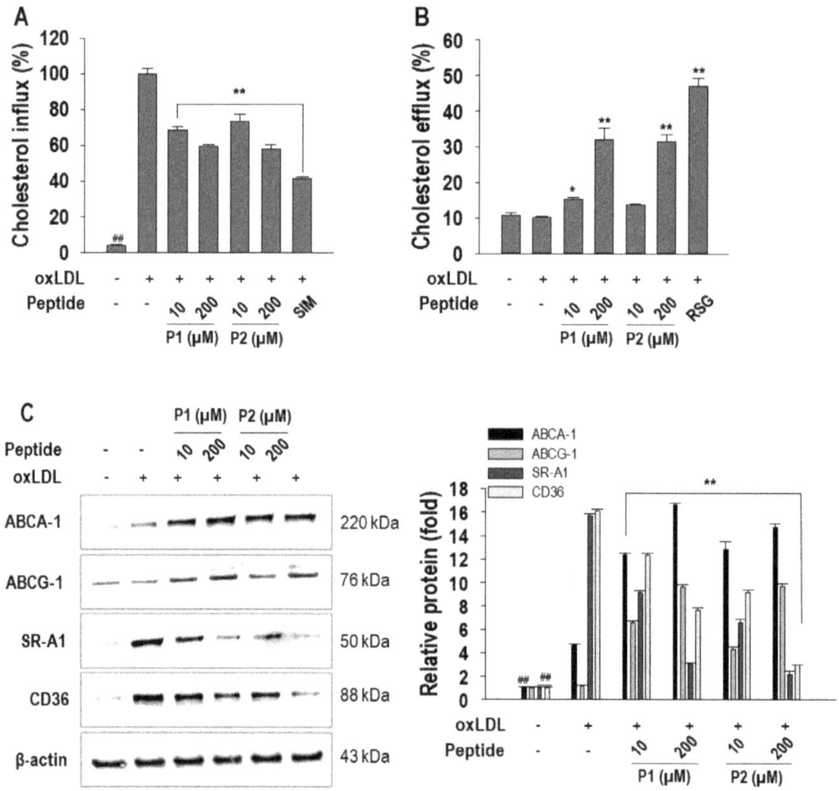

Figure 4. Effect of 10~200 μM of P1 and P2 peptides on (**A**) cholesterol influx, (**B**) cholesterol efflux, (**C**) ABCA-1, ABCG-1, SR-A1, and CD36 protein expressions in oxLDL-treated RAW264.7 macrophages. The macrophages were treated with P1 and P2 peptides for 1 h followed by oxLDL treatment for 24 h. Experiments consisted of three independent measurements ($n = 3$) with ± S.D. ** $p < 0.001$ and ## $p < 0.001$, compared to the oxLDL-treated group and non-treated group, respectively. * $p < 0.05$ compared to the oxLDL-treated group.

To further validate the role of P1 and P2 peptides in cholesterol flux, protein expressions associated with cholesterol influx and efflux were investigated. As shown in Figure 4C, the protein expression of ABCA-1 and ABCG-1, integral to cholesterol efflux, was elevated by P1 and P2 peptides. On the contrary, the levels of SR-A1 and CD36, which are associated with cholesterol influx, were dose-dependently suppressed by P1 and P2 peptides. In addition, the effects of P1 and P2 peptides on PPAR-γ and LXR-α protein expression, which are associated with cholesterol metabolism and flux, were investigated. Both P1 and P2 peptides significantly enhanced the expression of PPAR-γ and LXR-α. At a concentration of 200 μM, P1 treatment resulted in a 4.8 ± 0.1-fold increase in PPAR-γ expression and 2.9 ± 0.1-fold increase in LXR-α expression. Similarly, P2 treatment exhibited an increase in these transcription factor expressions, with 4.1 ± 0.1-fold enhancement in PPAR-γ expression and 1.6 ± 0.1-fold of enhancement of LXR-α expression at 200 μM concentration (Figure 5A).

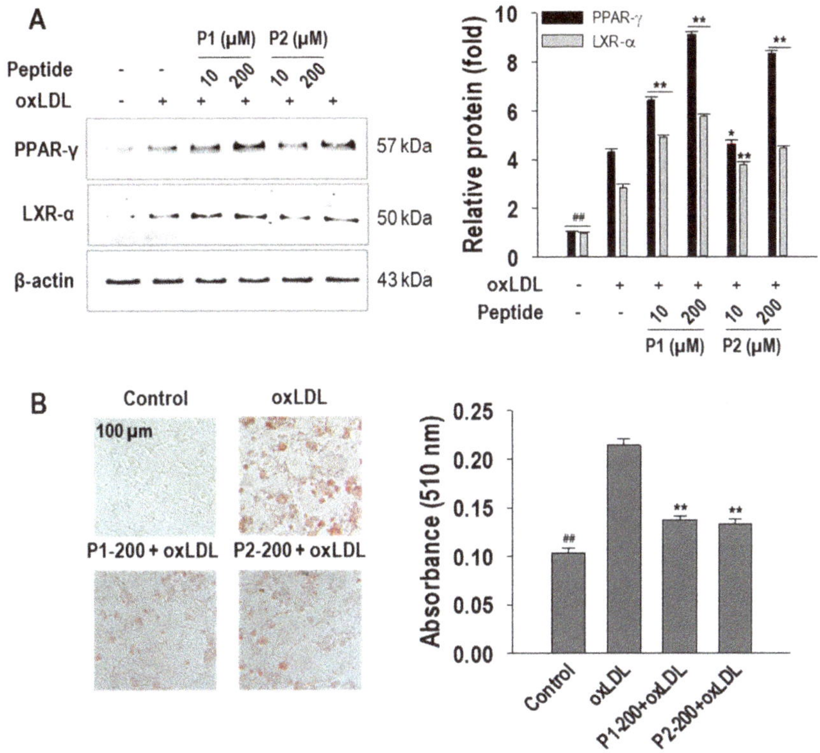

Figure 5. Effect of 10~200 μM of P1 and P2 peptides on (**A**) PPAR-γ and LXR-α protein expressions in oxLDL-treated RAW264.7 macrophages and (**B**) foam cell formation inhibition in hASMCs. The macrophages and hASMCs were treated with P1 and P2 peptides for 1 h followed by oxLDL treatment for 24 h. Relevant images are taken at 20× magnification. Experiments consisted of three independent measurements (n = 3) with ± S.D. ** $p < 0.001$ and ## $p < 0.001$, compared to the oxLDL-treated group and non-treated group, respectively. * $p < 0.05$ compared to the oxLDL-treated group. In images, numbers behind letters represent concentrations in μM.

Furthermore, this study extended its investigation into the foam cell formation inhibitory activities of P1 and P2 peptides using human models, especially human aortic smooth muscle cells (hASMCs). As depicted in Figure 5B, oxLDL induced a progressive increase in intracellular lipid accumulation in hASMCs. However, consistent with expectations, both P1 and P2 peptides effectively inhibited this lipid accumulation, achieving inhibition rates of approximately 69.1 ± 3.9% and 72.5 ± 4.3%, respectively. These findings underscore the potential of P1 and P2 peptides in mitigating foam cell formation not only in murine cells but also in human cells.

2.4. Effect of P1 and P2 Peptides on oxLDL-Induced Inflammation

Given the association of atherosclerosis with inflammatory responses, this study delved into the anti-inflammatory effect of P1 and P2 peptides. Pro-inflammatory cytokine levels, including TNF-α, IL-6, and IL-1β, were assessed following treatment with P1 and P2 peptides. OxLDL treatment induced higher production of these three pro-inflammatory cytokines, and both P1 and P2 peptides significantly ($p < 0.05$) suppressed their levels (Figure 6A~C). Especially, at a concentration of 200 μM, P1 treatment inhibited TNF-α, IL-6, and IL-1β levels by 86.1 ± 0.8%, 87.9 ± 5.0%, and 78.2 ± 3.2%, respectively. Similarly, P2 treatment exhibited inhibition levels of 90.3 ± 0.7%, 87.9 ± 6.6%, and 83.1 ± 4.5% for TNF-α, IL-6, and IL-1β, respectively.

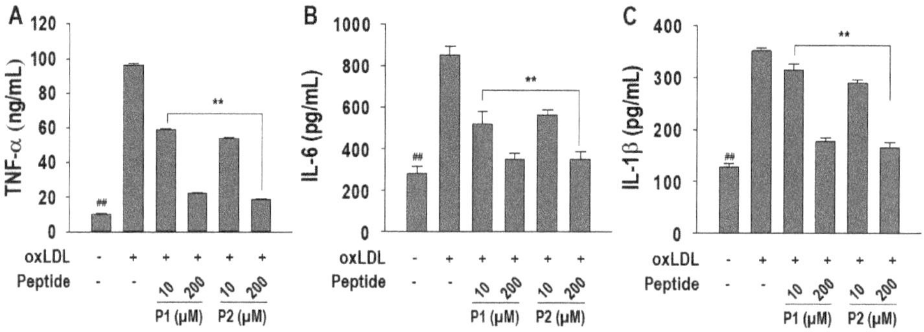

Figure 6. Effect of P1 and P2 peptides on pro-inflammatory cytokine production (**A**) TNF-α, (**B**) IL-6, and (**C**) IL-1β in oxLDL-treated RAW264.7 macrophages. The macrophages were treated with P1 and P2 peptides for 1 h followed by oxLDL treatment for 24 h. Experiments consisted of three independent measurements ($n = 3$) with ± S.D. ** $p < 0.001$ and ## $p < 0.001$, compared to the oxLDL-treated group and non-treated group, respectively.

Moreover, NO and PGE_2 levels, which are elevated in atherosclerosis and contribute to pro-inflammatory processes, were measured in culture media after treatment with P1 and P2 peptides. Both peptides significantly ($p < 0.05$) suppressed oxLDL-induced NO and PGE_2 levels. At a concentration of 200 μM, P1 and P2 peptides suppressed NO levels by 55.5 ± 7.2% and 64.5 ± 11.0%, respectively (Figure 7A). Additionally, P1 and P2 peptides decreased PGE_2 levels by 29.8 ± 2.0% and 36.4 ± 3.3%, respectively (Figure 7B). This study further investigated iNOS and COX-2 expression, which are linked to the production of NO and PGE_2. As shown in Figure 7C, both peptides exhibited a dose-dependent suppressive effect on iNOS and COX-2 expressions. In addition, further analysis revealed that both peptides increased HO-1 expression. Finally, the effects of P1 and P2 peptides on the nuclear translocation of NF-κB and Nrf2, transcription factors for iNOS and COX-2 and HO-1, were investigated. As shown in Figure 7D, immunostaining results demonstrated that macrophages treated with oxLDL alone exhibited strong fluorescence intensity for NF-κB in the cytoplasmic and the nuclear regions, indicating inflammatory response. However, the fluorescence intensity w P1 and P2 peptides was dramatically reduced in both cytoplasmic and nuclear regions, indicating anti-inflammatory action. In addition, Nrf2 translocation was not observed in macrophages treated with oxLDL alone. However, P1 and P2 peptide-treated macrophages exhibited strong fluorescence intensity, indicating Nrf2 translocation (Figure 7E).

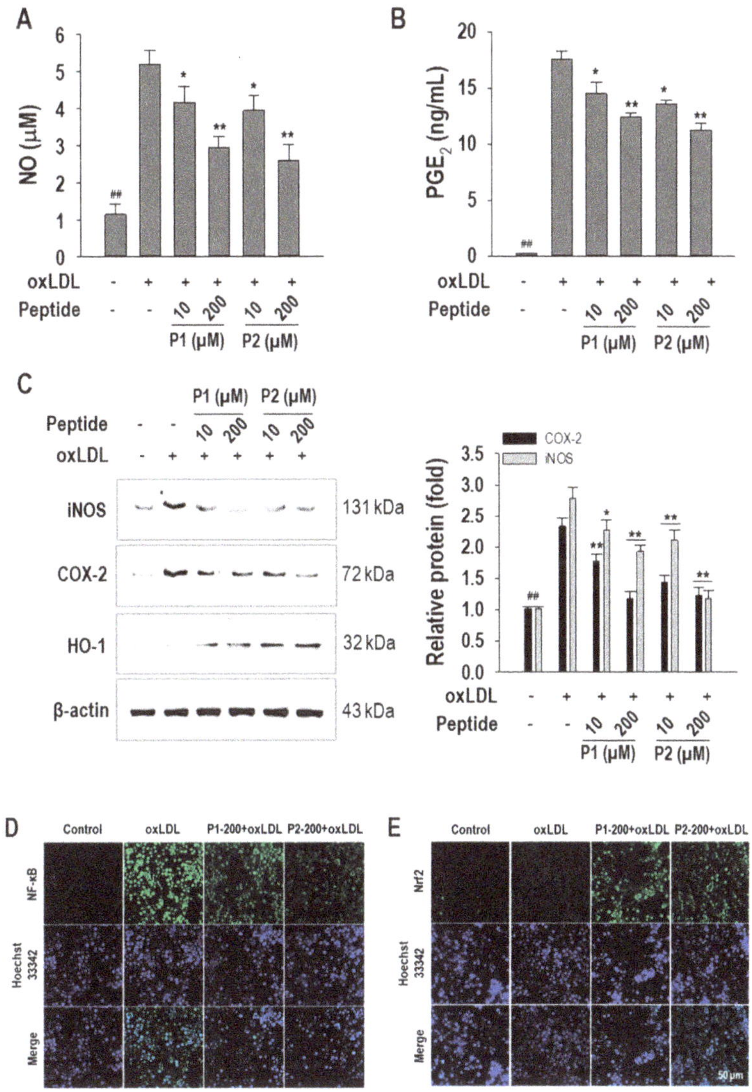

Figure 7. Effect of P1 and P2 peptides on (**A**) NO production, (**B**) PGE_2 production, (**C**) iNOS, COX-2, and HO-1 protein expression in oxLDL-treated RAW264.7 macrophages. The macrophages were treated with P1 and P2 peptides for 1 h followed by oxLDL treatment for 24 h. Experiments consisted of three independent measurements ($n = 3$) with ± S.D. ** $p < 0.001$ and ## $p < 0.001$, compared to the oxLDL-treated group and non-treated group, respectively. * $p < 0.05$ compared to the oxLDL-treated group. (**D**) NF-κB nuclear activation and (**E**) Nrf2 nuclear translocation in oxLDL-treated RAW264.7 macrophages. The macrophages were treated with peptides for 1 h followed by oxLDL (50 μg/mL) treatment for 2 h for NF-κB and Nrf2 immunostaining. The numbers behind letters in images denote concentrations in μM.

3. Discussion

Scientific evidence consistently shows that BAPs from marine sources have various biological activities, including antioxidant, anti-inflammatory, anti-cancer, and anti-diabetic properties, due to their unique environmental origins [13,27]. Despite this wealth of evidence, there is still a significant gap in research on the effects of marine BAPs in inhibiting macrophage foam cell formation and their potential athero-protective benefits. In a recent contribution to this developing field, our research team recently identified the foam cell formation inhibitory and anti-inflammatory activities of blue mussel hydrolysate in oxLDL-treated RAW264.7 macrophages [25]. Building on previous research that highlighted the anti-apoptotic, antioxidant, and anti-osteoporotic effects of blue mussel-derived P1 and P2 peptides [28–30], this study explores their novel role in inhibiting foam cell formation and their anti-inflammatory and anti-oxidative stress activities in oxLDL-treated RAW264.7 macrophages. The aim is to further understand the potential therapeutic benefits of these marine-derived peptides for atherosclerosis and related metabolic diseases.

Foam cell formation is recognized as a pivotal step in the pathogenesis of atherosclerosis, driven by excessive oxLDL, which leads macrophages to become foam cells [6]. Even in the early stages of atherosclerosis, many macrophages engulf oxLDL and adopt a foam cell phenotype. The vascular accumulation of these foam cells leads to arterial narrowing, further promoting the advancement of atherosclerosis [31]. Consequently, inhibiting foam cell formation is vital for combating the disease. Several studies, including our own, have reported anti-atherosclerotic effects achieved through the inhibition of foam cell formation [32–34]. Thus, as the primary focus in this study, we investigated the effect of P1 and P2 peptides on inhibiting foam cell formation in oxLDL-treated RAW264.7 macrophages. Consistent with our previous findings with blue mussel hydrolysates [25], the blue mussel-derived P1 and P2 peptides exhibited foam cell formation inhibitory activities, thereby indicating their anti-atherosclerotic effects.

Statin drugs, including atorvastatin, rosuvastatin, simvastatin, pravastatin, fluvastatin, lovastatin, and pitavastatin, are commonly used to lower cholesterol and treat CVDs. However, finding an accurate positive control for assessing foam cell formation inhibition has been difficult. In this study, simvastatin and rosiglitazone were chosen as positive controls, based on evidence from previous research [35–37]. Notably, peptides P1 and P2 demonstrated approximately equivalent levels of intracellular cholesterol inhibition compared to simvastatin and rosiglitazone, highlighting their potential in inhibiting foam cell formation.

Scavenger receptors, such as SR-A1 and CD36, are integral in the internalization of oxLDL by macrophages, leading to cellular cholesterol accumulation. Once oxLDL is internalized, oxLDL is broken down by liposomal acid lipase into free fatty acids and cholesterol [38]. To maintain cellular homeostasis, excess cholesterol is removed via ATP-binding cassettes transporters as ABCA-1 and ABCG-1 in macrophages, facilitating cholesterol efflux to Apo-A1 and HDL, respectively [8]. However, disruption in this process, with excessive cholesterol uptake and impaired efflux, causes abnormal cholesterol trafficking and foam cell formation. Research indicates that reducing cholesterol influx, while increasing cholesterol efflux, helps inhibit foam cell formation [39–41]. Building upon these insights, our study assessed the effects of P1 and P2 peptides on these mechanisms and found that they increased cholesterol efflux, decreased cholesterol influx, and reduced TC, FC, and CE in cells. However, the decrease in cholesterol influx and the increase in cholesterol efflux are relatively lower compared to the respective positive controls. Additionally, TG, TG-rich lipoproteins (TRL), and TRL remnants are recognized risk factors for cardiovascular diseases (CVDs) [42,43]. Interestingly, peptides P1 and P2 also inhibited TG levels, suggesting that they may contribute to the regulation of both cholesterol and lipid homeostasis.

In light of the higher rates of cholesterol efflux observed with P1 and P2 peptides compared to cholesterol influx, this study further extended to elucidating the molecular mechanism underlying cholesterol efflux. Building on previous findings where ark shell-derived peptides inhibited foam cell formation via the PPAR-γ/LXR-α signaling pathway [44], we focused on the activation of these transcription factors by P1 and P2 peptides. PPAR-γ, a nuclear receptor that forms heterodimers with Retinoid X receptor, regulates lipid metabolism genes and is a known therapeutic target for lipid disorders [45]. Similarly, LXR-α has been identified as a potential treatment for atherosclerosis [46]. However, PPAR-γ has a dual role in cholesterol metabolism: it can increase cholesterol influx by promoting CD36 expression and simultaneously enhance cholesterol efflux by upregulating ABC transporters. Despite this paradox, PPAR-γ generally reduces foam cell formation by promoting cholesterol efflux [47]. Our study found that P1 and P2 peptides increased the protein expression of both PPAR-γ and LXR-α, indicating their role in regulating lipid metabolism. Further extending our research to hASMCs, which are prominent in atherosclerotic lesions, we observed that P1 and P2 peptides reduced oxLDL-induced lipid accumulation. These results highlight the anti-atherogenic potential of P1 and P2 peptides in both murine and human cells by inhibiting cholesterol accumulation and foam cell formation.

Foam cells are linked with chronic inflammation observed in certain metabolic and autoimmune disorders. The formation of foam cells establishes a connection with inflammatory processes [48]. In particular, oxLDL induces a pro-inflammatory phenotype in macrophages, contributing to atherosclerosis [49]. Given the recognized correlation between foam cell formation and inflammation in atherosclerosis, this study aimed to clarify the role of P1 and P2 peptides in inflammatory responses. Studies have reported that oxLDL internalization leads to elevated levels of pro-inflammatory cytokines and inflammatory molecules [50]. In line with these findings, our study found that oxLDL treatment increased inflammatory responses. However, P1 and P2 peptides significantly reduced oxLDL-induced pro-inflammatory cytokines, NO, and PGE_2 production, demonstrating their anti-inflammatory effects. Additionally, the peptides inhibited the expression of iNOS and COX-2, which are responsible for producing NO and PGE_2, respectively.

Based on these findings, this study explored the molecular mechanisms of P1 and P2 peptides in anti-inflammation, focusing on the NF-κB pathway, which plays a key role in atherosclerosis and inflammation. Normally, NF-κB is kept inactive in the cytoplasm by binding to IκB proteins. However, inflammatory stimuli trigger the degradation of IKBα, allowing NF-κB to move to the nucleus and promote pro-inflammatory cytokines and proteins such as iNOS and COX-2 [51]. Inhibiting NF-κB signaling has been shown to reduce foam cell formation and inflammation [52]. This study found that P1 and P2 peptides inhibit NF-κB signaling in oxLDL-treated macrophages, potentially reducing inflammation and foam cell formation. Additionally, since P1 and P2 peptides increase HO-1 expression, we also examined their effect on Nrf2 activation. Nrf2, which is normally bound to Keap1 in the cytoplasm, dissociates and moves to the nucleus under oxidative stress, where it activates genes like HO-1 that have antioxidant and anti-inflammatory roles [53]. Our results showed that P1 and P2 peptides enhance Nrf2 nuclear translocation, suggesting their potential in modulating oxidative stress and inflammation in atherosclerosis. (Figure 8).

The biological activities of peptides are intricately associated with their amino acid compositions. Certain amino acids including glutamic acid, leucine, glycine, proline, lysine, and arginine have been recognized for their antiatherogenic properties [54–56]. P1 and P2 peptides, which share these amino acids, likely benefit from these compositions, contributing to their observed anti-atherosclerotic and anti-inflammatory activities.

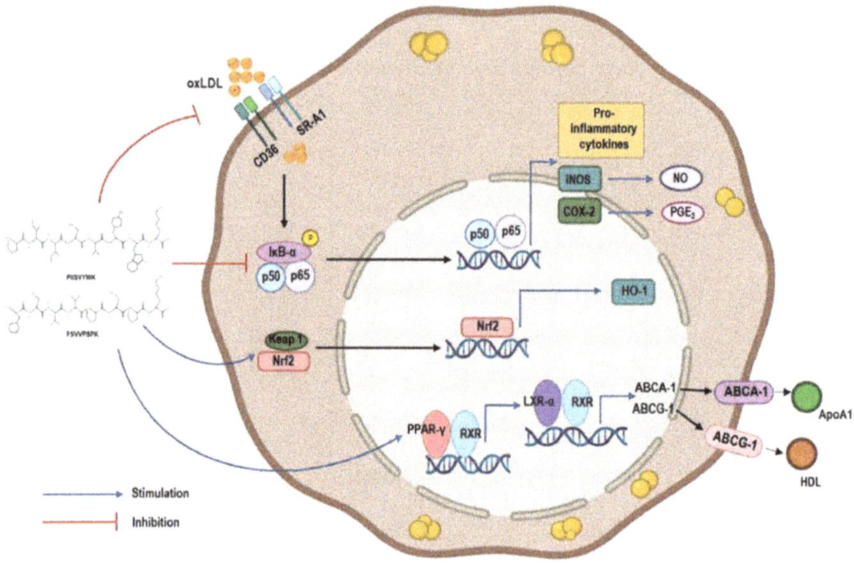

Figure 8. Schematic diagram for proposed mechanism.

4. Materials and Methods

4.1. Materials

PIISVYWK (P1) and FSVVPSPK (P2) peptides were chemically synthesized by Peptron Inc. (Dae-jeon, Korea) based on the sequences identified in our previous study [16]. The synthesized peptides were confirmed to have >95% purity, with molecular weights of 1005.2 for P1 and 860.05 for P2, respectively. Human plasma LDL was purchased from LEE BioSolutions (360-10, Lee BioSolution, Maryland Heights, MO, USA). Gibco BRL (Grand Island, NY, USA) provided all cell culture reagents. Primary and secondary antibodies were obtained from Santa Cruz Biotechnology Inc. (Santa Cruz, CA, USA), NovusBio ®, Colorada, USA, and Abcam (Dawinbio Inc, Seoul, Korea). All other reagents employed in this study were obtained from Sigma-Aldrich (St. Louis, MO, USA).

4.2. Oxidation of LDL and Determination of Thiobarbituric Acid-Reactive Substances (TBARS)

To induce oxidation, LDL (1 mg/mL) was oxidized with $CuSO_4$ (10 μM) for 4 h at 37 °C, and the extent of oxidation was assessed by conducting TBARS assay according to our previous study [25]. In brief, the resulting oxLDL was mixed with TCA (25% *w*/*v*) and TBA (1% *w*/*v* in 0.3% NaOH) in equal parts, then boiled at 92 °C for 40 min in the dark. The absorbance was measured at 532 nm with a microplate reader (Multiskan™ GO, Thermo Fisher Scientific, Rockford, IL, USA). The degree of LDL modification was quantified using a standard curve of malondialdehyde (MDA), expressed as nanomoles of MDA per milligram of LDL protein. For the experiments, TBARS values ranging from 165 to 200 nM/MDA were utilized.

4.3. Cell Culture and Treatment

RAW264.7 macrophages (American Type Culture Collection, ATCC, Manassas, VA, USA) were cultured in a DMEM culture medium under standard conditions. Cell densities of 1×10^5 or 1×10^6 cells/mL were utilized for 96-well plates or 6 cm culture dishes, respectively. Primary human aorta vascular smooth muscle cells (HASMC) were procured from ScienCell Research Laboratories (Carlsbad, CA, USA) and cultured in smooth muscle cell medium (SMCM, 1101, ScienCell Research Laboratories) under standard conditions.

Macrophages or hASMCs were treated with P1 or P2 for 1 h followed by exposure to oxLDL for an additional 24 h.

4.4. MTT Assay

Cytotoxicity of P1 and P2 in RAW264.7 macrophages and HASMC was evaluated using MTT assay according to our previous study [25]. In brief, cells were treated with P1 and P2 (10~200 μM) for 24 h, followed by a 4 h incubation with MTT working reagent. Once the formazan crystals formed, DMSO was added to dissolve them and the absorbance was measured at 570 nm using a microplate reader (Multiskan™ GO, Thermo Scientific™, Waltham, MA, USA).

4.5. Determination of Intracellular Lipid Accumulation Using ORO Staining Assay

RAW264.7 macrophages or HASMCs were exposed to P1 or P2 (10~200 μM) as detailed above, and ORO staining was performed to determine the effect of intracellular lipid accumulation following the protocol in our previous study [25]. 4% paraformaldehyde was added to each well for 1 h to fix the cells, followed by washing with 60% isopropanol. The cells were then stained with a freshly prepared filtered ORO solution for 1 h and washed twice with distilled water. Images were captured using an inverted microscope (DMI6000, Leica, Wetzlar, Germany) and quantification was performed by measuring absorbance at 510 nm with a microplate reader (Multiskan™ GO, Thermo Scientific™, Waltham, MA, USA).

4.6. Determination of TC, FC, CE, and TG Content

RAW264.7 macrophages were seeded in 12-well plates for 24 h and treated with P1 and P2 (10~200 μM) as detailed above. TC and FC were determined using BioVision (Inc., Mountain View, CA) total cholesterol and cholesteryl ester colorimetric assay kit II according to the manufacturer's instructions and cellular TG content was quantified by a commercially available colorimetric TG assay kit (Biomax, Seoul, Republic of Korea) after the treatment of peptides. The protein concentration of treated cells was determined by the BCA assay. CE amount was calculated by subtracting FC from TC.

4.7. Determination of Cholesterol Influx and Efflux

RAW264.7 macrophages were treated with P1 or P2 (10~200 μM) for 1 h followed by 24 h treatment of oxLDL in 96-black well plates, and cholesterol influx and efflux effects were determined using 25-NBD-cholesterol following the protocol in our previous study [25]. To determine cholesterol influx, cells were labeled with 25-NBD cholesterol (5 μg/mL) in serum-free DMEM for 6 h after the 24 h treatment, and the cholesterol content in the cells was measured at excitation (485 nm) and emission (535 nm) wavelengths using a GENios microplate reader (GENios, TECAN, Männedorf, Switzerland).

For cholesterol efflux assessment, treated cells were equilibrated with 25-NBD cholesterol (1 μg/mL) for 6 h. After incubation, the 25-NBD cholesterol-labeled cells were washed with PBS and incubated in DMEM for an additional 6 h. The fluorescence of the cholesterol released into the culture medium was measured as described above. Cholesterol efflux was expressed as the percentage of fluorescence intensity in the medium relative to the total fluorescence (fluorescence intensity of cells + fluorescence intensity of medium).

4.8. Determination of TNF-α, IL-1β, IL-6, and PGE_2 Levels

Macrophages were treated with P1 or P2 (10~200 μM) as detailed above, and the level of inflammatory mediators (TNF-α, IL-1β, IL-6, and PGE_2) were quantified using BioLegend ELISAMAX™ Deluxe kit, USA, and ELISA kit (Cayman Chem. Co., Ann Arbor, MI, USA) according to the manufacturer's instructions.

4.9. Determination of NO Level

NO level in the culture medium was quantified using the Griess reagent assay. Macrophages were treated with P1 and P2 as detailed above, and NO level in the culture medium was determined following the protocol in our previous study [57]. A 50 μL sample of the culture supernatant was combined with 50 μL of Griess reagent and incubated for 20 min. The absorbance was then measured at 540 nm using a microplate reader. The NO concentration was calculated using a standard curve derived from sodium nitrite.

4.10. Western Blot Analysis

Western blot analysis was conducted following a standard protocol. Briefly, whole cell lysates were prepared using RIPA buffer with protease and phosphatase inhibitors (Roche Diagnostics, Seoul, Korea) after treating the cells as previously described. The nuclear fraction was extracted using the NE-PER Nuclear and Cytoplasmic Extraction Reagents kit (NE-PER Nuclear and Cytoplasmic Extraction Reagents, Thermo Scientific) according to the manufacturer's instructions. Bands were visualized using a chemiluminescence ECL assay kit (Life Technologies, Seoul, Republic of Korea) and imaged with a Davinch-Chemi Imager™ (CAS400SM, Core Bio, Seoul, Korea).

4.11. Statistical Analysis

Sigma Plot 12.0 (Systat Software Inc., San Jose, CA, USA) was used to perform a one-way ANOVA and data are presented as means ± SD (n = 3). Student's t-test was performed and values with $p < 0.05$ were regarded as statistically significant.

5. Conclusions

Multifunctional marine-derived BAPs with anti-inflammatory properties represent an attractive strategy for mitigating foam cell formation preventing atherosclerosis. Hence, in this study, we investigated the foam cell formation inhibitory activity and associated anti-inflammatory activities of two blue mussel-derived peptides PIISVYWK (P1) and FSVVPSPK (P2). P1 and P2 peptides demonstrated promising effects on foam cell formation inhibition and maintaining cholesterol flux processes. They attenuated cholesterol influx, enhanced cholesterol efflux, and led to increased activation of transcription factors PPAR-γ and LXR-α. Moreover, P1 and P2 peptides inhibited foam cell formation in hASMCs. They also demonstrated anti-inflammatory effects by inhibiting the nuclear activation of NF-κB and showed anti-oxidative stress properties through the activation of Nrf2 nuclear translocation. These results suggest that P1 and P2 peptides from blue mussels may offer therapeutic potential in the prevention and treatment of atherosclerosis and related metabolic diseases. However, further in vivo studies are necessary to confirm and expand upon these findings.

Author Contributions: Conceptualization, C.K.M. and J.-Y.J.; Methodology, C.K.M. and J.-Y.J.; Investigation, C.K.M.; Data curation, C.K.M.; Supervision, J.-Y.J.; Writing—original draft, review and editing, J.-Y.J. All authors have read and agreed to the published version of the manuscript.

Funding: This research was supported by grants (2021R1I1A3047702) of the Basic Science Research Program through the National Research Foundation (NRF) funded by the Ministry of Education, Republic of Korea.

Data Availability Statement: The data presented in this study are available on request from the corresponding authors.

Acknowledgments: Authors would like to thank the Basic Science Research Program through the National Research Foundation (NRF) funded by the Ministry of Education, Republic of Korea.

Conflicts of Interest: The authors have no conflicts of interest relevant to this study to disclose.

Abbreviations

BAPs: bioactive peptides, P1: PIISVYWK, P2: FSVVPSPK, CVDs: cardiovascular diseases, CD36: cluster differentiation 36, SR-A1: class A1 scavenger receptor, ABCA-1: ATP-binding cassette transporter A1, ABCG-1: ATP-binding cassette subfamily G member 1, PPAR-γ: peroxisome proliferator-activated receptor-gamma, LXR-α: liver X receptor-alpha, TNF-α: tumor necrosis factor alpha, IL-6: Interleukin 6, IL-1β: interleukin-1β, NO: nitric oxide, PGE_2: prostaglandin E_2, iNOS: inducible nitric oxide synthase, COX-2: cyclooxygenase-2, NF-κB: Nuclear factor kappa B, HO-1: heme oxygenase-1, Nrf2: nuclear factor erythroid 2-related factor 2, LDL: low-density lipoproteins, oxLDL: oxidized-low density lipoproteins, BAPs: bio-active peptides, DMEM: Dulbecco's modified eagle medium, HASMC: human aorta vascular smooth muscle cells, ORO: Oil Red O, TC: total cholesterol, FC: free cholesterol, CE: cholesterol ester, TG: triglycerides, SIM: simvastatin, RSG: rosiglitazone, MDA: Malondialdehyde

References

1. Kim, H.; Kim, S.; Han, S.; Rane, P.P.; Fox, K.M.; Qian, Y.; Suh, H.S. Prevalence and incidence of atherosclerotic cardiovascular disease and its risk factors in Korea: A nationwide population-based study. *BMC Public Health* **2019**, *19*, 1112. [CrossRef] [PubMed]
2. Libby, P. The changing landscape of atherosclerosis. *Nature* **2021**, *592*, 524–533. [CrossRef]
3. Coca, A.; Castellano, J.M.; Camafort, M.; Fuster, V. Polypill in cardiovascular disease prevention: Recent Advances. *Pol. Arch. Intern. Med.* **2023**, *133*, 16460. [CrossRef]
4. Maguire, E.M.; Pearce, S.W.; Xiao, Q. Foam cell formation: A new target for fighting atherosclerosis and cardiovascular disease. *Vasc. Pharmacol.* **2019**, *112*, 54–71. [CrossRef]
5. Quinn, M.T.; Parthasarathy, S.; Fong, L.G.; Steinberg, D. Oxidatively modified low density lipoproteins: A potential role in recruitment and retention of monocyte/macrophages during atherogenesis. *Proc. Natl. Acad. Sci. USA* **1987**, *84*, 2995–2998. [CrossRef] [PubMed]
6. Chistiakov, D.A.; Melnichenko, A.A.; Myasoedova, V.A.; Grechko, A.V.; Orekhov, A.N. Mechanisms of foam cell formation in atherosclerosis. *J. Mol. Med.* **2017**, *95*, 1153–1165. [CrossRef] [PubMed]
7. Shashkin, P.; Dragulev, B.; Ley, K. Macrophage differentiation to foam cells. *Curr. Pharm. Des.* **2005**, *11*, 3061–3072. [CrossRef]
8. Hopkins, P.N. Molecular biology of atherosclerosis. *Physiol. Rev.* **2013**, *93*, 1317–1542. [CrossRef]
9. Libby, P.; Ridker, P.M.; Maseri, A. Inflammation and atherosclerosis. *Circulation* **2002**, *105*, 1135–1143. [CrossRef]
10. Hamed, I.; Özogul, F.; Özogul, Y.; Regenstein, J.M. Marine bioactive compounds and their health benefits: A review. *Compr. Rev. Food Sci. Food Saf.* **2015**, *14*, 446–465. [CrossRef]
11. Suleria, H.A.R.; Gobe, G.; Masci, P.; Osborne, S.A. Marine bioactive compounds and health promoting perspectives; innovation pathways for drug discovery. *Trends Food Sci. Technol.* **2016**, *50*, 44–55. [CrossRef]
12. Ngo, D.H.; Vo, T.S.; Ngo, D.N.; Wijesekara, I.; Kim, S.K. Biological activities and potential health benefits of bioactive peptides derived from marine organisms. *Int. J. Biol. Macromol.* **2012**, *51*, 378–383. [CrossRef] [PubMed]
13. Macedo, M.W.F.S.; Cunha, N.B.d.; Carneiro, J.A.; Costa, R.A.d.; Alencar, S.A.d.; Cardoso, M.H.; Franco, O.L.; Dias, S.C. Marine organisms as a rich source of biologically active peptides. *Front. Mar. Sci.* **2021**, *8*, 667764. [CrossRef]
14. Liu, H.; Yang, Y.; Liu, Y.; Cui, L.; Fu, L.; Li, B. Various bioactive peptides in collagen hydrolysate from salmo salar skin and the combined inhibitory effects on atherosclerosis in vitro and in vivo. *Food Res. Int.* **2022**, *157*, 111281. [CrossRef]
15. Wang, Y.M.; Pan, X.; He, Y.; Chi, C.F.; Wang, B. Hypolipidemic activities of two pentapeptides (VIAPW and IRWWW) from miiuy croaker (*Miichthys miiuy*) muscle on lipid accumulation in HepG2 cells through regulation of AMPK pathway. *Appl. Sci.* **2020**, *10*, 817. [CrossRef]
16. Sun, K.L.; Gao, M.; Wang, Y.Z.; Li, X.R.; Wang, P.; Wang, B. Antioxidant peptides from protein hydrolysate of marine red algae Eucheuma cottonii: Preparation, identification, and cytoprotective mechanisms on H_2O_2 oxidative damaged HUVECs. *Front. Microbiol.* **2022**, *13*, 791248. [CrossRef]
17. Zhao, Y.Q.; Zhang, L.; Tao, J.; Chi, C.-F.; Wang, B. Eight antihypertensive peptides from the protein hydrolysate of Antarctic krill (*Euphausia superba*): Isolation, identification, and activity evaluation on human umbilical vein endothelial cells (HUVECs). *Food Res. Int.* **2019**, *121*, 197–204. [CrossRef]
18. Venugopal, V.; Gopakumar, K. Shellfish: Nutritive value, health benefits, and consumer safety. *Compr. Rev. Food Sci. Food Saf.* **2017**, *16*, 1219–1242. [CrossRef]
19. Wang, B.; Li, L.; Chi, C.F.; Ma, J.H.; Luo, H.Y.; Xu, Y.F. Purification and characterisation of a novel antioxidant peptide derived from blue mussel (*Mytilus edulis*) protein hydrolysate. *Food Chem.* **2013**, *138*, 1713–1719. [CrossRef]
20. Park, S.Y.; Kim, Y.S.; Ahn, C.B.; Je, J.Y. Partial purification and identification of three antioxidant peptides with hepatoprotective effects from blue mussel (*Mytilus edulis*) hydrolysate by peptic hydrolysis. *J. Funct. Foods* **2016**, *20*, 88–95. [CrossRef]

21. Oh, Y.; Ahn, C.B.; Nam, K.H.; Kim, Y.K.; Yoon, N.Y.; Je, J.Y. Amino acid composition, antioxidant, and cytoprotective effect of blue mussel (*Mytilus edulis*) hydrolysate through the inhibition of caspase-3 activation in oxidative stress-mediated endothelial cell injury. *Mar. Drugs* **2019**, *17*, 135. [CrossRef]
22. Kim, Y.S.; Ahn, C.B.; Je, J.Y. Anti-inflammatory action of high molecular weight Mytilus edulis hydrolysates fraction in LPS-induced RAW264. 7 macrophage via NF-κB and MAPK pathways. *Food Chem.* **2016**, *202*, 9–14. [CrossRef] [PubMed]
23. Xu, Z.; Zhao, F.; Chen, H.; Xu, S.; Fan, F.; Shi, P.; Tu, M.; Wang, Z.; Du, M. Nutritional properties and osteogenic activity of enzymatic hydrolysates of proteins from the blue mussel (*Mytilus edulis*). *Food Funct.* **2019**, *10*, 7745–7754. [CrossRef] [PubMed]
24. Suo, S.K.; Zhao, Y.Q.; Wang, Y.M.; Pan, X.Y.; Chi, C.F.; Wang, B. Seventeen novel angiotensin converting enzyme (ACE) inhibitory peptides from the protein hydrolysate of Mytilus edulis: Isolation, identification, molecular docking study, and protective function on HUVECs. *Food Funct.* **2022**, *13*, 7831–7846. [CrossRef]
25. Marasinghe, C.K.; Yoon, S.D.; Je, J.Y. Blue mussel (*Mytilus edulis*) hydrolysates attenuate oxidized-low density lipoproteins (ox-LDL)-induced foam cell formation, inflammation, and oxidative stress in RAW264. 7 macrophages. *Process Biochem.* **2023**, *134*, 131–140. [CrossRef]
26. Daliri, E.B.M.; Oh, D.H.; Lee, B.H. Bioactive peptides. *Foods* **2017**, *6*, 32. [CrossRef]
27. Cheung, R.C.F.; Ng, T.B.; Wong, J.H. Marine peptides: Bioactivities and applications. *Mar. Drugs* **2015**, *13*, 4006–4043. [CrossRef]
28. Oh, Y.; Ahn, C.B.; Je, J.Y. Blue mussel-derived peptides PIISVYWK and FSVVPSPK trigger Wnt/β-catenin signaling-mediated osteogenesis in human bone marrow mesenchymal stem cells. *Mar. Drugs* **2020**, *18*, 510. [CrossRef]
29. Oh, Y.; Jung, W.K.; Je, J.Y. Protective effect of multifunctional peptides PIISVYWK and FSVVPSPK on oxidative stress-mediated HUVEC injury through antioxidant and anti-apoptotic action. *Process Biochem.* **2023**, *125*, 121–129. [CrossRef]
30. Oh, Y.; Ahn, C.B.; Cho, W.H.; Yoon, N.Y.; Je, J.Y. Anti-osteoporotic effects of antioxidant peptides PIISVYWK and FSVVPSPK from Mytilus edulis on ovariectomized mice. *Antioxidants* **2020**, *9*, 866. [CrossRef]
31. Wang, D.; Yang, Y.; Lei, Y.; Tzvetkov, N.T.; Liu, X.; Yeung, A.W.K.; Xu, S.; Atanasov, A.G. Targeting foam cell formation in atherosclerosis: Therapeutic potential of natural products. *Pharmacol. Rev.* **2019**, *71*, 596–670. [CrossRef] [PubMed]
32. Lu, S.; Luo, Y.; Sun, G.; Sun, X. Ginsenoside compound K attenuates ox-LDL-mediated macrophage inflammation and foam cell formation via autophagy induction and modulating NF-κB, p38, and JNK MAPK signaling. *Front. Pharmacol.* **2020**, *11*, 567238. [CrossRef] [PubMed]
33. Wang, S.; Zhang, X.; Liu, M.; Luan, H.; Ji, Y.; Guo, P.; Wu, C. Chrysin inhibits foam cell formation through promoting cholesterol efflux from RAW264. 7 macrophages. *Pharm. Biol.* **2015**, *53*, 1481–1487. [CrossRef]
34. Marasinghe, C.K.; Jung, W.K.; Je, J.Y. OxLDL-Induced Foam Cell Formation Inhibitory Activity of Pepsin Hydrolysate of Ark Shell (*Scapharca subcrenata* (Lischke, 1869)) in RAW264. 7 Macrophages. *J. Food Biochem.* **2023**, *2023*, 6905673. [CrossRef]
35. Wu, C.; Chen, R.; Liu, M.; Liu, D.; Li, X.; Wang, S.; Niu, S.; Guo, P.; Lin, W. Spiromastixones inhibit foam cell formation via regulation of cholesterol efflux and uptake in RAW264. 7 macrophages. *Mar. Drugs* **2015**, *13*, 6352–6365. [CrossRef]
36. Zhou, Y.; Chen, R.; Liu, D.; Wu, C.; Guo, P.; Lin, W. Asperlin inhibits LPS-evoked foam cell formation and prevents atherosclerosis in ApoE$^{-/-}$ mice. *Mar. Drugs* **2017**, *15*, 358. [CrossRef]
37. Gao, L.N.; Zhou, X.; Lu, Y.R.; Li, K.; Gao, S.; Yu, C.Q.; Cui, Y.L. Dan-Lou prescription inhibits foam cell formation induced by ox-LDL via the TLR4/NF-κB and PPARγ signaling pathways. *Front. Physiol.* **2018**, *9*, 323814. [CrossRef]
38. Yu, X.H.; Fu, Y.C.; Zhang, D.W.; Yin, K.; Tang, C.K. Foam cells in atherosclerosis. *Clin. Chim. Acta* **2013**, *424*, 245–252. [CrossRef]
39. Babaev, V.R.; Gleaves, L.A.; Carter, K.J.; Suzuki, H.; Kodama, T.; Fazio, S.; Linton, M.F. Reduced atherosclerotic lesions in mice deficient for total or macrophage-specific expression of scavenger receptor-A. *Arterioscler. Thromb. Vasc. Biol.* **2000**, *20*, 2593–2599. [CrossRef]
40. Febbraio, M.; Podrez, E.A.; Smith, J.D.; Hajjar, D.P.; Hazen, S.L.; Hoff, H.F.; Sharma, K.; Silverstein, R.L. Targeted disruption of the class B scavenger receptor CD36 protects against atherosclerotic lesion development in mice. *J. Clin. Investig.* **2000**, *105*, 1049–1056. [CrossRef]
41. Wang, X.; Collins, H.L.; Ranalletta, M.; Fuki, I.V.; Billheimer, J.T.; Rothblat, G.H.; Tall, A.R.; Rader, D.J. Macrophage ABCA1 and ABCG1, but not SR-BI, promote macrophage reverse cholesterol transport in vivo. *J. Clin. Investig.* **2007**, *117*, 2216–2224. [CrossRef] [PubMed]
42. Ginsberg, H.N.; Packard, C.J.; Chapman, M.J.; Borén, J.; Aguilar-Salinas, C.A.; Averna, M.; Ference, B.A.; Gaudet, D.; Hegele, R.A.; Kersten, S. Triglyceride-rich lipoproteins and their remnants: Metabolic insights, role in atherosclerotic cardiovascular disease, and emerging therapeutic strategies—A consensus statement from the European Atherosclerosis Society. *Eur. Heart J.* **2021**, *42*, 4791–4806. [CrossRef] [PubMed]
43. Varbo, A.; Nordestgaard, B.G. Remnant cholesterol and triglyceride-rich lipoproteins in atherosclerosis progression and cardiovascular disease. *Am. Heart Assoc.* **2016**, *36*, 2133–2135. [CrossRef] [PubMed]
44. Marasinghe, C.K.; Yoon, S.D.; Je, J.Y. Two peptides LLRLTDL and GYALPCDCL inhibit foam cell formation through activating PPAR-γ/LXR-α signaling pathway in oxLDL-treated RAW264. 7 macrophages. *BioFactors* **2024**. *ahead of print*. [CrossRef] [PubMed]
45. Monsalve, F.A.; Pyarasani, R.D.; Delgado-Lopez, F.; Moore-Carrasco, R. Peroxisome proliferator-activated receptor targets for the treatment of metabolic diseases. *Mediat. Inflamm.* **2013**, *2013*, 549627. [CrossRef]
46. Lund, E.G.; Menke, J.G.; Sparrow, C.P. Liver X receptor agonists as potential therapeutic agents for dyslipidemia and atherosclerosis. *Arterioscler. Thromb. Vasc. Biol.* **2003**, *23*, 1169–1177. [CrossRef]

47. Lazar, M.A. Progress in cardiovascular biology: PPAR for the course. *Nat. Med.* **2001**, *7*, 23–24. [CrossRef]
48. Guerrini, V.; Gennaro, M.L. Foam cells: One size doesn't fit all. *Trends Immunol.* **2019**, *40*, 1163–1179. [CrossRef]
49. Rhoads, J.P.; Major, A.S. How oxidized low-density lipoprotein activates inflammatory responses. *Crit. Rev. Immunol.* **2018**, *38*, 333–342. [CrossRef]
50. Mushenkova, N.V.; Bezsonov, E.E.; Orekhova, V.A.; Popkova, T.V.; Starodubova, A.V.; Orekhov, A.N. Recognition of oxidized lipids by macrophages and its role in atherosclerosis development. *Biomedicines* **2021**, *9*, 915. [CrossRef]
51. Wan, F.; Lenardo, M.J. The nuclear signaling of NF-κB: Current knowledge, new insights, and future perspectives. *Cell Res.* **2010**, *20*, 24–33. [CrossRef] [PubMed]
52. Ferreira, V.; van Dijk, K.W.; Groen, A.K.; Vos, R.M.; Van Der Kaa, J.; Gijbels, M.J.; Havekes, L.M.; Pannekoek, H. Macrophage-specific inhibition of NF-κB activation reduces foam-cell formation. *Atherosclerosis* **2007**, *192*, 283–290. [CrossRef] [PubMed]
53. Zhang, Q.; Liu, J.; Duan, H.; Li, R.; Peng, W.; Wu, C. Activation of Nrf2/HO-1 signaling: An important molecular mechanism of herbal medicine in the treatment of atherosclerosis via the protection of vascular endothelial cells from oxidative stress. *J. Adv. Res.* **2021**, *34*, 43–63. [CrossRef] [PubMed]
54. Chen, J.; Zhang, S.; Wu, J.; Wu, S.; Xu, G.; Wei, D. Essential role of nonessential amino acid glutamine in atherosclerotic cardiovascular disease. *DNA Cell Biol.* **2020**, *39*, 8–15. [CrossRef]
55. Ivanov, V.; Roomi, M.W.; Kalinovsky, T.; Niedzwiecki, A.; Rath, M. Anti-atherogenic effects of a mixture of ascorbic acid, lysine, proline, arginine, cysteine, and green tea phenolics in human aortic smooth muscle cells. *J. Cardiovasc. Pharmacol.* **2007**, *49*, 140–145. [CrossRef] [PubMed]
56. Zaric, B.L.; Radovanovic, J.N.; Gluvic, Z.; Stewart, A.J.; Essack, M.; Motwalli, O.; Gojobori, T.; Isenovic, E.R. Atherosclerosis linked to aberrant amino acid metabolism and immunosuppressive amino acid catabolizing enzymes. *Front. Immunol.* **2020**, *11*, 551758. [CrossRef]
57. Hyung, J.H.; Ahn, C.B.; Kim, B.I.; Kim, K.; Je, J.Y. Involvement of Nrf2-mediated heme oxygenase-1 expression in anti-inflammatory action of chitosan oligosaccharides through MAPK activation in murine macrophages. *Eur. J. Pharmacol.* **2016**, *793*, 43–48. [CrossRef]

marine drugs

MDPI

Article

Pilot-Scale Enzymatic Conversion of Low Stability, High Free Fatty, Squid Oil to an Oxidatively Stable Astaxanthin-Rich Acylglyceride Oil Suitable for Nutritional Applications

Asavari Joshi [1,2], Brendan Holland [2], Moninder Sachar [3] and Colin J. Barrow [1,2,4,*]

1 ARC Industrial Transformation Training Centre for Green Chemistry in Manufacturing, Deakin University, Waurn Ponds, Geelong, VIC 3216, Australia
2 Centre for Sustainable Bioproducts, Deakin University, Waurn Ponds, Geelong, VIC 3216, Australia; brendan.holland@deakin.edu.au
3 Australian Omega Oils Pty Ltd., North Geelong, Geelong, VIC, 3215, Australia; monindersachar@gmail.com
4 Distinguished Visiting Research Fellow, College of Engineering, Abu Dhabi University, Zayed City 59911, Abu Dhabi, United Arab Emirates
* Correspondence: colin.barrow@deakin.edu.au

Abstract: Squid viscera, a byproduct of squid processing, contains oil rich in omega-3 fatty acids (up to 10% by mass) and the antioxidant astaxanthin. However, its high free fatty acid (FFA) content compromises stability. To address this, pilot-scale (200 L) enzymatic re-esterification of squid oil using immobilized lipase (Lipozyme RMIM) was demonstrated, resulting in high acylglyceride yields. The processed oil was analyzed for oxidation kinetics and thermodynamics using Rancimat, fatty acid composition using GC, omega-3 fatty acid positional distribution in the acylglyceride product using ^{13}C NMR, and astaxanthin content. Lipase treatment reduced FFA levels from 44% to 4% and increased acylglycerides to 93% in squid oil. This reduction in FFA was accompanied by significantly increased stability (0.06 to 18.9 h by Rancimat). The treated oil showed no loss in astaxanthin (194.1 μg/g) or omega-3 fatty acids, including docosahexaenoic acid (DHA). DHA remaining predominantly at sn-2 indicated that the naturally occurring positional distribution of this omega-3 FFA was retained in the product. Lipase treatment significantly enhanced oxidative stability, evidenced by improved thermodynamic parameters (E_a 94.15 kJ/mol, ΔH 91.09 kJ/mol, ΔS −12.6 J/mol K) and extended shelf life (IP_{25} 74.42 days) compared to starting squid oil and commercial fish/squid oils lacking astaxanthin. Thus, lipase treatment offers an effective strategy for reducing FFA levels and producing oxidatively stable, astaxanthin-rich acylglyceride squid oil with DHA retained at the nutritionally favored sn-2 position.

Keywords: enzyme-processed squid oil; rancimat; lipid oxidation kinetics; astaxanthin

1. Introduction

Squid cephalopods are an important marine food, while the non-edible parts, such as viscera, are usually discarded [1]. Squid viscera contains high levels of anti-inflammatory marine oils, particularly omega-3 fatty acids, such as docosahexaenoic acid (DHA) and eicosapentaenoic acid (EPA), which account for about 25% of the total lipid content [2]. EPA and DHA have potent anti-inflammatory properties and are precursors to anti-inflammatory mediators such as resolvins and protectins and have been shown to have cardiovascular benefits, be important for normal brain development, and benefit a range of inflammatory mediated conditions [3–5]. However, due to their polyunsaturated nature, omega-3 fatty acids are susceptible to auto-oxidation and photosensitized oxidation [6]. The auto-oxidation of these fatty acids leads to free radicals that continue to react during exponential oxidation [7]. The primary products generated during oxidation are called hydroperoxides, which are highly unstable and give rise to the formation of secondary oxidation products, such as ketones, aldehydes, hydrocarbons, alcohols, and acids [7–9]. In addition to decreasing omega-3 levels in oil, oxidation causes the formation of sensory, unpleasant aldehyde, making these oils taste bad even after relatively small levels of oxidation [10–12]. Squid viscera naturally contains a high level of free fatty acids, most likely due to lipase activity in the gut [13], with high FFA oils being particularly susceptible to oxidation. Squid viscera oil also contains highly colored astaxanthin, making normal colorimetric methods for determining oxidation levels problematic [14].

Astaxanthin is a xanthophyll carotenoid that is found naturally in a variety of marine species, such as shrimp, krill, salmon, squid, and crab, and is a powerful antioxidant [15–18] that is used in aquaculture, cosmetics, food, feed, nutraceuticals, and pharmaceuticals. Reports have suggested that astaxanthin has the ability to cross the blood-brain barrier, thereby working to reduce free radical-induced neurotoxicity and memory loss, and its anti-inflammatory properties indicate it has cardioprotective benefits and has wound-healing, neuroprotective, hepatoprotective, and osteoprotective properties [18–21]. The natural form of astaxanthin is normally esterified and has been observed to exhibit higher bioactivity than synthetic astaxanthin [22–26]. Astaxanthin incorporated into omega-3-rich products can provide synergistic antioxidative and anti-inflammatory benefits [27–29] and also improve omega-3 oil storage stability [30–33].

The Rancimat technique offers accelerated oxidation analysis by measuring volatile oxidation products through electrical conductivity, providing an induction period before accelerated oxidation occurs. It can be used for the rapid determination of oxidative stability and is particularly useful for oils where standard colorimetric methods for oxidation products (peroxide value, PV and p-anisidine values, pAV) are not accurate, such as colored oils or oils containing astaxanthin [34]. The Rancimat technique, including the determination of kinetic and thermodynamic parameters to predict lipid oxidation, has been applied to a range of oils, including vegetable oils [35–38] and fish oils [39–42], but only a few studies have investigated non-fish seafood-derived omega-3 oils, such as krill [43], shrimp [15], and squid oil. The current study aims to re-esterify squid visceral oil at the pilot scale (200 L) in order to reduce the levels of free fatty acid content while retaining astaxanthin by employing the in-house enzymatic method [44]. The processed squid visceral oil was then subjected to accelerated oxidation using the Rancimat method to investigate its oxidative stability toward developing this waste oil into a nutritional oil that can be used for nutritional supplements or functional foods. Since there has been no study that has reported kinetic and thermodynamic parameter determination for enzymatically processed squid viscera-derived omega-3-rich oil, lipid oxidation parameters are determined that further aid in understanding the oxidative stability of squid visceral oil. An overview of the study is depicted in Figure 1. The stability of the ESO was then compared with commercially available calamari and fish oil.

The results demonstrate that the reduced free fatty acid content of the oil, together with the retention of natural astaxanthin, produces a more oxidatively stable squid viscera-derived oil compared to other commercially available omega-3 oil sources.

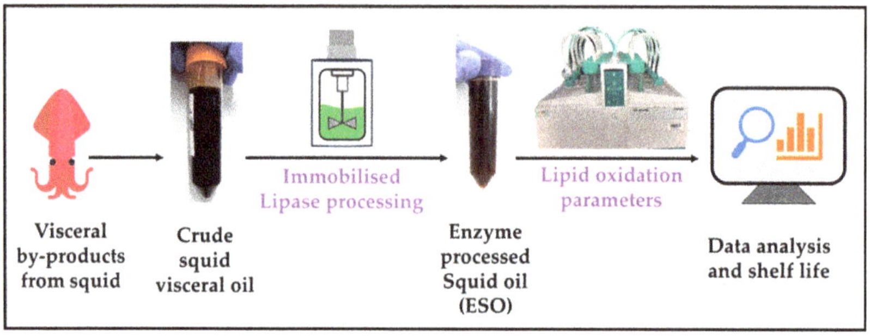

Figure 1. Lipid oxidation parameters of enzyme-processed squid oil using Rancimat.

2. Results and Discussion

2.1. Free Fatty Acid Content in Crude Squid Visceral Oil During Enzymatic Processing

The enzymatic processing of crude squid visceral oil was carried out at the pilot scale using immobilized lipase. The crude squid visceral oil had an initial free fatty acid content of 44 ± 0.39%, which was significantly reduced during the lipase treatment period, as depicted in Figure 2. The free fatty acid content decreased steeply in the initial 9 h, followed by a slow decline to a free fatty acid content of 4 ± 0.5% between 24 h and 54 h. This was attributed to the initial abundance of free fatty acid substrate available for the lipase, resulting in a higher esterification rate during the initial 9 h. As the reaction progressed, the concentration of free fatty acid substrate decreased, leading to a reduced esterification rate beyond 9 h. These findings suggest that future batches of lipase treatment could be halted after 24 h of processing to decrease the reaction time and improve the cost of production.

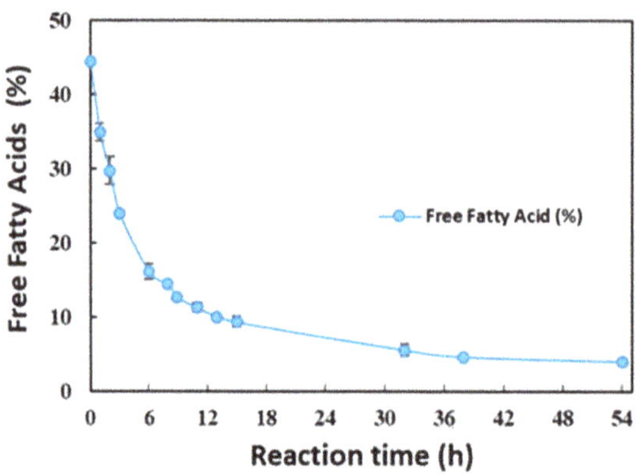

Figure 2. Free fatty acid reduction profile of lipase-processed squid visceral oil (ESO). Results are presented as mean ± SD.

We determined the lipid class profile of squid visceral oil, including the content of acylglycerides and fatty acid ethyl esters, both before and after lipase treatment. Nutritional oils with a high acylglyceride content exhibit superior stability, sensory acceptance, and bioavailability [45]. In contrast, elevated levels of fatty acid ethyl esters can hinder the digestion and absorption of fatty acids [45] and are associated with an increased risk of arrhythmia and atrial fibrillation [46]. The total acylglyceride content of squid visceral oil increased significantly after lipase treatment from 53.20 ± 0.5% to 93.16 ± 0.5%, while the ethyl ester content remained consistently low, with values of 2.71 ± 0.3% prior to lipase treatment and 2.63 ± 0.2% after lipase treatment. The final product squid visceral oil obtained after pilot-scale lipase treatment consisted of 20.8 ± 1.2% triacylglycerides, 45.6 ± 2.0% diacylglycerides, and 26.8 ± 2.9% monoacylglycerides. This lipid class profile showed a similar trend to the results obtained during the laboratory-scale demonstration in a previous study [44] and to the results reported for the de-acidification of vegetable oil [47]. These findings highlight the potential of immobilized lipase treatment for the large-scale processing of crude squid visceral oil.

2.2. Fatty Acid Composition in Crude Squid Visceral Oil During Lipase Processing

The fatty acid composition of the squid oil during enzymatic processing was determined using gas chromatography with a (GC)-flame ionization detector (FID). The results are shown in Table 1.

Table 1. Fatty acid composition of squid visceral oil during lipase processing. The results are presented as mean ± SD. The columns not showing common lowercase subscript for each row of fatty acid categories are significantly different ($p < 0.05$).

Fatty Acids (%) (Average of Three Replicates)	Lipase-Processed Crude Squid Oil			
	0 h	2 h	10 h	54 h
Saturated fatty acids total	25.6 ± 0.0 $_a$	24.4 ± 0.1 $_b$	23.4 ± 0.1 $_c$	22.9 ± 0.4 $_c$
Monounsaturated fatty acids total	26.9 ± 0.1 $_a$	27.4 ± 0.1 $_b$	27.5 ± 0.0 $_b$	27.8 ± 0.1 $_c$
Eicosapentaenoic acid (EPA)	20.2 ± 0.0 $_a$	20.2 ± 0.0 $_a$	20.8 ± 0.0 $_b$	20.7 ± 0.1 $_b$
Docosahexaenoic acid (DHA)	20.8 ± 0.0 $_a$	20.9 ± 0.1 $_a$	21.4 ± 0.0 $_b$	21.3 ± 0.1 $_b$
Omega-3 total	43.0 ± 0.1 $_a$	43.1 ± 0.1 $_a$	44.2 ± 0.0 $_b$	44.1 ± 0.2 $_b$
Omega-6 total	4.5 ± 0.0 $_a$	4.60 ± 0.0 $_b$	4.7 ± 0.0 $_c$	4.7 ± 0.0 $_c$
Polyunsaturated fatty acids total	47.3 ± 0.1 $_a$	47.5 ± 0.2 $_a$	48.7 ± 0.0 $_b$	48.5 ± 0.0 $_c$

The results indicate that the fatty acid profile remains relatively stable throughout the enzymatic processing, despite showing statistically significant differences at p-value < 0.05. The average total omega-3 (43.0%), eicosapentaenoic acid (20.2%), and docosahexaenoic acid (20.8%) content were higher than those achieved in a previous study [13].

2.3. Positional Distribution of Omega-3 Fatty Acids in Lipase-Treated Squid Visceral Oil

The bioavailability of omega-3 fatty acids is influenced by their positional distribution within the acylglycerol, specifically between the sn-2 and sn-1,3 positions. Omega-3 fatty acids in the sn-2 position exhibit higher bioavailability compared to those in the sn-1,3 positions [48]. Supplementation with EPA in the sn-2 position has been shown to enhance the brain levels of EPA and DHA, offering a potential therapeutic approach for brain and mental health conditions [49]. In this study, we utilized ^{13}C NMR spectroscopy to investigate the positional distribution of omega-3 fatty acids in the squid viscera oil obtained after lipase treatment. The carbonyl region of the resulting ^{13}C NMR spectra was specifically analyzed (Figure 3), as it encompasses the distribution of key omega-3 fatty acids such as EPA and DHA [50,51].

As presented in Table 2, ETA is predominantly (>78%) positioned at the sn-1,3 locations, whereas MUFA, DPA, and SDA exhibit a more randomized distribution, with 44–61% located at the sn-1,3 positions and 38–56% at the sn-2 position. SFA is distributed at a 1:1 ratio over sn-2 and sn-1,3. EPA is preferentially distributed, with 72.5% at the sn-2 position and 27.5% at the sn-1 position. A similar preferential enrichment of EPA at the sn-2 position has been observed in oils derived from tuna [52], shrimp [53], and squid [54], as well as in lipase-treated salmon oil [55]. In contrast, DHA is predominantly found at the sn-2 position, with 92.9% of the total DHA at sn-2 and only 7.1% at the sn-1,3 positions. This predominant placement enhances its bioavailability and oxidative stability and is consistent with the position of DHA in naturally acylglyceride marine oils. For example,

DHA is predominantly located at the sn-2 position in the triacylglycerides (TAGs) of salmon, mackerel, cod liver, and herring, while EPA tends to be more randomly distributed in these oils, as well as in those derived from hoki [50].

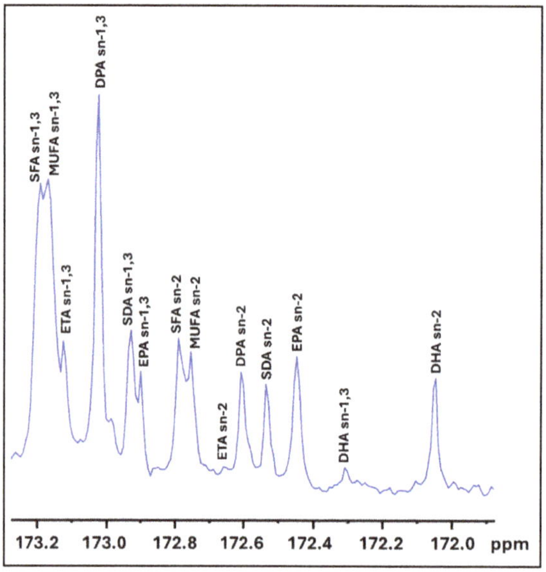

Figure 3. Carbonyl region of ^{13}C NMR of lipase-treated squid visceral oil illustrating positional distribution of fatty acids. Abbreviations: DHA (docosahexaenoic acid), EPA (eicosapentaenoic acid), SDA (stearidonic acid), DPA (docosapentaenoic acid), ETA (eicosatetraenoic acid), MUFA (monounsaturated fatty acids), and SFA (saturated fatty acids).

Table 2. Positional distribution of EPA and DHA within the acylglycerides of lipase-treated squid visceral oils. [a] Values represent the mean of three independent spectral analyses performed using ^{13}C NMR. Each spectrum was acquired with 12,000 scans to ensure accuracy.

Position	Fatty Acid	Molar Percentage (%) [a]
sn-2	EPA	17.5 ± 1.0
	DHA	12.0 ± 0.1
	SDA	13.7 ± 1.2
	DPA	16.8 ± 0.0
	ETA	2.9 ± 0.5
	MUFA	16.3 ± 1.4
	SFA	20.8 ± 0.7
sn-1,3	EPA	6.6 ± 1.1
	DHA	0.9 ± 0.1
	SDA	10.8 ± 0.2
	DPA	23.8 ± 0.4
	ETA	10.5 ± 0.0
	MUFA	25.9 ± 2.1
	SFA	21.4 ± 1.0

2.4. *Rancimat Analysis, Lipid Oxidation Kinetics, and Shelf Life Prediction*

The oxidative stability of the enzymatically converted squid visceral oil (ESO) studied at four different temperatures was compared to that of commercial calamari oil (CCO) and commercial fish oil (CFO), as shown in Figure 4a.

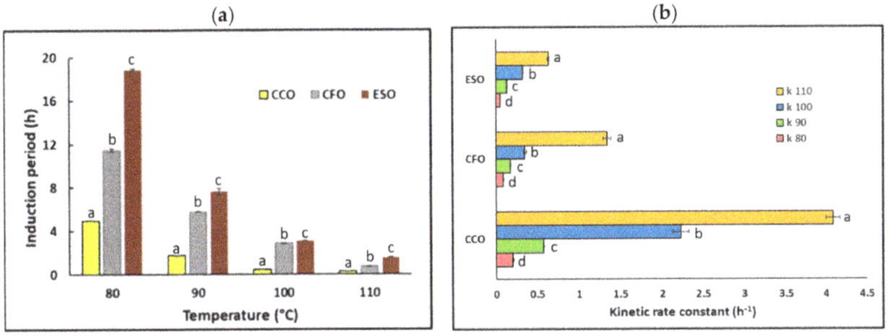

Figure 4. (**a**) Induction period (IP) of the oils against temperature (CCO—commercial calamari oil; CFO—commercial fish oil; ESO—enzymatically re-esterified squid output oil); (**b**) kinetic rate constant (k) of lipid oxidation of the CCO, CFO, and SE. Results are presented as mean ± SD. The bars not sharing common lowercase letters (labelled on the top of each bar) for each temperature in (**a**) and each oil in (**b**) are significantly different ($p < 0.05$).

Crude squid oil showed induction periods of less than 0.1 h at all studied temperatures, which can be attributed to the high free fatty acid content (44%), making this oil very susceptible to autooxidation (with an induction period of 0.06 ± 0.01 h for FFA 44.5 ± 0.4% at 80 °C and 20 L/h air flow in Rancimat). Enzymatic re-esterification to convert most of the free fatty acid to acylglyceride produced a more stable oil (ESO) at tested temperatures (slightly higher at 100 °C), which was also more stable than CCO and CFO. Oil stability decreased with temperature for all oils. After 54 h, FFA was 4.0 ± 0.5% and the induction period was 18.9 ± 0.1% h at 80 °C and 20 L/h air flow in the Rancimat. The induction period changed from 0.06 to 18.9 h when FFA decreased from 44.5 to 4%, which illustrates the importance of low FFA for squid oil stability.

Changes in the induction period (IP) were demonstrated using first-order kinetics. The kinetic rate constant (k) increased as a function of temperature (80–110 °C) ($p < 0.05$), which indicated an increased rate of oxidation with temperature (Figure 4b). The lipid oxidation rate was in the order CCO > CFO > ESO. The lowest values for 'k' were observed for ESO at all tested temperatures, indicating greater thermo-oxidative stability compared to CCO and CFO.

Another lipid oxidation kinetic parameter, the activation energy for lipid oxidation (E_a), showed substantial variation amongst the oils ($p < 0.05$) (Table 3). E_a had a range between 94.15 to 116.95 kJ/mol, with a lower value for ESO than for CCO or CFO. E_a indicates the energy required for initial oxidation and correlates with the production of primary oxidation products [39]. A lower E_a value indicates a delayed onset of rancidity [36] and confirms ESO is more stable than CCO and CFO.

The thermodynamic parameters of lipid oxidation, including activation enthalpies (ΔH) and activation entropies (ΔS), are given in Table 3. The regression coefficients ($R^2 > 0.95$) indicated good suitability to models describing how the temperature affects lipid oxidation. Overall, the positive values of change in activation enthalpies indicate the endothermic process requiring elevated energy to initiate the reaction. While activation enthalpies (ΔH) and entropies (ΔS) indicated that the ESO and CFO shared closer rates compared to CCO, ESO exhibited the slowest lipid oxidation. Nonetheless, the negative value of entropy couples with the positive activation enthalpy for ESO signals for a non-spontaneous reaction. Unlike CCO and CFO, ESO showed a negative value of ΔS, indicating the formation of an ordered activated complex desirable for improved oxidative stability [35,36,56].

Table 3. Kinetic and thermodynamic parameters of oils oxidation and shelf life (IP_{25}) prediction using Rancimat. The columns not sharing a common lowercase subscript for each parameter are significantly different ($p < 0.05$).

Parameters	ESO $^{\dagger}{}_{a}$	CCO $^{\dagger}{}_{b}$	CFO $^{\dagger}{}_{c}$
Arrhenius constant (A, h − 1)	$(4.57 \pm 0.03) \times 10^{12}$ $_{a}$	$(4.11 \pm 0.16) \times 10^{16}$ $_{b}$	$(4.52 \pm 1.5) \times 10^{13}$ $_{c}$
Activation energy for lipid oxidation (Ea, kJ/mol)	94.15 ± 0.04 $_{a}$	116.95 ± 0.04 $_{b}$	99.76 ± 0.95 $_{c}$
Activation enthalpies (ΔH, kJ/mol)	91.09 ± 0.04 $_{a}$	113.89 ± 0.04 $_{b}$	96.7 ± 0.95 $_{c}$
Activation entropies (ΔS, J/mol K)	-12.6 ± 0.05 $_{a}$	63.08 ± 0.34 $_{b}$	5.96 ± 2.88 $_{c}$
Temperature coefficient ($T_{coeff} \times 10^{-2}$, K^{-1})	-8.36 ± 0.0 $_{a}$	-10.38 ± 0.0 $_{b}$	-8.91 ± 0.0 $_{c}$
Temperature acceleration factor (Q_{10})	2.31 ± 0.0 $_{a}$	2.82 ± 0.0 $_{b}$	2.44 ± 0.02 $_{c}$
Shelf life (IP_{25}, days) ‡	74.42 ± 1.13 $_{a}$	58.93 ± 1.7 $_{b}$	72.97 ± 1.86 $_{c}$

† Coefficient of determination > 0.99 and ‡ Coefficient of determination > 0.95.

The influence of heating on lipid oxidation can be expressed by a temperature acceleration factor (Q_{10}) (Table 3) ranging between 2.31 and 2.82 in the current study, being the maximum for CCO and the minimum for ESO. The lower value of Q_{10} for ESO indicates a slower rate of oxidation with a 10 °C rise in temperature. Similarly, the temperature coefficient (T_{coeff}) with the minimum value for ESO, -8.36×10^{-2} K^{-1}, is also consistent with slower oxidation for ESO compared to other oils.

The application of Rancimat enables the rapid determination of oxidative stability at multiple temperatures, along with the application of Equation (3), which enables extrapolation to other temperatures [36,56]. The shelf life of oils (Table 3) in the order ESO > CFO > CCO ($p < 0.05$) was consistent with the kinetic parameters. The high shelf life of the ESO could be attributed to stabilization by the natural presence of astaxanthin antioxidant together with low levels of free fatty acids after enzymatic esterification [57].

2.5. Astaxanthin Content

The astaxanthin content in the dark-brown-colored ESO was found to be 194.1 ± 0.2 μg/g of lipid, whereas no astaxanthin was detected in either CCO or CFO. Most fish oils do not contain astaxanthin, and both CFO and CCO squid oil undergo bleaching during the refining process. Bleaching is known to remove colored components, including astaxanthin. Astaxanthin is a naturally occurring carotenoid with a potent antioxidant capacity 10 times higher than β-carotene and 300 times higher than α-tocopherol [30]. The astaxanthin structure consists of two terminal six-membered rings with hydroxyl and carbonyl groups, joined by a polyene chain with eleven conjugated carbon-carbon double bonds, which endow it with exceptional capacity for scavenging reactive oxygen species (ROS) [58]. Therefore, astaxanthin contributes to the improvement of the oxidative stability of oils by neutralizing free radicals and reactive oxygen species. Its incorporation into oils delays lipid oxidation by scavenging free radicals, interrupting the chain reactions that lead to oxidative degradation [32,59,60]. Furthermore, natural astaxanthin is widely utilized as a nutraceutical approved by the United States Food and Drug Administration (USFDA) owing to its diverse bioactivities, including antioxidant, anti-cancer, neuroprotective, cardioprotective, osteoprotective, hepatoprotective, anti-inflammatory, and anti-diabetic properties [19]. Therefore, astaxanthin-rich oils are used as specialty oils in nutraceutical applications [61]. Considering this, oil processing methods should aim to preserve natural astaxanthin to enhance oil stability and leverage its associated health benefits. A notable commercial example is krill oil, which undergoes processing methods that intentionally avoid bleaching to preserve astaxanthin, resulting in a stable and high-nutritional-value oil [50]. This study highlights the role of astaxanthin in improving the oxidative stability of oil. Our analysis of oxidation kinetics and thermodynamics revealed that squid visceral oil containing astaxanthin exhibits a delayed onset of oxidation compared to commercial oils, CCO and CFO, which lack astaxanthin. Thus, the astaxanthin-rich lipase-treated squid visceral oil (ESO) obtained in this study demonstrates potential suitability for nutraceutical applications due to both improved stability and health benefits associated with astaxanthin.

3. Materials and Methods

3.1. Materials

Crude squid visceral oil was procured from Mantzaris Fisheries, North Geelong, Victoria, Australia. Immobilized *Rhizomucor miehei* lipase (Lipozym RMIM) was purchased from Oppenheimer Pty Ltd., Victoria, Australia. Commercial calamari oil and commercial fish oil were purchased from the market and used before their date of expiry. All other chemicals used were of analytical grade unless otherwise specified.

3.2. Lipase Processing of Crude Squid Visceral Oil

The crude squid visceral oil was processed using an immobilized enzyme lipase, as previously described in laboratory-scale studies [44]. In the present study, the pilot-scale processing of crude squid visceral oil was undertaken. A custom-built pilot scale reactor (200 L) was loaded with crude squid oil and glycerol at a ratio of 3:1, with a known amount of immobilized enzyme and molecular sieves at the bottom of the reactor. The reactor contents were pumped from top to bottom. The reactor contents were recirculated at 500 mL/min, held at 50 °C, and stirred at 500 rpm. Processed samples were taken intermittently up to 54 h to check the free fatty acid (FFA) content of the enzyme-processed squid visceral output oil (ESO).

3.3. Free Fatty Acid Content (%) and Other Lipid Classes by Capillary Chromatography with a Flame Ionisation Detector (Iatroscan)

The oil samples were analyzed using capillary chromatography connected to a flame ionization detector (Iatroscan MK-6, Iatron Laboratories Inc., Tokyo, Japan) with the three replicates of the samples, as previously reported [62], with slight modifications. The instrument was set at an air flow rate of 2 L/min, a hydrogen flow rate of 160 mL/min, and a scanning speed of 0.5 min/scan. The oil samples were then spotted onto the precleaned chromarods and developed in a tank containing a solvent mixture of heptane:diethyl ether:acetic acid (30:8.5:0.1, *v*/*v*/*v*) for 22 min and analyzed in an Iatroscan. The FFA percentage content and other lipid classes were determined by integration using SIC-480 II software Version 1.0.

3.4. Analysis of Fatty Acid Composition Using Gas Chromatography with a Flame Ionisation Detector (GC-FID)

The fatty acids in the oil samples were converted to methyl esters before analysis using gas chromatography. The method of analysis required 10 mg of oil samples dissolved in 1 mL of toluene, followed by the addition of 0.2 mL of internal standard (5 µg/µL methyl nonadecanoate (Sigma–Aldrich, Melbourne, Australia) in toluene) and 0.2 mL (1 µg/µL 2,6-di-tert-butyl-4-methylphenol (butylated hydroxytoluene; BHT, Sigma–Aldrich) in toluene) as the antioxidant in each of the oil samples. Then, 2 mL of acidic methanol (prepared by adding 1 mL of acetyl chloride (Sigma–Aldrich) dropwise to 10 mL of methanol on ice) was added to each of the samples, mixed well, and incubated overnight at 50 °C in a sealed tube. The mixture in each of the tubes was cooled, and 5 mL of sodium chloride solution (5% *m*/*v*) was added. The fatty acid methyl esters were extracted twice with 5 mL of heptane, and the heptane layer was washed with 5 mL of potassium bicarbonate solution (2% *m*/*v*). The heptane layer was then dried over sodium sulfate, followed by rotary evaporation to remove hexane, and the samples were then taken for analysis [59,62].

The samples were analyzed using a previously reported method [63] with minor modifications. An Agilent 6890 gas chromatograph (GC) with a flame ionization detector (FID) (Agilent, Mulgrave, Australia), equipped with a BPX70 SGE column (30 m length × 0.25 mm column ID × 0.25 μm film thickness; Supelco, Sigma–Aldrich, Melbourne, Australia), was used to analyze the samples. The oven was set to run at a rate of 4 °C/min from 140 °C (5 min hold) to 220 °C (5 min hold) for a total run period of 30 min. Then, 1 μL of the sample solution was injected with a split ratio of 50:1 (injector temperature, 250 °C). Helium was employed as the carrier gas with a constant flow of 1.5 mL/min. The detector gases were 30 mL/min hydrogen, 400 mL/min air, and 30 mL/min nitrogen. ChemStation B.04.03 software was used to integrate the peak areas, which were corrected using theoretical relative FID response factors.

3.5. Positional Distribution of Omega-3 Fatty Acids in Lipase-Treated Squid Visceral Oil by ^{13}C-Nuclear Magnetic Resonance (NMR)

^{13}C NMR analysis was performed to determine the positional distribution of omega-3 fatty acids in lipase-treated squid visceral oil by following the previous method [64]. An oil sample (250 mg ± 0.01 mg) was dissolved in deuterated chloroform (600 μL) and transferred into an NMR tube (5 mm) for analysis. The ^{13}C NMR spectra were acquired using a Bruker 400 MHz instrument (Bruker, Avance III HD, Billerica, MA, USA), employing the following acquisition conditions: 12,000 scans, a spectral width of 238 ppm, and an acquisition time of 1.36 s. The DHA (C22:6 sn-2) peak was assigned at 172.0497 ppm, with other peaks in the carbonyl region referenced to the DHA sn-2 spectra [50]. The quantification of fatty acids in the carbonyl region was performed based on the area percentage of fatty acids obtained from the integrator response of the NMR spectra using TopSpin (version 4.3.0, Bruker).

3.6. Rancimat Test and Lipid Oxidation Kinetics

The oil samples were exposed at higher temperatures (80 °C, 90 °C, 110 °C, and 110 °C) in a saturated air flow of 20 L/h using Rancimat (743 model, Metrohm, Switzerland). The stability of the oil samples was expressed as an induction period (IP) in hours.

A kinetic rate constant (k) for lipid oxidation was assessed as an inverse of the induction period (k = 1/IP, h^{-1}). The activation energies (E_a, kJ/mol) and frequency factors (A, h^{-1}) for lipid oxidation in the oil samples were determined using the Arrhenius Equation (1), as shown below:

$$\ln(k) = \ln(A) - (E_a/RT), \quad (1)$$

where k is the kinetic rate constant (h^{-1}) and R is the molar gas constant (8.314 J/mol K). The activation enthalpies (ΔH) and entropies (ΔS) of lipid oxidation in the oil samples were calculated using the activated complex theory (Equation (2)), as shown below:

$$\ln(k/T) = \ln(k_B/h) + (\Delta S/R) - (\Delta H/RT), \quad (2)$$

where k_B is the Boltzmann constant (1.380×10^{-23} J/K) and h is the Planck's constant (6.63×10^{-34} J s). ΔH and ΔS were determined using the slope and intercept of Equation (2) [11].

3.7. Prediction of Shelf Life

The shelf life of the oil samples was predicted by plotting the natural logarithm of the induction period (IP) against the absolute temperature (K) using Equation (3):

$$\ln(IP) = a(T) + b, \quad (3)$$

where 'a' represents slope and 'b' indicates the intercept of Equation (3). The slope was used for the determination of the temperature coefficients ($T_{coeff.}$, K^{-1}). The temperature acceleration factor (Q_{10} number) was calculated using the ratio of the induction period (IP) at T and T + 10. The semi-logarithmic plots were extrapolated for calculating the shelf life at 25 °C.

3.8. Astaxanthin Quantification

Astaxanthin quantification (μg/g of lipid) in the oil samples was carried out using the method by Takeungwongtrakul and Benjakul [65], with minor modifications. A 0.3% (*w*/*v*) of the oil sample was mixed with petroleum ether and incubated at room temperature for 30 min. After appropriate dilution, the absorbance of the sample was measured at 468 nm using a Cary series UV-Vis spectrophotometer (Agilent Technologies, Mulgrave, Australia).

3.9. Statistical Analysis

The experiments were performed in duplicate (Rancimat, GC-FID, and NMR) or triplicate (all other tests) with data expressed as mean values ± standard deviation. Statistically significant differences between the datasets were evaluated ($p < 0.05$) using analysis of variance (ANOVA) carried out with the help of Minitab (Release 21.4.2. for Microsoft Windows) and Microsoft Excel software 2016. All graphs were drawn with Microsoft Excel software 2016.

4. Conclusions

An immobilized lipase-based process was successfully used at the pilot scale (200 L) to reduce the naturally occurring high levels of free fatty acid in squid visceral oil to produce acylglyceride-rich squid oil. The produced acylglyceride squid oil was rich in astaxanthin and the omega-3 fatty acids EPA and DHA, with EPA preferentially distributed at the sn-2 position and DHA predominantly retained at the naturally occurring sn-2 position, which generally improved bioavailability and stability. Since traditional colorimetric methods (PV and PAV methods) are not accurate for colored oils, including those containing astaxanthin, the Rancimat method was applied for investigating the oxidative stability of the squid visceral oil, which was compared with two commercial omega-3-rich oils. The kinetic and thermodynamic oxidation parameters were determined from the Rancimat data. The enzymatically processed high-acylglyceride product oil exhibited a much slower oxidation rate compared to the unprocessed input oil, commercial fish oil, and commercial calamari oil. This enhanced stability was attributed to both the retention of natural astaxanthin and lower FFA levels in the oil following enzymatic processing.

Some limitations of the current method include (a) challenges in obtaining high levels of triacylglyceride versus mono- and diacylglycerides and (b) difficulty in determining oil quality due to the presence of astaxanthin, which is colored and interferes with the standard PV and PAV colorimetric testing. For (a), it is necessary to remove water as it forms during the reaction to drive the reaction forward, since it is an equilibrium reaction. This is done using a high vacuum but becomes more challenging as the scale increases. Furthermore, the reaction requires the oil and water to remain in an emulsion during contact with the enzyme bed, which is more challenging as the scale increases. The presence of astaxanthin means that Rancimat is a better method for measuring stability than standard colorimetric methods. New and improved methods for detecting low levels of oxidation in colored oils are required for astaxanthin-containing oils.

Overall, this investigation shows that squid visceral oil can be converted to a relatively stable, low free fatty acid oil containing high natural levels of the antioxidant astaxanthin and omega-3 fatty acids, with retention of DHA positional distribution. The lower FFA and high astaxanthin and omega-3 levels, together with the high stability and natural DHA positional distribution retained at sn-2, make this oil an excellent nutritional oil with potential in nutritional supplements or functional foods.

Author Contributions: Conceptualization, A.J., B.H. and C.J.B.; methodology, A.J.; analysis, A.J.; investigation, A.J.; resources, M.S. and C.J.B.; data curation, A.J.; writing—original draft preparation, A.J., B.H. and C.J.B.; writing—review and editing, A.J, B.H., M.S. and C.J.B.; supervision, B.H., M.S. and C.J.B.; project administration, B.H., M.S. and C.J.B.; funding acquisition, M.S. and C.J.B. All authors have read and agreed to the published version of the manuscript.

Funding: This work was funded by the Australian Research Council Industrial Transformation Training Centre for Green Chemistry in Manufacturing project number IC190100034.

Institutional Review Board Statement: Not applicable.

Informed Consent Statement: Not applicable.

Data Availability Statement: Data will be provided upon request.

Acknowledgments: This work was supported by the Centre for Sustainable Bioproducts, Deakin University, Australia. Asavari Joshi acknowledges a PhD scholarship from the ARC Industrial Transformation Training Centre for Green Chemistry in Manufacturing at Deakin University.

Conflicts of Interest: Author Moninder Sachar was employed by the company Australian Omega Oils Pty Ltd. The remaining authors declare that the research was conducted in the absence of any commercial or financial relationships that could be construed as a potential conflict of interest.

References

1. Moovendhan, M.; Seedevi, P.; Vairamani, S.; Shanmugam, A. Exploring the chemical composition and anticancer potential of oil from squid (*Loligo duvauceli*) liver waste from fish processing industry. *Waste Biomass Valorization* **2019**, *10*, 2967–2973. [CrossRef]
2. Cho, S.-Y.; Joo, D.-S.; Choi, H.-G.; Nara, E.; Miyashita, K. Oxidative stability of lipids from squid tissues. *Fish. Sci.* **2001**, *67*, 738–743. [CrossRef]
3. Kaushik, P.; Dowling, K.; Barrow, C.J.; Adhikari, B. Microencapsulation of omega-3 fatty acids: A review of microencapsulation and characterization methods. *J. Funct. Foods* **2015**, *19*, 868–881. [CrossRef]
4. Jain, P.; Mandal, S.; Minhas, A.K.; Puri, M.; Barrow, C.J. Concentrating omega-3 fatty acids in Nannochloropsis oceanica oil by using enzyme immobilized nano-silica systems. *J. Clean. Prod.* **2023**, *406*, 137030. [CrossRef]
5. Xuan, J.; Xia, Q.; Tu, Y.; Luo, T.; Mao, Q.; Han, Z.; Barrow, C.J.; Liu, S.; Wang, B. Effect of enzymatically produced tuna oil acylglycerol on the characteristics of gelatin O/W emulsion during microencapsulation using complex coacervation. *LWT* **2023**, *190*, 115580. [CrossRef]
6. Wang, J.; Han, L.; Wang, D.; Sun, Y.; Huang, J.; Shahidi, F. Stability and stabilization of omega-3 oils: A review. *Trends Food Sci. Technol.* **2021**, *118*, 17–35. [CrossRef]
7. Jacobsen, C.; García-Moreno, P.J.; Yesiltas, B.; Sørensen, A.-D.M. Lipid oxidation and traditional methods for evaluation. In *Omega-3 Delivery Systems*; Elsevier: Amsterdam, The Netherlands, 2021; pp. 183–200.
8. Albert, B.B.; Cameron-Smith, D.; Hofman, P.L.; Cutfield, W.S. Oxidation of marine omega-3 supplements and human health. *BioMed Res. Int.* **2013**, *2013*, 464921. [CrossRef] [PubMed]
9. Du, Q.; Zhou, L.; Li, M.; Lyu, F.; Liu, J.; Ding, Y. Omega-3 polyunsaturated fatty acid encapsulation system: Physical and oxidative stability, and medical applications. *Food Front.* **2022**, *3*, 239–255. [CrossRef]
10. Kolanowski, W.; Jaworska, D.; Weißbrodt, J. Importance of instrumental and sensory analysis in the assessment of oxidative deterioration of omega-3 long-chain polyunsaturated fatty acid-rich foods. *J. Sci. Food Agric.* **2007**, *87*, 181–191. [CrossRef]
11. Nogueira, M.S.; Scolaro, B.; Milne, G.L.; Castro, I.A. Oxidation products from omega-3 and omega-6 fatty acids during a simulated shelf life of edible oils. *LWT* **2019**, *101*, 113–122. [CrossRef]
12. Yenipazar, H.; Şahin-Yeşilçubuk, N. Effect of packaging and encapsulation on the oxidative and sensory stability of omega-3 supplements. *Food Sci. Nutr.* **2023**, *11*, 1426–1440. [CrossRef] [PubMed]
13. Li, D.; Liu, P.; Wang, W.; Yang, B.; Ou, S.; Wang, Y. An efficient upgrading approach to produce n-3 polyunsaturated fatty acids-rich edible grade oil from high-acid squid visceral oil. *Biochem. Eng. J.* **2017**, *127*, 167–174. [CrossRef]
14. Lin, C.-C.; Hwang, L.S. A comparison of the effects of various purification treatments on the oxidative stability of squid visceral oil. *J. Am. Oil Chem. Soc.* **2002**, *79*, 489–494. [CrossRef]

15. Scurria, A.; Fabiano Tixier, A.-S.; Lino, C.; Pagliaro, M.; D'Agostino, F.; Avellone, G.; Chemat, F.; Ciriminna, R. High yields of shrimp oil rich in omega-3 and natural astaxanthin from shrimp waste. *ACS Omega* **2020**, *5*, 17500–17505. [CrossRef]
16. Phadtare, I.; Vaidya, H.; Hawboldt, K.; Cheema, S.K. Shrimp oil extracted from shrimp processing by-product is a rich source of omega-3 fatty acids and astaxanthin-esters, and reveals potential anti-adipogenic effects in 3T3-L1 adipocytes. *Mar. Drugs* **2021**, *19*, 259. [CrossRef] [PubMed]
17. Calvo, N.S.; Reynoso, C.M.; Resnik, S.; Cortés-Jacinto, E.; Collins, P. Thermal stability of astaxanthin in oils for its use in fish food technology. *Anim. Feed Sci. Technol.* **2020**, *270*, 114668. [CrossRef]
18. Barros, M.P.; Poppe, S.C.; Bondan, E.F. Neuroprotective properties of the marine carotenoid astaxanthin and omega-3 fatty acids, and perspectives for the natural combination of both in krill oil. *Nutrients* **2014**, *6*, 1293–1317. [CrossRef]
19. Aneesh, P.; Ajeeshkumar, K.; Lekshmi, R.K.; Anandan, R.; Ravishankar, C.; Mathew, S. Bioactivities of astaxanthin from natural sources, augmenting its biomedical potential: A review. *Trends Food Sci. Technol.* **2022**, *125*, 81–90. [CrossRef]
20. Aneesh, P.; Anandan, R.; Kumar, L.R.; Ajeeshkumar, K.; Kumar, K.A.; Mathew, S. A step to shell biorefinery—Extraction of astaxanthin-rich oil, protein, chitin, and chitosan from shrimp processing waste. *Biomass Convers. Biorefinery* **2023**, *13*, 205–214. [CrossRef]
21. Rajasekaran, B.; Gulzar, S.; Gopalrajan, S.; Karunanithi, M.; Benjakul, S. Omega-3 Enriched Fish and Shellfish Oils: Extraction, Preservation, and Health Benefits. In *Fish Waste to Valuable Products*; Springer: Berlin/Heidelberg, Germany, 2024; pp. 195–229.
22. Tizkar, B.; Seidavi, A.; Ponce-Palafox, J.T.; Pourashoor, P. The effect of astaxanthin on resistance of juvenile prawns Macrobrachium nipponense (Decapoda: Palaemonidae) to physical and chemical stress. *Rev. Biol. Ía Trop.* **2014**, *62*, 1331–1341. [CrossRef] [PubMed]
23. Dhankhar, J.; Kadian, S.S.; Sharma, A. Astaxanthin: A potential carotenoid. *Int. J. Pharm. Sci. Res.* **2012**, *3*, 1246.
24. Miki, W. Biological functions and activities of animal carotenoids. *Pure Appl. Chem.* **1991**, *63*, 141–146. [CrossRef]
25. Yamashita, E. Let astaxanthin be thy medicine. *PharmaNutrition* **2015**, *3*, 115–122. [CrossRef]
26. Nishida, Y.; Berg, P.C.; Shakersain, B.; Hecht, K.; Takikawa, A.; Tao, R.; Kakuta, Y.; Uragami, C.; Hashimoto, H.; Misawa, N. Astaxanthin: Past, present, and future. *Mar. Drugs* **2023**, *21*, 514. [CrossRef] [PubMed]
27. Saw, C.L.L.; Yang, A.Y.; Guo, Y.; Kong, A.-N.T. Astaxanthin and omega-3 fatty acids individually and in combination protect against oxidative stress via the Nrf2–ARE pathway. *Food Chem. Toxicol.* **2013**, *62*, 869–875. [CrossRef] [PubMed]
28. Jiang, X.; Pan, K.; Yang, Y.; Shu-Chien, A.C.; Wu, X. Dietary DHA oil supplementation promotes ovarian development and astaxanthin deposition during the ovarian maturation of Chinese mitten crab Eriocheir sinensis. *Aquac. Nutr.* **2022**, *2022*, 9997317. [CrossRef]
29. Zhang, L.; Zhang, R.; Jiang, X.; Wu, X.; Wang, X. Dietary supplementation with synthetic astaxanthin and DHA interactively regulates physiological metabolism to improve the color and odor quality of ovaries in adult female Eriocheir sinensis. *Food Chem.* **2024**, *430*, 137020. [CrossRef] [PubMed]
30. Wang, H.; He, W.; Dansou, D.M.; Zhang, H.; Nugroho, R.D.; Tang, C.; Guo, X.; Yu, Y.; Zhao, Q.; Qin, Y. Astaxanthin improved the storage stability of docosahexaenoic acid-enriched eggs by inhibiting oxidation of non-esterified poly-unsaturated fatty acids. *Food Chem.* **2022**, *381*, 132256. [CrossRef]
31. Spotti, M.L.; Acosta, C.A.; Carrara, C.R.; Fioramonti, S.A. Influence of storage temperature and natural antioxidants addition on chia oil nutraceutical blends shelf life. *Eur. J. Lipid Sci. Technol.* **2024**, *126*, 2300179. [CrossRef]
32. Espinaco, B.Y.; Niizawa, I.; Marino, F.; Zorrilla, S.E.; Sihufe, G.A. Storage stability of chia (*Salvia hispanica* L.) oil incorporated with astaxanthin. *J. Food Process. Preserv.* **2021**, *45*, e15184. [CrossRef]
33. Colletti, A.; Cravotto, G.; Citi, V.; Martelli, A.; Testai, L.; Cicero, A.F. Advances in technologies for highly active omega-3 fatty acids from krill oil: Clinical applications. *Mar. Drugs* **2021**, *19*, 306. [CrossRef] [PubMed]
34. Symoniuk, E.; Łapińska, A.; Ratusz, K.; Wroniak, M. Influence of the Rancimat Apparatus Operating Parameters on Oxidative Stability Determination of Cold-Pressed Camelina and Hemp Seed Oil. *Eur. J. Lipid Sci. Technol.* **2023**, *125*, 2200062. [CrossRef]
35. Gülmez, Ö.; Şahin, S. Evaluation of oxidative stability in hazelnut oil treated with several antioxidants: Kinetics and thermodynamics studies. *LWT* **2019**, *111*, 478–483. [CrossRef]
36. Ghosh, M.; Upadhyay, R.; Mahato, D.K.; Mishra, H.N. Kinetics of lipid oxidation in omega fatty acids rich blends of sunflower and sesame oils using Rancimat. *Food Chem.* **2019**, *272*, 471–477. [CrossRef] [PubMed]
37. Farhoosh, R.; Niazmand, R.; Rezaei, M.; Sarabi, M. Kinetic parameter determination of vegetable oil oxidation under Rancimat test conditions. *Eur. J. Lipid Sci. Technol.* **2008**, *110*, 587–592. [CrossRef]
38. Farhoosh, R.; Hoseini-Yazdi, S.Z. Evolution of oxidative values during kinetic studies on olive oil oxidation in the Rancimat test. *J. Am. Oil Chem. Soc.* **2014**, *91*, 281–293. [CrossRef]
39. Yang, K.-M.; Chiang, P.-Y. Variation quality and kinetic parameter of commercial n-3 PUFA-rich oil during oxidation via Rancimat. *Mar. Drugs* **2017**, *15*, 97. [CrossRef]
40. Méndez, E.; Sanhueza, J.; Speisky, H.; Valenzuela, A. Validation of the Rancimat test for the assessment of the relative stability of fish oils. *J. Am. Oil Chem. Soc.* **1996**, *73*, 1033–1037. [CrossRef]

41. Pazhouhanmehr, S.; Farhoosh, R.; Sharif, A.; Kenari, R.E. Oxidation kinetics of common Kilka (*Clupeonella cultiventris* caspia) oil in presence of bene oils' unsaponifiable matter. *Food Chem.* **2016**, *190*, 748–754. [CrossRef] [PubMed]
42. Yeşilsu, A.F.; Özyurt, G. Oxidative stability of microencapsulated fish oil with rosemary, thyme and laurel extracts: A kinetic assessment. *J. Food Eng.* **2019**, *240*, 171–182. [CrossRef]
43. Shen, Y.; Guo, C.; Lu, T.; Ding, X.-Y.; Zhao, M.-T.; Zhang, M.; Liu, H.-L.; Song, L.; Zhou, D.-Y. Effects of gallic acid alkyl esters and their combinations with other antioxidants on oxidative stability of DHA algae oil. *Food Res. Int.* **2021**, *143*, 110280. [CrossRef] [PubMed]
44. Haque, M.A.; Akanbi, T.O.; Holland, B.J.; Sachar, M.; Barrow, C.J. Sustainable Enzymatic Production of Omega-3 Oil from Squid Viscera. *Sustainability* **2024**, *16*, 4243. [CrossRef]
45. Yang, Z.; Jin, W.; Cheng, X.; Dong, Z.; Chang, M.; Wang, X. *Enzymatic enrichment* of n-3 polyunsaturated fatty acid glycerides by selective hydrolysis. *Food Chem.* **2021**, *346*, 128743. [CrossRef] [PubMed]
46. Yan, J.; Liu, M.; Yang, D.; Zhang, Y.; An, F. Efficacy and safety of omega-3 fatty acids in the prevention of cardiovascular disease: A systematic review and meta-analysis. *Cardiovasc. Drugs Ther.* **2024**, *38*, 799–817. [CrossRef]
47. von der Haar, D.; Stäbler, A.; Wichmann, R.; Schweiggert-Weisz, U. Enzymatic esterification of free fatty acids in vegetable oils utilizing different immobilized lipases. *Biotechnol. Lett.* **2015**, *37*, 169–174. [CrossRef]
48. Zhang, H.; Zhao, H.; Zhang, Y.; Shen, Y.; Su, H.; Jin, J.; Jin, Q.; Wang, X. Characterization of Positional Distribution of Fatty Acids and Triacylglycerol Molecular Compositions of Marine Fish Oils Rich in Omega-3 Polyunsaturated Fatty Acids. *BioMed Res. Int.* **2018**, *2018*, 3529682. [CrossRef] [PubMed]
49. Yalagala, P.R.; Sugasini, D.; Dasarathi, S.; Pahan, K.; Subbaiah, P.V. Dietary lysophosphatidylcholine-EPA enriches both EPA and DHA in the brain: Potential treatment for depression [S]. *J. Lipid Res.* **2019**, *60*, 566–578. [CrossRef] [PubMed]
50. Tengku-Rozaina, T.M.; Birch, E.J. Positional distribution of fatty acids on hoki and tuna oil triglycerides by pancreatic lipase and 13C NMR analysis. *Eur. J. Lipid Sci. Technol.* **2014**, *116*, 272–281. [CrossRef]
51. Akanbi, T.O.; Barrow, C.J. Lipase-catalysed incorporation of EPA into emu oil: Formation and characterisation of new structured lipids. *J. Funct. Foods* **2015**, *19*, 801–809. [CrossRef]
52. Lee-Chang, K.J.; Taylor, M.C.; Drummond, G.; Mulder, R.J.; Mansour, M.P.; Brock, M.; Nichols, P.D. Docosahexaenoic acid is naturally concentrated at the sn-2 position in triacylglycerols of the Australian thraustochytrid *Aurantiochytrium* sp. strain TC 20. *Mar. Drugs* **2021**, *19*, 382. [CrossRef] [PubMed]
53. Ando, Y.; Samoto, H.; Murayama, Y. Positional distribution of DHA and EPA in triacyl-sn-glycerols (TAG) of Artemia franciscana nauplii enriched with fish oils ethyl esters and TAG. *Aquaculture* **2004**, *233*, 321–335. [CrossRef]
54. Ikeda, I.; Yoshida, H.; Tomooka, M.; Yosef, A.; Imaizumi, K.; Tsuji, H.; Seto, A. Effects of long-term feeding of marine oils with different positional distribution of eicosapentaenoic and docosahexaenoic acids on lipid metabolism, eicosanoid production, and platelet aggregation in hypercholesterolemic rats. *Lipids* **1998**, *33*, 897–904. [CrossRef]
55. Dovale-Rosabal, G.; Rodríguez, A.; Espinosa, A.; Barriga, A.; Aubourg, S.P. Synthesis of EPA-and DHA-enriched structured acylglycerols at the sn-2 position starting from commercial salmon oil by enzymatic lipase catalysis under supercritical conditions. *Molecules* **2021**, *26*, 3094. [CrossRef] [PubMed]
56. Upadhyay, R.; Mishra, H.N. Multivariate optimization of a synergistic blend of oleoresin sage (*Salvia officinalis* L.) and ascorbyl palmitate to stabilize sunflower oil. *J. Food Sci. Technol.* **2016**, *53*, 1919–1928. [CrossRef]
57. Roy, V.C.; Getachew, A.T.; Cho, Y.-J.; Park, J.-S.; Chun, B.-S. Recovery and bio-potentialities of astaxanthin-rich oil from shrimp (Penaeus monodon) waste and mackerel (*Scomberomous niphonius*) skin using concurrent supercritical CO_2 extraction. *J. Supercrit. Fluids* **2020**, *159*, 104773. [CrossRef]
58. Liu, X.; Luo, Q.; Rakariyatham, K.; Cao, Y.; Goulette, T.; Liu, X.; Xiao, H. Antioxidation and anti-ageing activities of different stereoisomeric astaxanthin in vitro and in vivo. *J. Funct. Foods* **2016**, *25*, 50–61. [CrossRef]
59. Akanbi, T.O.; Adcock, J.L.; Barrow, C.J. Selective concentration of EPA and DHA using Thermomyces lanuginosus lipase is due to fatty acid selectivity and not regioselectivity. *Food Chem.* **2013**, *138*, 615–620. [CrossRef] [PubMed]
60. Wang, L.; Yang, B.; Yan, B.; Yao, X. Supercritical fluid extraction of astaxanthin from Haematococcus pluvialis and its antioxidant potential in sunflower oil. *Innov. Food Sci. Emerg. Technol.* **2012**, *13*, 120–127. [CrossRef]
61. Hernandez, E.M. Specialty oils: Functional and nutraceutical properties. *Funct. Diet. Lipids* **2016**, 69–101. [CrossRef]
62. Thyagarajan, T. Fermentation of Omega-3 and Carotenoid Producing Marine Microorganisms. Ph.D. Dissertation, Deakin University, Geelong, Australia, 2015.
63. Ackman, R.G. The gas chromatograph in practical analyses of common and uncommon fatty acids for the 21st century. *Anal. Chim. Acta* **2002**, *465*, 175–192. [CrossRef]

64. Ahmmed, M.K.; Ahmmed, F.; Stewart, I.; Carne, A.; Tian, H.S.; Bekhit, A.E.-D.A. Omega-3 phospholipids in Pacific blue mackerel (*Scomber australasicus*) processing by-products. *Food Chem.* **2021**, *353*, 129451. [CrossRef] [PubMed]
65. Takeungwongtrakul, S.; Benjakul, S. Astaxanthin degradation and lipid oxidation of Pacific white shrimp oil: Kinetics study and stability as affected by storage conditions. *Int. Aquat. Res.* **2016**, *8*, 15–27. [CrossRef]

marine drugs

MDPI

Article

Proteomics Analysis of the Protective Effect of Polydeoxyribonucleotide Extracted from Sea Cucumber (*Apostichopus japonicus*) Sperm in a Hydrogen Peroxide-Induced RAW264.7 Cell Injury Model

Zhiqiang Shu [1,2,†], Yizhi Ji [1,2,†], Fang Liu [2,3], Yuexin Jing [2,3], Chunna Jiao [2,3], Yue Li [1,2], Yunping Zhao [2,3], Gongming Wang [2,3,*] and Jian Zhang [2,3,*]

1 Department of Food Science and Technology, Shanghai Ocean University, Shanghai 200120, China; s13970318519@163.com (Z.S.)
2 Shandong Marine Resource and Environment Research Institute, Yantai 264006, China
3 Yantai Key Laboratory of Quality and Safety Control and Deep Processing of Marine Food, Yantai 264006, China
* Correspondence: wgmsd105@163.com (G.W.); zjsd408@163.com (J.Z.)
† These authors contributed equally to this work.

Abstract: Sea cucumber viscera contain various naturally occurring active substances, but they are often underutilized during sea cucumber processing. Polydeoxyribonucleotide (PDRN) is an adenosine A_{2A} receptor agonist that activates the A_{2A} receptor to produce various biological effects. Currently, most studies on the activity of PDRN have focused on its anti-inflammatory, anti-apoptotic, and tissue repair properties, yet relatively few studies have investigated its antioxidant activity. In this study, we reported for the first time that PDRN was extracted from the sperm of *Apostichopus japonicus* (AJS-PDRN), and we evaluated its antioxidant activity using 2,2-diphenyl-1-picrylhydrazyl (DPPH), 2,2′-azino-bis-3-ethylbenzothiazoline-6-sulphonic acid (ABTS), and hydroxyl radical scavenging assays. An in vitro injury model was established using H_2O_2-induced oxidative damage in RAW264.7 cells, and we investigated the protective effect of AJS-PDRN on these cells. Additionally, we explored the potential mechanism by which AJS-PDRN protects RAW264.7 cells from damage using iTRAQ proteomics analysis. The results showed that AJS-PDRN possessed excellent antioxidant activity and could significantly scavenge DPPH, ABTS, and hydroxyl radicals. In vitro antioxidant assays demonstrated that AJS-PDRN was cytoprotective and significantly enhanced the antioxidant capacity of RAW264.7 cells. The results of GO enrichment and KEGG pathway analysis indicate that the protective effects of AJS-PDRN pretreatment on RAW264.7 cells are primarily achieved through the regulation of immune and inflammatory responses, modulation of the extracellular matrix and signal transduction pathways, promotion of membrane repair, and enhancement of cellular antioxidant capacity. The results of a protein–protein interaction (PPI) network analysis indicate that AJS-PDRN reduces cellular oxidative damage by upregulating the expression of intracellular selenoprotein family members. In summary, our findings reveal that AJS-PDRN mitigates H_2O_2-induced oxidative damage through multiple pathways, underscoring its significant potential in the prevention and treatment of diseases caused by oxidative stress.

Keywords: sea cucumber sperm; polydeoxyribonucleotide; antioxidant; proteomics; RAW264.7 cell; oxidative stress

1. Introduction

Sea cucumbers, which are classified within the phylum Echinodermata and the class Holothuroidea, have long been recognized as a traditional nutritious food in China and other Asian countries. Currently, more than 1700 species of sea cucumbers have been identified worldwide, with the majority found in temperate and tropical regions. The Asia–Pacific region, in particular, boasts the greatest diversity and abundance of sea cucumber species and resources [1]. In recent years, sea cucumbers have received significant attention as a valuable source for drug development. This is due to their rich composition of unique bioactive substances, including polysaccharides, saponins, lipids, peptides, and others [2]. These active ingredients have important physiological functions in the human body. For example, sea cucumber polysaccharides have various biological benefits such as antitumor [3], antioxidant [4], and anticoagulant activities [5]. Small molecule peptides extracted from sea cucumbers demonstrate antidiabetic [6], enhancing immunity [7], anticancer [8], and antibacterial functions [9]. Sea cucumber saponins have various physiological benefits such as antitumor [10], anti-Parkinson's disease [11], and immune regulation functions [12]. Therefore, sea cucumbers, as a precious marine food, have great potential in promoting drug research and development.

Under normal physiological conditions, the body has an antioxidant defense system that helps maintain a balance between the generation and elimination of free radicals. However, when this balance is disrupted, excessive free radicals can cause cellular damage, leading to oxidative stress. This oxidative stress can result in dysfunction and lesions within the body [13,14]. Numerous studies have shown that oxidative stress is commonly associated with the pathogenesis of diseases such as aging, diabetes, cancer, ischemia–reperfusion injury, and atherosclerosis [15–17]. Therefore, it is crucial to intake sufficient antioxidants to prevent or mitigate oxidative stress induced by free radicals for maintaining normal physiological functions and reducing the occurrence of diseases. However, research has indicated that some commonly used synthetic antioxidants, such as tert-butylhydroquinone (TBHQ), butyl hydroxyanisole (BHA), and propyl gallate (PG), tend to be toxic and carcinogenic [18]. As a result, the search for safe and effective natural antioxidants has become a prominent focus in antioxidant research in recent years.

Polydeoxyribonucleotide is a mixture of nucleotides with molecular weights ranging from 50 to 1500 kDa [19]. Currently, PDRN is primarily derived from the human placenta, salmon sperm, and trout sperm [20]. Research has shown that PDRN is an adenosine A_{2A} receptor agonist, which exerts antioxidant activity by activating the Keap1-Nrf2/HO-1 pathway, thereby increasing the activity of endogenous antioxidant enzymes and promoting the clearance of free radicals [21]. Additionally, PDRN exhibits various biological activities, including anti-inflammatory and anti-apoptotic effects, the promotion of angiogenesis, and the facilitation of tissue repair [22].

Proteomics is a powerful analytical technology that detects the structure, function, and content of all proteins in organisms at the molecular level. It has been widely used in studying the antioxidant mechanisms of various natural active substances [23,24]. To investigate the antioxidant effects of specific active compounds or drugs, RAW264.7 macrophages are often used as an in vitro model. This study evaluated the in vitro antioxidant capacity of AJS-PDRN through DPPH, ABTS, and hydroxyl radical scavenging tests. We used H_2O_2 to induce oxidative damage in RAW264.7 cells to establish an in vitro oxidative damage model. By measuring the survival rate and biomarker content of RAW264.7 cells under different treatment conditions, we investigated the protective effect of AJS-PDRN on the oxidative damage model. Additionally, proteomic analysis was performed using isobaric tags for relative and absolute quantification (iTRAQ) to elucidate the specific mechanisms through which AJS-PDRN exerts its protective effect and prevents RAW264.7 cell damage.

2. Results

2.1. In Vitro Antioxidant Experiment of AJS-PDRN

DPPH, ABTS, and hydroxyl radical scavenging assays were used to assess the antioxidant capacity of AJS-PDRN. The same concentration of vitamin C (VC) was chosen as a control, and the results are shown in Figure 1.

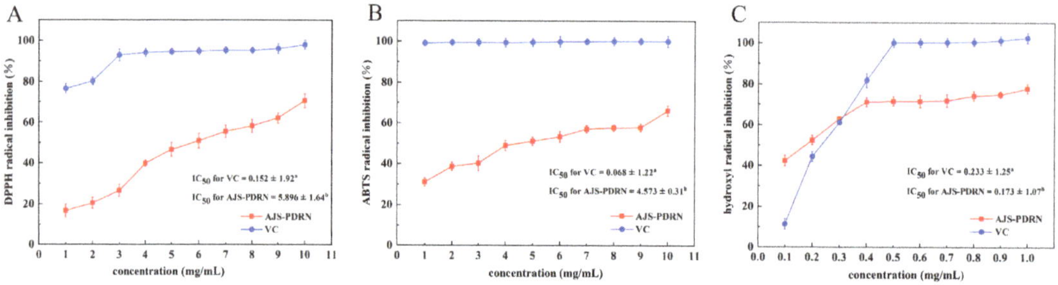

Figure 1. AJS-PDRN scavenging assays for DPPH, ABTS, and hydroxyl radicals. (**A**) AJS-PDRN scavenging assay of DPPH radicals; (**B**) AJS-PDRN scavenging assay of ABTS radicals; and (**C**) AJS-PDRN scavenging assay of hydroxyl radicals. ^{a,b} IC_{50} data with different alphabets show significantly different values ($p < 0.05$).

As the concentration of AJS-PDRN increases, there is a corresponding increase in the scavenging rate of DPPH radicals (Figure 1A). Specifically, at a concentration of 10 mg/mL, the DPPH radical scavenging rate reaches 70.6%, representing a 53.92% increase compared to a concentration of 1 mg/mL. Furthermore, the IC_{50} values of AJS-PDRN and VC for scavenging DPPH radicals are 5.896 ± 1.64 mg/mL and 0.152 ± 1.92 mg/mL, respectively. Similarly, the ability of AJS-PDRN to scavenge ABTS radicals increases with higher concentrations (Figure 1B). At a concentration of 10 mg/mL, the scavenging rate of ABTS radicals by AJS-PDRN is 66.2%, indicating a 35.0% increase compared to 1 mg/mL. The IC_{50} values of AJS-PDRN and VC for scavenging ABTS radicals are 4.573 ± 0.31 mg/mL and 0.068 ± 1.22 mg/mL, respectively. In the hydroxyl radical scavenging assay, a similar trend was observed. As the concentration of AJS-PDRN increased, its ability to scavenge hydroxyl radicals also increased (Figure 1C). The IC_{50} values for hydroxyl radical scavenging by AJS-PDRN and VC were 0.173 ± 1.07 mg/mL and 0.233 ± 1.25 mg/mL, respectively. In general, the lower the IC_{50} value of a natural antioxidant, the stronger its inhibitory activity. Therefore, AJS-PDRN exhibited a stronger inhibitory effect on hydroxyl radicals than VC, indicating a highly potent hydroxyl radical scavenging activity. However, its inhibitory capacity for DPPH and ABTS radicals was moderate. We speculate that this may be related to the chemical structure of AJS-PDRN. DPPH and ABTS are relatively stable radicals, and their scavenging mechanisms primarily rely on the hydrogen-donating ability of the antioxidant [25]. In contrast, hydroxyl radicals are highly reactive and unstable, and scavenging them usually requires antioxidants with high electron-donating capacity and rapid reactivity [26]. Overall, the total antioxidant activity of AJS-PDRN was lower than that of VC. Compared to other identified natural antioxidants, AJS-PDRN demonstrated stronger hydroxyl radical inhibitory activity than the polysaccharide PPP-2 extracted from persimmon peels (IC_{50}: 4.08 mg/mL) [27]. Similarly, AJS-PDRN exhibited greater radical scavenging activity compared to PDRN extracted from salmon sperm [28]. In summary, the results of the three assays indicated that within a specific concentration range, the radical scavenging ability of AJS-PDRN showed a dose-dependent increase, demonstrating significant antioxidant activity.

2.2. *Protective Effect of AJS-PDRN on H_2O_2-Induced RAW264.7 Cell Injury Model*

2.2.1. Effect of AJS-PDRN on RAW264.7 Cell Viability

Hydrogen peroxide can induce various oxidative stresses in cells. By treating cells with exogenous hydrogen peroxide to induce oxidative damage, researchers can investigate the protective effects of active substances on cells. However, higher doses often cause cell death [29]. The cell survival rate is the most intuitive indicator reflecting the degree of cell damage and death caused by external redox imbalances. Therefore, it is a crucial indicator for establishing an oxidative stress model [30]. As shown in Figure 2A, within the concentration range of 100–600 μmol/L, there is a negative correlation between H_2O_2 concentration and cell survival rate. At an H_2O_2 concentration of 400 μmol/L, the cell survival rate is 52 ± 1.8%, meeting the standard for an oxidative damage model (50–70% cell survival rate). Therefore, 400 μmol/L was chosen as the optimal concentration to induce the damage model.

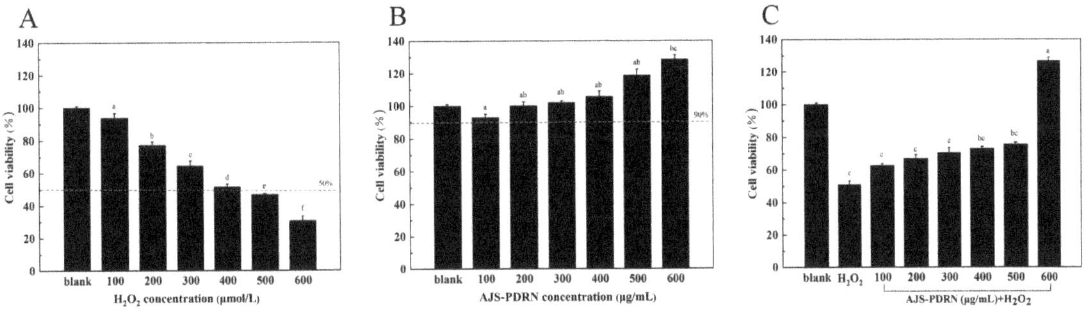

Figure 2. Effects of AJS-PDRN on RAW264.7 cell viability with/without H_2O_2 induction. (**A**) Cells treated with the indicated concentrations of H_2O_2 for 4 h; (**B**) cells treated with the indicated concentrations of AJS-PDRN for 6 h; and (**C**) cells pretreated with the indicated concentrations of AJS-PDRN for 6 h and then stimulated with 400 μM H_2O_2 for 4 h. The results are presented as the mean ± SD of three replicates. Different letters at the top of the columns indicate statistically significant differences.

Following treatment of RAW264.7 cells with varying concentrations (100–600 μg/mL) of AJS-PDRN for 6 h, the survival rate of the cells was above 90%, which indicated that AJS-PDRN was essentially non-toxic to the cells in this range. At a concentration of 200 μg/mL or higher, the survival rate of RAW264.7 cells exceeded 100%, suggesting that AJS-PDRN promotes cell proliferation (Figure 2B).

By determining the effects of different concentrations of AJS-PDRN pretreatment on the viability of RAW264.7 cells induced by H_2O_2, we observed that AJS-PDRN had a significant protective effect on damaged cells in the selected concentration range (100–600 μg/mL). As depicted in Figure 2C, following treatment with 400 μmol/L H_2O_2, the cell survival rate was 52.0 ± 3.6% of the normal control. Pretreatment of oxidatively damaged RAW264.7 cells with different concentrations of AJS-PDRN significantly increased cell survival. At a concentration of 600 μg/mL, the cell survival rate reached 126.8%. Their results indicate that AJS-PDRN could protect the cells from oxidative damage and thus improve cell viability.

2.2.2. Oxidative Stress Biomarker Levels in RAW264.7 Cells

To evaluate the antioxidant effect of AJS-PDRN on H_2O_2-induced RAW264.7 cell injury, cells cultured in blank, H_2O_2, and AJS-PDRN groups were collected, and the levels of antioxidant indexes, such as superoxide dismutase (SOD), catalase (CAT), glutathione (GSH), and malondialdehyde (MDA), were determined in cells of each group. The results are shown in Figure 3.

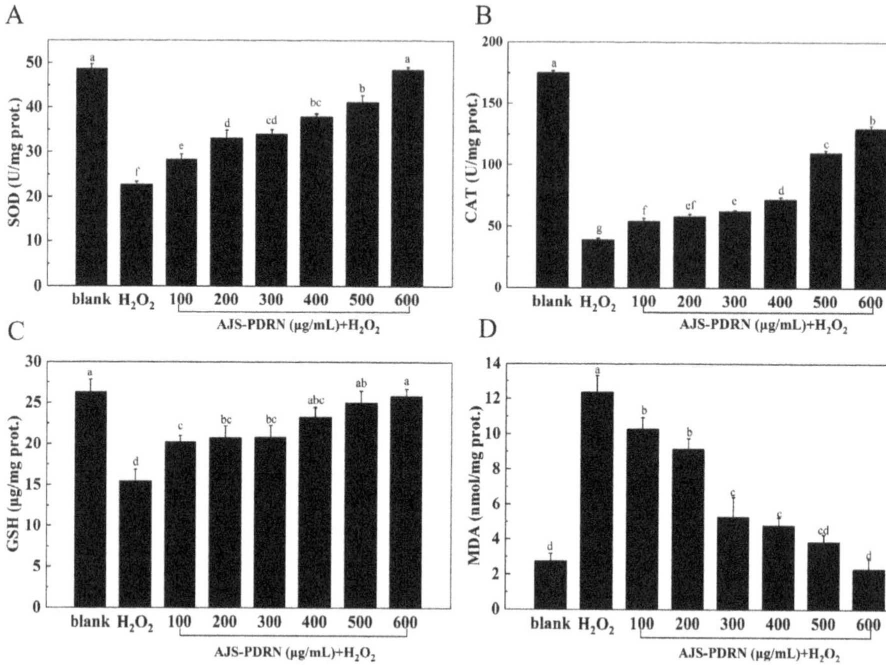

Figure 3. Effects of AJS-PDRN on the levels of oxidative stress biomarkers in H_2O_2-induced RAW264.7 cells. (**A**) SOD activity; (**B**) CAT activity; (**C**) GSH content; and (**D**) MDA content. The results are presented as the mean ± SD of three replicates. Different letters at the top of the columns indicate statistically significant differences.

SOD is one of the most effective intracellular enzymes that scavenges superoxide anions ($O_2^{\bullet-}$) free radicals and H_2O_2. This enzyme reduces oxidative damage and cytotoxicity, thus alleviating intracellular oxidative stress [31]. As shown in Figure 3A, the SOD content in the H_2O_2 group was significantly lower than in the normal group, indicating that H_2O_2 damaged RAW264.7 cells and reduced SOD activity. Compared to the H_2O_2 group, the intracellular SOD content significantly increased after pretreatment with AJS-PDRN. Additionally, as the concentration of AJS-PDRN increased, the intracellular SOD content proportionally increased. At an AJS-PDRN concentration of 600 μg/mL, the intracellular SOD content increased by 53.18% compared to the H_2O_2 group. This indicates that AJS-PDRN can enhance the SOD activity in RAW264.7 cells, protect them from H_2O_2 damage, and strengthen the cellular antioxidant system.

CAT maintains the body's redox balance by scavenging excess free radicals and catalyzing the decomposition of H_2O_2 into H_2O and O_2 [32]. As shown in Figure 3B, the CAT content in the H_2O_2 group was significantly lower than that in the blank group, indicating that H_2O_2 damaged RAW264.7 cells and reduced CAT activity. Compared to the H_2O_2 group, the intracellular CAT content significantly increased after pretreatment with AJS-PDRN. Moreover, as the concentration of AJS-PDRN increased, the intracellular CAT content also increased. At an AJS-PDRN concentration of 600 μg/mL, the intracellular CAT content increased by 69.77% compared to the H_2O_2 group. This demonstrates that AJS-PDRN can enhance the CAT activity in RAW264.7 cells and protect them against H_2O_2-induced damage.

GSH is an endogenous antioxidant that effectively eliminates lipid peroxides in the body [33]. As shown in Figure 3C, the GSH content in the H_2O_2 group was significantly lower than in the blank group, indicating that H_2O_2 damaged RAW264.7 cells and reduced GSH content. Compared to the H_2O_2 group, the intracellular GSH content significantly increased after pretreatment with AJS-PDRN. Additionally, as the concentration of AJS-PDRN increased, the intracellular GSH content also increased. At an AJS-PDRN concentration of 600 μg/mL, the intracellular GSH content increased by 38.76% compared to the H_2O_2 group. This demonstrates that AJS-PDRN can enhance GSH content in RAW264.7 cells and protect them from H_2O_2-induced damage.

MDA is a product of lipid peroxidation caused by oxidative stress. It reacts with biological macromolecules, causing cytotoxicity and serving as an indicator of the body's peroxidation levels [34]. As shown in Figure 3D, the MDA content in RAW264.7 cells was significantly higher in the H_2O_2 group. In comparison to the H_2O_2 group, the MDA levels in RAW264.7 cells pretreated with AJS-PDRN were significantly reduced, gradually returning to the level of the normal group with increasing AJS-PDRN concentration. Therefore, AJS-PDRN can reduce the lipid peroxidation caused by H_2O_2 and exert antioxidant activity.

2.3. *Effect of AJS-PDRN on Protein Expression Profiles in RAW264.7 Cells Induced by H_2O_2*

2.3.1. Screening of Differentially Expressed Proteins

To investigate the protective effects of AJS-PDRN against oxidative stress-induced damage in RAW264.7 cells, we conducted a proteomic analysis utilizing iTRAQ tag quantification technology. Samples from three replicates of each subgroup (normal, H_2O_2, and AJS-PDRN-H_2O_2) were pooled and subjected to mass spectrometry for protein isolation. Leveraging the mouse (mmu) protein database, we identified a total of 7631 proteins (1% FDR and protein-level FDR). Principal component analysis (PCA) was performed on the expression levels of reliable proteins. The results showed a high level of quantitative repeatability in the degree of aggregation among repeated samples, with significant differences observed between various samples (Figure 4A). Proteins meeting the criteria of having at least one peptide, a fold change of ≥1.5 or ≤0.67, and a p-value < 0.05 were considered differentially expressed proteins (DEPs).

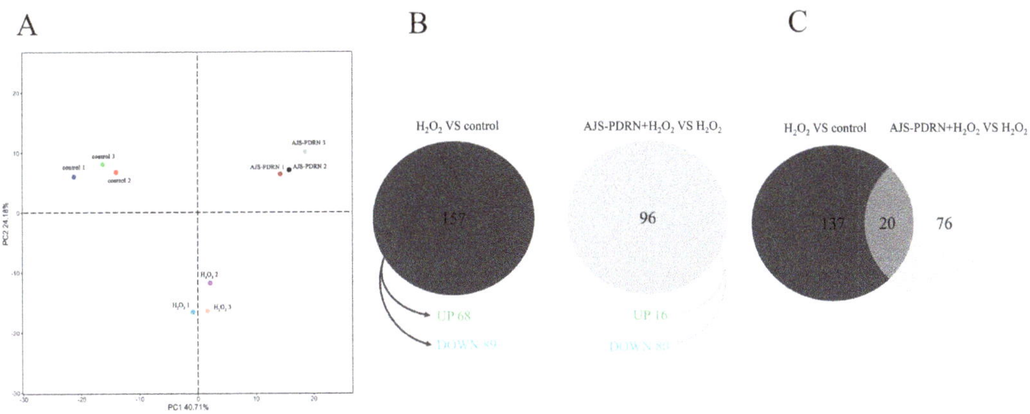

Figure 4. Effect of AJS-PDRN on H_2O_2-induced protein expression profile in RAW264.7 cells. (**A**) PCA based on quantitative data of the selected proteins in each group (n = 3 for each group); (**B**) Venn diagram of DEPs in the H_2O_2 group and the AJS-PDRN group; and (**C**) Venn diagram demonstrating the number of DEPs identified in each comparison.

To identify the proteins whose expression was influenced by AJS-PDRN, we analyzed the DEPs that were either increased or decreased in both the H_2O_2 group and the AJS-PDRN-H_2O_2 group using Venn diagram analysis (Figure 4B). Our results showed that the H_2O_2 group had 157 DEPs compared to the normal group, with 68 upregulated and 89 downregulated. The AJS-PDRN-H_2O_2 group had 96 DEPs compared to the H_2O_2 group, of which 16 were upregulated and 80 were downregulated. Intriguingly, among the 20 DEPs screened in both comparisons, six were upregulated in the H_2O_2 group and downregulated in the AJS-PDRN-H_2O_2 group. Only one DEP was downregulated in the H_2O_2 group and upregulated in the AJS-PDRN-H_2O_2 group (Figure 4C, Table 1).

Table 1. List of the 20 selected differentially expressed proteins in RAW264.7 cells.

Accession	Protein Description	Gene Symbol	H_2O_2/Control [a]	PDRN/H_2O_2 [b]
P01942	Hemoglobin subunit alpha	Hba	1.718	0.607
Q64669	NAD(P)H dehydrogenase [quinone] 1	Nqo1	1.641	0.515
Q9D0U6	Repressor of RNA polymerase III transcription MAF1 homolog	Maf1	2.329	0.035
P51667	Myosin regulatory light chain 2, ventricular/cardiac muscle isoform	Myl2	5.929	0.453
Q9CXT6	Bifunctional peptidase and arginyl-hydroxylase JMJD5	Kdm8	1.551	0.485
Q66JY6	Rho guanine nucleotide exchange factor 39	Arhgef39	1.546	0.578
Q64445	Cytochrome c oxidase subunit 8A, mitochondrial	Cox8a	0.069	1.979
P08905	Lysozyme C-2	Lyz2	0.647	0.581
Q05117	Tartrate-resistant acid phosphatase type 5	Acp5	0.404	0.463
O88199	Carbohydrate sulfotransferase 3	Chst3	45.981	67.64
Q9D722	Oxidative stress-responsive serine-rich protein 1	Oser1	10.169	16.966
P54987	Cis-aconitate decarboxylase	Acod1	0.392	0.571
O70167	Phosphatidylinositol 3-kinase C2 domain-containing subunit gamma	Pik3c2g	0.168	0.069
P05555	Integrin alpha-M	Itgam	0.638	0.642
Q9CPU9	Probable low-affinity copper uptake protein 2	Slc31a2	0.6	0.661
P11835	Integrin beta-2	Itgb2	0.663	0.661
Q61704	Inter-alpha-trypsin inhibitor heavy chain H3	Itih3	1.933	2.489
P54830	Tyrosine protein phosphatase non-receptor type 5	Ptpn5	0.408	0.464
O88531	Palmitoyl protein thioesterase 1	Ppt1	0.653	0.628
P31809	Carcinoembryonic antigen-related cell adhesion molecule 1	Ceacam1	0.543	0.538

[a] Fold changes in the proteins in the H_2O_2 group vs. the control group. [b] Fold changes in the proteins in the AJS-PDRN group vs. the H_2O_2 group.

2.3.2. Gene Ontology (GO) Functional Annotation Enrichment Analysis of DEPs

In order to comprehensively understand the functional classification of the DEPs, we used DAVID bioinformatics resource 6.8 to conduct GO functional annotation analysis of the DEPs. Enrichment analysis was performed from the aspects of biological process (BP), cellular component (CC), and molecular function (MF). The top 10 terms that were significantly enriched ($p < 0.05$) in each category are listed in Figure 5. In the comparison between the control and H_2O_2 groups (Figure 5A), GO BP analysis revealed that the DEPs induced by H_2O_2 were enriched in processes such as cellular response to interferon-beta, response to the bacterium, defense response to the virus, and response to the virus. Under oxidative stress conditions, cells activate a series of defense mechanisms, including the enhancement of interferon-β-related antiviral responses and immune responses against bacteria. GO CC analysis showed that these proteins are mainly involved in CCs such as the Golgi apparatus, lysosome, plasma membrane, and mitochondrion. These alterations in protein levels suggest that oxidative stress impacts multiple critical cellular sites, encompassing protein processing and degradation (Golgi apparatus and lysosome), cell signaling and material exchange (plasma membrane), and energy metabolism (mitochondria). GO MF analysis revealed that the MFs primarily involved in this group of differential proteins include 2′-5′-oligoadenylate synthetase activity, tapasin binding, linoleoyl-CoA desaturase activity, peptide transmembrane transporter activity, etc. These functions are associated with antiviral responses, antigen presentation, fatty acid metabolism, and transmembrane substance transport, which indicate that cells maintain function and survival through various pathways in response to oxidative stress.

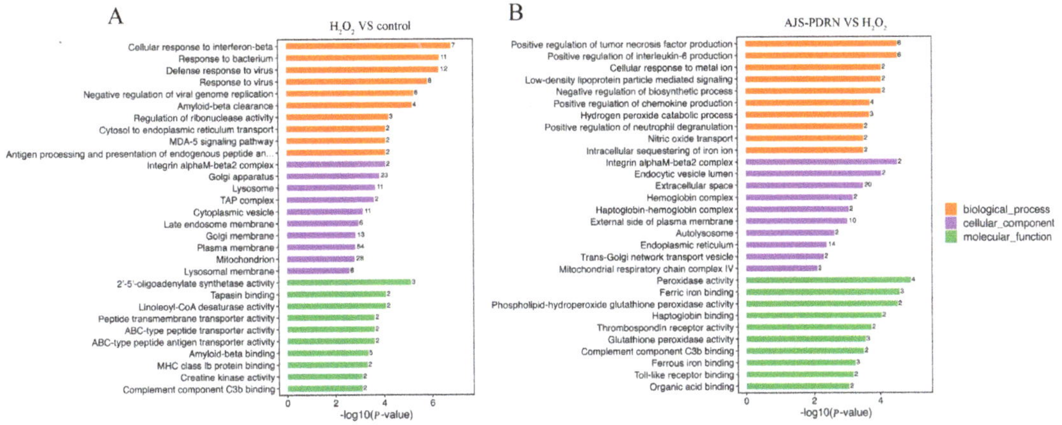

Figure 5. GO enrichment analysis of DEPs. (**A**) The H_2O_2 group vs. the control group; (**B**) the AJS-PDRN group vs. the H_2O_2 group. The number after each term represents the number of differential proteins annotated to that term.

In the comparative analysis of the AJS-PDRN and H_2O_2 groups (Figure 5B), GO BP analysis revealed that the differentially expressed proteins between the AJS-PDRN and H_2O_2 groups were primarily enriched in the processes of positive regulation of tumor necrosis factor production, positive regulation of interleukin-6 production, and positive regulation of chemokine production, as well as the hydrogen peroxide catabolic process. The upregulation of tumor necrosis factor, interleukin-6, and the production of chemokines suggests that AJS-PDRN may alleviate oxidative stress-induced damage by modulating these key inflammatory mediators. Moreover, the enrichment of hydrogen peroxide decomposition processes indicates that AJS-PDRN may mitigate oxidative damage by enhancing the cells' capacity to eliminate H_2O_2. GO CC analysis showed that these differential proteins were primarily enriched in CCs such as integrin alphaM-beta2 complex, extracellular space, external side of the plasma membrane, and endoplasmic reticulum. Research indicates that proteins within integrin complexes and on the extracellular side of the plasma membrane typically participate in cell adhesion and signal transduction processes [35]. This suggests that AJS-PDRN likely exerts its protective effects by enhancing intercellular interactions and signal transduction. Moreover, the enrichment of proteins in the endoplasmic reticulum suggests that AJS-PDRN may alleviate endoplasmic reticulum stress by modulating protein synthesis and folding. GO MF analysis showed that the differentially expressed proteins in this group were primarily involved in MFs, including peroxidase activity, ferric iron binding, glutathione peroxidase activity, and ferrous iron binding. These MFs indicate that AJS-PDRN exerts its protective effects primarily by enhancing the antioxidant capacity of cells. In summary, AJS-PDRN safeguards RAW264.7 cells from H_2O_2-induced oxidative damage through multiple mechanisms. AJS-PDRN not only regulates the production of inflammatory mediators and enhances anti-inflammatory responses but also exerts its protective effects by boosting the cells' antioxidant capacity and modulating the extracellular matrix and signal transduction pathways.

2.3.3. KEGG Pathway Enrichment Analysis of DEPs

In order to further analyze the mechanism of action of AJS-PDRN, the KEGG database was used to perform enrichment analysis on the selected metabolic pathways of DEPs, screening for enriched metabolic terms with a p-value of less than 0.05. The results demonstrated that the metabolic pathways that exhibited significant enrichment for the differential proteins in the H_2O_2 and control groups included arginine and proline metabolism, biosynthesis of unsaturated fatty acids, glutathione metabolism, and NOD-like receptor signaling pathway (Figure 6A). The accumulation of these DEPs in the aforementioned metabolic pathways illustrates the cell's multifaceted response to H_2O_2-induced oxidative stress. These pathways encompass the regulation of metabolism, the repair of damaged cell membranes, the elimination of reactive oxygen species, and the activation of immune and inflammatory responses. The synergistic action of these mechanisms aids cells in maintaining survival and function in response to oxidative damage. In the comparison between the AJS-PDRN group and the H_2O_2 group, the signaling pathways enriched by differential proteins were primarily glutathione metabolism, fatty acid elongation, complement and coagulation cascades, and lysosome (Figure 6B). Studies suggest that fatty acid elongation plays a critical role in the construction and repair of cell membranes [36]. Oxidative stress may damage cell membranes, leading to impaired cellular function. Therefore, AJS-PDRN might improve cell survival under oxidative stress by promoting fatty acid elongation and assisting in the repair of damaged membrane structures. Furthermore, the complement and coagulation cascades are crucial defense mechanisms in the body, involved in immune and inflammatory responses [37]. In summary, AJS-PDRN mitigates H_2O_2-induced oxidative damage through multiple pathways. The enrichment results of DEPs in the above pathways suggest that AJS-PDRN protects cells from oxidative damage by enhancing antioxidant capacity, promoting membrane repair, regulating immune and inflammatory responses, and augmenting intracellular degradation functions.

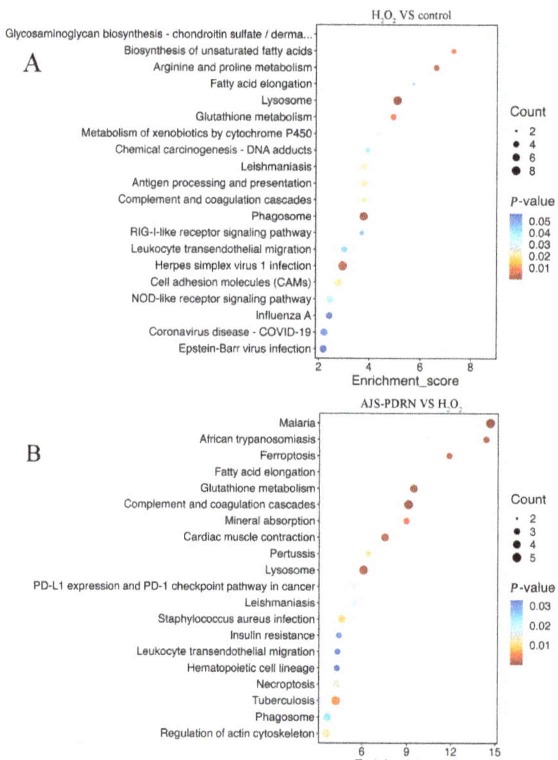

Figure 6. The bubble diagram of KEGG pathway analysis of DEPs. (**A**) The H_2O_2 group vs. the control group; (**B**) the AJS-PDRN group vs. the H_2O_2 group. The larger the bubble the greater the number of differential proteins contained in the entry. The color of the bubbles changes from blue to red, indicating that the smaller the enrichment *p*-value, the greater the degree of significance.

2.3.4. Analysis of Protein Interaction Network

Research has shown that most proteins do not operate independently in organisms, but rather need to interact with other proteins in order to fulfill their functions [38]. Consequently, we conducted a network analysis of the two groups of differential proteins using a protein–protein interaction network. The PPI network of differential proteins between two different groups was constructed using the STRING database and Cytoscape software (version 3.10.2). In the comparison of the H_2O_2 group with the control group, the differential protein PPI network contained 59 nodes and 298 interactions. Each node was ranked according to the Betweenness Centrality (BC) using the Cytoscape plugin CytoNCA. The proteins with more interactions are displayed in the inner circle of the PPI network map (Figure 7A). Furthermore, we also used molecular complex detection (MCODE) algorithm analysis for DEPs to establish PPI networks. MCODE is a density-based non-overlapping clustering algorithm that utilizes seed nodes as the center to expand to neighboring nodes, which are then screened to construct complexes in a protein–protein interaction network. This approach enables the identification of potential biological mechanisms related to the network [39]. We screened the top cluster with the highest clustering score (score: 9.4), and the results are shown in Figure 7B. This cluster comprises a total of 11 protein nodes and 94 interactions. To gain further understanding of the function of these proteins, we performed biological process enrichment and KEGG pathway analysis using ClueGO and CluePedia, and the result is shown in Figure 7C. The proteins are primarily engaged in biological processes such as the regulation of viral genome replication (Gbp7, Ifih1, Oas2, Oas3, and Oasl2) and the response to interferon-beta (Gbp7, Ifih1, Irgm1, and Xaf1).

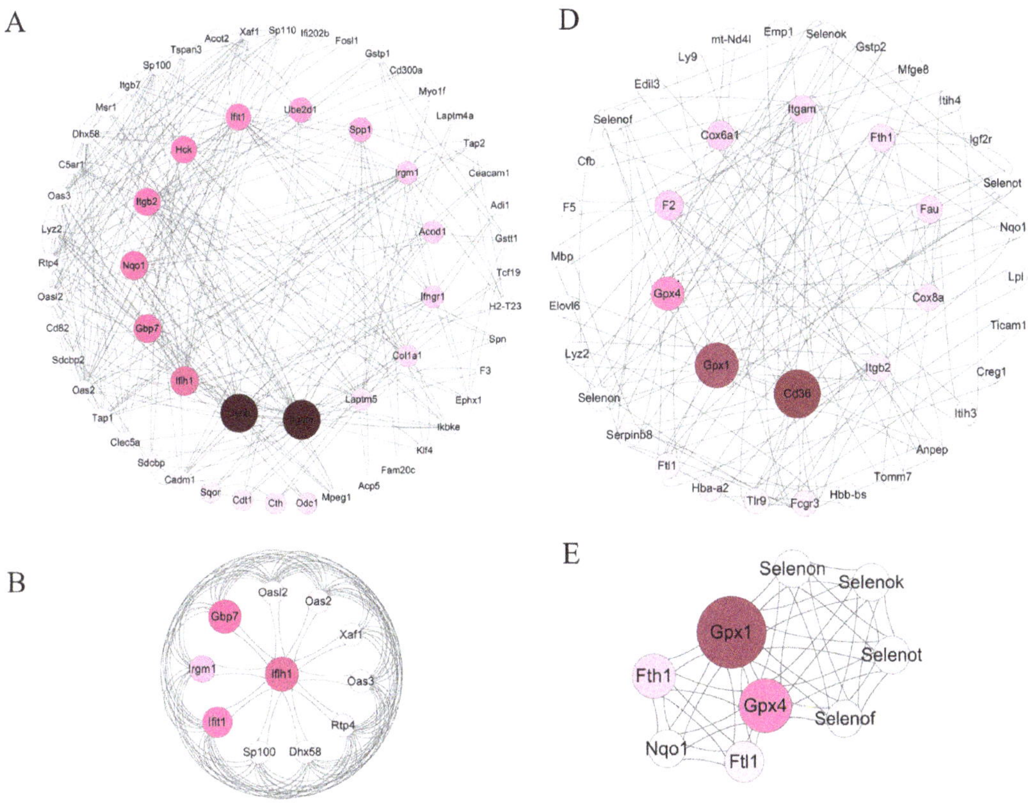

Figure 7. *Cont.*

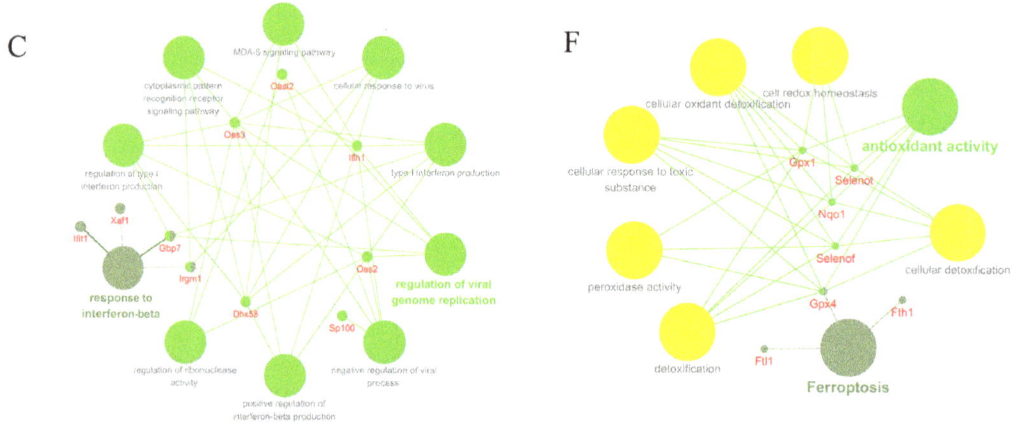

Figure 7. PPI network analysis of DEPs. (**A**) PPI network diagram of all DEPs with interactions in the H_2O_2 group vs. the control group. (**B**) The highest-scoring sub-network in the H_2O_2 group was selected using the MCODE algorithm. (**C**) The major GO BP terms were significantly enriched by 11 proteins in the sub-network, as well as the related DEPs. (**D**) PPI network diagram of all DEPs with interactions in the AJS-PDRN group vs. the H_2O_2 group. (**E**) The highest-scoring sub-network in the AJS-PDRN group was selected using the MCODE algorithm. (**F**) The major GO BP terms and KEGG pathway were significantly enriched by 9 proteins in the sub-network, as well as the related DEPs.

In the comparison of the AJS-PDRN group and the H_2O_2 group, the differential protein PPI network contained a total of 40 protein nodes and 160 interactions (Figure 7D). Additionally, the module with the highest clustering score, identified using the MCODE algorithm, is shown in Figure 7E. This cluster comprises nine protein nodes and 48 interactions, most of which are members of the selenoprotein family. It is well known that selenium is an essential trace element for the human body, with strong antioxidant properties. The physiological functions of selenium are primarily realized through selenoproteins [40]. Numerous studies have demonstrated that selenoproteins play a crucial role in regulating the body's redox balance [41,42]. Furthermore, the results of ClueGO and CluePedia enrichment analysis are shown in Figure 7F. The GO biological processes involving these proteins are all related to antioxidant activity (Gpx1, Gpx4, Nqo1, Selenot, and Selenof), and the only associated KEGG signaling pathway is Ferroptosis (Gpx4, Fth1, and Ftl1).

3. Discussion

As a traditional health food, sea cucumber has high nutritional and medicinal value. The main edible part of the sea cucumber is its body wall; therefore, most research focuses on this component [43]. During sea cucumber processing, viscera byproducts, such as sea cucumber sperm, are often underutilized. Studies have shown that sea cucumber viscera are rich in taurine, polydeoxyribonucleotides, arginine, unsaturated fatty acids, trace elements, and other active compounds, in addition to those similar to the body wall [44,45]. Therefore, sea cucumber viscera also possess various biological activities, including antioxidant, antitumor, anticancer, and immunomodulatory effects [46,47]. The lack of awareness and neglect of the active substances in sea cucumber viscera lead to significant resource wastage and loss. Additionally, research on the active substances of sea cucumber viscera, both domestically and internationally, remains limited, and few relevant products have been developed. Therefore, sea cucumber sperm was chosen as the raw material for this study to extract PDRN, which exhibits various biological activities.

It is well known that H_2O_2 is highly susceptible to diffusion through cell membranes, reaching nuclear tissues and initiating a series of oxidative stress reactions. Moreover, H_2O_2 is readily obtainable and relatively stable chemically. Therefore, exogenous H_2O_2

has become an important tool for studying cellular oxidative damage [29]. This is of great significance for researchers to study the cytoprotective and reparative roles of bioactive substances. Studies have shown that oxidative stress is usually associated with the development of various diseases, and the excess reactive oxygen species it induces can cause extensive damage to DNA and cellular macromolecules, such as altering membrane fluidity, destroying the cytoskeleton, and promoting protein denaturation, etc., which ultimately causes a series of cellular dysfunction phenomena such as apoptosis and cancer [17]. Therefore, the search for natural active substances with high antioxidant properties is crucial to protect the body cells from oxidative stress damage.

PDRN is a naturally occurring low-molecular-weight DNA derivative extracted and prepared primarily from the sperm cells of trout or salmon [20]. PDRN is commonly used as an adenosine A_{2A} receptor activator, which exerts various physiological effects [48]. Currently, most studies on PDRN activity have focused on anti-inflammatory, anti-apoptotic, and tissue repair properties [22]. However, there are relatively few studies on its antioxidant activity. In this study, we report for the first time that PDRN was extracted from *Apostichopus japonicus* sperm, and its antioxidant activity was investigated using DPPH, ABTS, and hydroxyl radical scavenging assays. The results of all three assays showed that AJS-PDRN exhibits excellent antioxidant properties.

The excellent antioxidant activity of AJS-PDRN suggests that AJS-PDRN may have the ability to protect cells from oxidative stress damage. Therefore, in this study, we successfully constructed a cell injury model using exogenous H_2O_2 to induce oxidative damage in RAW264.7 cells. The cytoprotective and reparative abilities of AJS-PDRN were evaluated in vitro. The results showed that AJS-PDRN had superior protective abilities, as demonstrated by its promotion of cell proliferation and reduction in H_2O_2-induced cellular damage (Figure 2B,C).

To maintain the balance of the body's redox system, the body relies on its antioxidant enzyme system, which consists of key enzymes such as SOD and CAT [49]. These enzymes protect cells from oxidative damage by scavenging excess ROS and free radicals from the cells. SOD is the enzyme that catalyzes the disproportionation of superoxide anion radicals to produce hydrogen peroxide and oxygen [31]. CAT is the antioxidant enzyme that is present in virtually all organisms and catalyzes the conversion of hydrogen peroxide to water and oxygen [32]. GSH is an important antioxidant that can scavenge lipid peroxides through Gpx4 and inhibit Ferroptosis [33]. MDA is a byproduct of lipid peroxidation and serves as a marker of oxidative stress [34]. In this study, we evaluated the reparative effect of AJS-PDRN on cellular damage by measuring the levels of these four biomarkers in RAW264.7 cells under different treatment conditions. The results showed that AJS-PDRN significantly increased the intracellular levels of SOD, CAT, and GSH, and decreased MDA content, attenuating H_2O_2-induced RAW264.7 cell injury in a dose-dependent manner. Currently, commonly used natural antioxidants also encompass polyphenolic compounds. Phenolic compounds extracted from fruit wines can significantly enhance the activity of antioxidant enzymes in cells and mitigate the levels of MDA in cells subjected to experimentally induced oxidative stress [50]. In conclusion, AJS-PDRN demonstrates potent antioxidant activity and exhibits superior protective and reparative effects on H_2O_2-induced RAW264.7 cell injury.

In order to elucidate the mechanism of the protective effect of AJS-PDRN on H_2O_2-induced RAW264.7 cells, DEPs in the cells were identified by the iTRAQ proteomics method in this study. The results showed that a total of 157 DEPs were identified in the H_2O_2 group versus the blank group, while 96 DEPs were identified in the AJS-PDRN group and the H_2O_2 group. Interestingly, six DEPs (Hba, Nqo1, Maf1, Myl2, Kdm8, and Arhgef39) were found to have upregulated expression in the H_2O_2 group, whereas their expression was downregulated after pretreatment with AJS-PDRN. Additionally, one DEP (Cox8a) exhibited the opposite expression pattern (Table 1).

Hemoglobin subunit alpha (Hba) is a crucial component of hemoglobin that is primarily responsible for oxygen transport. In addition, hemoglobin is involved in the detoxification of cellular oxidants and protects cells from oxidative damage. Studies have shown that hemoglobin not only transports oxygen in red blood cells but also has antioxidant functions in other cells. Hemoglobin can reduce oxidative damage by interacting with peroxides via its subunit α and reducing the production of free radicals [51]. This protective mechanism may explain the upregulation of hemoglobin subunit α expression in the H_2O_2 group after induction by H_2O_2. Nqo1 is a key antioxidant enzyme that reduces quinones to less toxic hydroquinones, thus reducing the generation of reactive oxygen species and decreasing oxidative stress-induced cellular damage [52]. Studies have shown that Nqo1 expression is regulated by the Nrf2 (nuclear factor E2-related factor 2)/ARE (antioxidant response element) signaling pathway. Under oxidative stress conditions, Nrf2 is released from the Keap1 complex, translocates to the nucleus, and binds to ARE, initiating the expression of various antioxidant genes such as Nqo1 [53]. Therefore, the increased expression of the Nqo1 protein in the H_2O_2 group is a self-protective mechanism of cells. Maf1 is a major repressor of RNA polymerase III. Under oxidative stress conditions, Maf1 reduces the metabolic burden of cells by inhibiting the transcriptional activity of RNA polymerase III, thus reducing oxidative damage [54]. Upregulation of Maf1 protein was detected in the H_2O_2 group, suggesting that cells may reduce oxidative damage by decreasing metabolic burden. Myl2 is a member of the myosin light chain family that is expressed mainly in cardiac and skeletal muscle and is involved in the regulation of muscle contraction [55]. Myl2 regulates the contraction and relaxation of muscle fibers by binding to myosin-heavy chains in cardiac and skeletal muscle. Upregulation of Myl2 expression after treatment with H_2O_2 enhances cellular resistance to oxidative damage, maintains cytoskeletal stability and function, and may promote cell survival by regulating oxidative stress-associated signaling pathways, such as the Nrf2 pathway. Kdm8 is a histone demethylase that can help cells repair DNA damage and maintain gene stability by regulating chromatin structure and gene expression [56]. In the H_2O_2 group, upregulation of Kdm8 expression may enhance the antioxidant capacity and DNA repair mechanism of cells, reducing oxidative stress-induced damage. The reduction in Kdm8 protein levels after pretreatment with AJS-PDRN indicates its potential repair role. Arhgef39 is a guanine nucleotide exchange factor belonging to the Rho GTPase-regulated protein family, affecting various cellular processes [57]. Oxidative stress activates a variety of signaling pathways, including the Rho family of GTPase signaling pathways. Arhgef39, through the activation of Rho GTPases, may regulate cell proliferation, survival, and migration during cellular response to oxidative stress.

Cox8a is a subunit of the mitochondrial respiratory chain complex IV (cytochrome c oxidase) involved in electron transfer and ATP synthesis [58]. Increased Cox8a expression may improve mitochondrial electron transfer efficiency, thereby reducing reactive oxygen species generation under oxidative stress and enhancing cell survival.

Regarding the analysis of GO and KEGG pathways, the present study revealed that AJS-PDRN significantly affects the positive regulation of tumor necrosis factor production, positive regulation of interleu-kin-6 production, hydrogen peroxide catabolic process, extracellular space, endoplasmic reticulum, peroxidase activity, and glutathione peroxidase activity, among other related GO terms (Figure 5B). These GO terms are closely related to the antioxidant function as well as the anti-inflammatory activity of the organism.

The KEGG signaling pathways enriched in the AJS-PDRN group compared with the H_2O_2 group mainly included glutathione metabolism, fatty acid elongation, complement and coagulation cascades, and lysosome. Glutathione is an important intracellular antioxidant that effectively scavenges free radicals and other reactive oxygen species [59]. Therefore, glutathione plays an important role in protecting cells from oxidative damage. The fatty acid extension process plays a key role in cell membrane synthesis and energy metabolism [36]. This suggests a possible role for AJS-PDRN in repairing and maintaining the integrity of membrane structure. In addition, studies have shown that the complement system and coagulation system have important roles in immune defense and damage repair processes in vivo [37]. The enrichment results of the AJS-PDRN pretreated group implied that AJS-PDRN might also have immunomodulatory and anti-inflammatory roles, which need to be further investigated in depth.

In order to further investigate the protection mechanism of AJS-PDRN on the RAW264.7 cell injury model, this study utilized the PPI network to analyze the two groups of DEPs in the experiment separately. Using the MCODE algorithm, we filtered out a sub-network with the highest clustering score from the AJS-PDRN group. The results showed that there were nine protein nodes and 48 interactions in this module. Six of these proteins (Gpx1, Gpx4, Selenon, Selenok, Selenot, and Selenof) are selenoprotein family members. Studies have shown that selenoproteins play an important role in regulating redox homeostasis in the human body [41]. The main mechanism involves the direct scavenging of hydrogen peroxide and organic peroxides through the catalysis of enzymes such as glutathione peroxidase, thioredoxin reductase, and selenoprotein P, which, in turn, attenuates oxidative damage [60]. Subsequently, we enriched and analyzed these nine proteins using ClueGO and CluePedia plugins. The results showed that these proteins were mainly involved in biological processes related to antioxidant activity. In addition, Fth1, Ftl1, and Gpx4 were enriched in the Ferroptosis KEGG signaling pathway. The studies showed that Ferroptosis is a novel mode of non-apoptotic cell death characterized by iron-dependent accumulation of lipid peroxides and altered redox homeostasis [61]. In summary, AJS-PDRN may attenuate cellular oxidative damage by promoting the expression of intracellular selenoprotein family members, enhancing the activity of various intracellular antioxidant enzymes. The proteomic analysis provided initial insights into the in vivo mechanism of action of AJS-PDRN, paving the way for comprehensive studies on its prospective application in oxidative stress-related conditions.

4. Materials and Methods

4.1. Materials

RAW264.7 cells were purchased from the Chinese Academy of Sciences Cell Bank. Fresh spermary of sea cucumber (*Apostichopus japonicus*) was purchased from Shanshui seafood Co., Ltd. (Yantai, China). Proteinase K (enzyme activity 43.6 U/mg), Spark 2000PDRN Marker, Spark 6× PDRN Loading Buffer, and Spark 5× TBE Buffer were purchased from Shandong SparkJade Biotechnology Co. (Jinan, China); Gelred nucleic acid dye was purchased from Shanghai Sangon Biotech Co. (Shanghai, China); Cell Counting Kit-8 (CCK-8) kit and phenylmethylsulfonyl fluoride (PMSF) were purchased from Shanghai Beyotime Biotechnology Co. (Shanghai, China); the SOD, CAT, MDA and GSH assay kits were all acquired from Beijing Solarbio Biotechnology Co. (Beijing, China); and other chemical reagents were purchased from Sinopharm (Beijing, China).

4.2. Extraction and Preparation of AJS-PDRN

Referring to the method of Cawthorn et al. [62], a 0.06 g sample of fresh sea cucumber sperm was placed into a 1.5 mL centrifuge tube using sterilized scissors. A volume of 0.3 mL of lysis buffer (10 mM Tris-HCl, pH 8.0; 2 mM EDTA, pH 8.0; 0.4 M NaCl) was added, followed by the addition of 10% SDS and 0.8 μL of proteinase K. The mixture was incubated in a 50 °C water bath for 12 h for enzymatic digestion. After digestion, the mixture was centrifuged at 10,000 r/min for 1 h. The supernatant was transferred to a new centrifuge tube and 0.5 volumes of 6 M NaCl along with an equal volume of phenol:chloroform:alcohol (25:24:1) were added and mixed thoroughly. After thorough mixing, the mixture was centrifuged at 10,000 r/min for 1 h and the supernatant was transferred to a new centrifuge tube. Subsequently, 0.6 volumes of isopropanol were added to precipitate the DNA, which was then washed twice with 70% (*v*/*v*) ethanol. Finally, the DNA precipitate was dried in an oven at 65 °C and stored at −20 °C for future use.

4.3. DPPH Radical Scavenging Assay by AJS-PDRN

The DPPH radical scavenging activity of AJS-PDRN was measured by referring to the method of Shao et al. with slight modifications [63]. In brief, 1 mL of a 0.2 mmol/L DPPH–

ethanol solution was combined with 1 mL of sample solutions of varying concentrations, followed by a 30 min reaction at room temperature in the dark. The absorbance value at 517 nm was measured and recorded as A_1. Subsequently, 1 mL of both the sample solution and anhydrous ethanol were thoroughly mixed and reacted in the dark at room temperature for 30 min, with the absorbance measured as A_2. Lastly, 1 mL of distilled water was substituted for the sample solution and mixed with 1 mL of DPPH–ethanol solution, allowing the reaction to proceed in the dark for 30 min. The absorbance was then measured, resulting in A_3. VC was used as a standard solution in a control experiment. The DPPH scavenging effect was calculated as follows:

$$\text{DPPH scavenging rate } (\%) = \left[\frac{1-(A_1-A_2)}{A_3}\right] \times 100\%.$$

4.4. ABTS Radical Scavenging Assay by AJS-PDRN

The ABTS free radical scavenging assay was also employed to assess the antioxidant activity of AJS-PDRN [64]. The working solution was prepared by combining an ABTS solution (7 mmol/L) with a potassium persulfate solution (2.45 mmol/L) in equal volumes and shielded from light for a period of 12 h. The absorbance at 734 nm was 0.700 ± 0.005 after dilution with ethanol. The diluted ABTS working solution (4 mL) was mixed with 100 μL of the sample solution and reacted for 10 min under the protection of light. The absorbance at 734 nm was designated as A_1, and the value of the absorbance measured by using the ethanol solution in lieu of the ABTS working solution was recorded as A_2. The absorbance measured by reacting a diluted ABTS working solution (4 mL) with 100 μL of an ethanol solution was recorded as A_3. A control experiment was conducted using VC. The ABTS scavenging effect was calculated as follows:

$$\text{ABTS scavenging rate } (\%) = \left[\frac{1-(A_1-A_2)}{A_3}\right] \times 100\%.$$

4.5. Hydroxyl Radical Scavenging Activity

The hydroxyl radical scavenging activity of AJS-PDRN was determined by the method of Souza et al. with slight modifications [65]. An amount of 1 mL of 9 mmol/L $FeSO_4$, 9 mmol/L of salicylic acid–ethanol solution, 8.8 mmol/L of hydrogen peroxide solution, and the sample solution were added to the test tube, respectively, and allowed to react for 30 min at 37 °C. The absorbance was measured at 510 nm and counted as A_1. The salicylic acid was replaced with distilled water, and the absorbance was counted as A_2. The sample was replaced with distilled water, and the absorbance was counted as A_3. VC was used as a control experiment. The hydroxyl radical scavenging effect was calculated as follows:

$$\bullet\text{OH scavenging rate } (\%) = \left[\frac{1-(A_1-A_2)}{A_3}\right] \times 100\%.$$

4.6. Cell Culture

The RAW264.7 cells were cultured in Dulbecco's Modified Eagle Medium (DEME) supplemented with 10% fetal bovine serum (FBS) and 1% dual-antibody reagent (consisting of 100 U/mL of penicillin and 100 mg/mL of streptomycin). The cells were cultured in a humidified environment at 5% CO_2 at 37 °C, with the medium being changed every two or three days.

4.7. Cell Viability Assay

The viability of the cells was determined using the Cell Counting Kit-8 (CCK-8) method. In brief, RAW264.7 cells (10,000 cells/well) were inoculated into 96-well plates, and then CCK-8 solution (10 μL per well) was added at 0, 24, 48, and 72 h, respectively. The cells were incubated at 37 °C for 2 h, and then the absorbance was measured at 450 nm using an enzyme-labeled instrument (ThermoFisher Scientific, Shanghai, China).

4.8. Establishment of H_2O_2-Induced Oxidative Stress Model of RAW264.7 Cells

RAW264.7 cells (10,000 cells/well) were seeded in 96-well plates and incubated for 24 h. Following this incubation period, 100 μL of varying concentrations of H_2O_2 solution (100 μM, 200 μM, 300 μM, 400 μM, 500 μM, and 600 μM) were added and incubated for an additional 4 h. Subsequently, 10 μL of CCK-8 solution was added, and the cells were further incubated for 1 h. The absorbance was measured at a wavelength of 450 nm and cell viability was calculated.

4.9. Toxic Effect of AJS-PDRN on RAW264.7 Cells

RAW264.7 cells (10,000 cells/well) were seeded in a 96-well plate and cultured for 24 h. Then, 100 μL of AJS-PDRN solution of different concentrations (100 μM, 200 μM, 300 μM, 400 μM, 500 μM, and 600 μM) was added, and after 6 h of action, 10 μL of CCK-8 solution was added and incubated for 1 h. The absorbance was measured at a wavelength of 450 nm and cell viability was calculated.

4.10. Protective Effect of AJS-PDRN on H_2O_2-Induced Cellular Oxidative Stress Model

In order to explore the protective effect of AJS-PDRN on cells, RAW264.7 cells (10,000 cells/well) were seeded in a 96-well plate and cultured for 24 h. The RAW264.7 cells were then treated with AJS-PDRN solution of different concentrations (100 μM, 200 μM, 300 μM, 400 μM, 500 μM, and 600 μM) for 6 h. Following two washes with PBS, the cells were then treated with a 400 μM H_2O_2 solution (IC_{50} concentration) for 4 h. Cell viability was assessed using the CCK-8 method.

4.11. CAT, SOD, GSH, and MDA in RAW264.7 Cells

RAW264.7 cells (10,000 cells/well) were seeded in a 96-well plate and cultured for 24 h, and a blank group, a control group, and an experimental group were set. The blank group consisted of normally growing cells; cells treated with 2 mL of 400 μM H_2O_2 solution served as the control group; and the experimental group added 2 mL of AJS-PDRN of different concentrations to normal cells and cultured them for 6 h, and then added 2 mL of 400 μM H_2O_2 solution for 4 h. Finally, according to the instructions of the CAT, SOD, GSH and MDA detection kits, the contents of CAT, SOD, GSH and MDA were measured on the 96-well plate.

4.12. Protein Preparation and iTRAQ Labelling

RAW264.7 cells were initially seeded in culture dishes at a density of 2×10^4 cells/cm^2 and incubated until reaching 80–90% confluence for subsequent iTRAQ-based proteomics analysis. Following the assessment of cell viability and biochemical assays, a high concentration of AJS-PDRN was chosen for the proteomic study. The RAW264.7 cells were then divided into nine groups, comprising three control groups, three H_2O_2 groups, and three AJS-PDRN+H_2O_2 groups. Cells in the control group underwent normal culture conditions, those in the H_2O_2 group were treated to 400 μM H_2O_2 for 6 h, and cells in the AJS-PDRN group were pretreated with 600 μM AJS-PDRN for 6 h before being treated with 400 μM H_2O_2 for an additional 6 h. Subsequently, cellular proteins were extracted using a protein extraction kit, and protein concentration was determined using a BCA protein assay kit (Solarbio, Beijing, China). All steps were performed in accordance with the manufacturer's instructions.

RAW264.7 cells in each group were collected by centrifugation and washed twice with PBS. The samples were sonicated three times in lysis buffer (8 M urea, 1% protease inhibitor cocktail) on ice using an ultrasonic cell crusher (Scientz, Shenzhen, China), and the supernatants were collected. Then, trypsin was added to the protein solution at a mass ratio of protein to the enzyme of 30:1, and enzymatic hydrolysis was carried out at 37 °C for 4 h. Subsequently, 2 μL of 0.2% trifluoroacetic acid was immediately added to terminate the enzymatic hydrolysis. Desalting was performed via solid-phase extraction cartridge

Sep-Pak C18, followed by drying under vacuum. The digested peptides were then labeled with iTRAQ using the 8-plex kit.

4.13. LC-MS/MS High-Resolution Mass Spectrometry Analysis

The labeled peptides were separated using high-pH reversed-phase high-performance liquid chromatography. The trypsin-digested peptides were then analyzed by LC-MS/MS using a timsTOF Pro mass spectrometer (Bruker Daltonics, Bremen, Germany). The mass spectrometry data were analyzed and processed using Spectronaut Pulsar 18.4 software (Biognosys, Zurich, Switzerland). The chromatographic column is an Eksigent C18 (75 μm × 250 mm, 1.7 μm), with mobile phase A being a 0.1% formaldehyde aqueous solution (v/v), and mobile phase B being a 0.1% formaldehyde in acetonitrile solution. The elution gradient was as follows: 0 min, 5% B; 48 min, 22% B; 53 min, 35% B; 56 min, 90% B; 57 min, 3% B; 60 min, 3% B; and the flow rate was 300 nL/min. Additionally, the external electrospray voltage is 1.5 kV, and the m/z scanning range of the full scan is from 100 to 1700.

4.14. Protein Identification and Bioinformatic Analysis

The mass spectrometry data were processed using Spectronaut Pulsar 18.4 software. Proteins possessing at least one unique peptide with an unused value of more than 2 were screened for further identification. Differentially expressed proteins were screened with a p-value < 0.05 and fold change $\geq$ 1.5 or fold change $\leq$ 0.67. Additionally, functional classification and annotation were performed using DAVID Bioinformatics Resource 6.8 with GO to determine enrichment in cellular components, biological processes, and molecular function. Pathway analysis was conducted using the KEGG database to determine enrichment in signaling pathways. Protein interaction analysis was carried out using the STRING database and Cytoscape software.

4.15. Statistical Processing and Analysis

The physiological indicators or proteomic analysis for all samples were repeated three times, and the results are presented as mean ± standard deviation (SD). Statistical analysis of the data was conducted using SPSS Statistics 26 software, and Duncan's multiple test was performed via one-way analysis of variance ($p < 0.05$ indicating significant differences).

5. Conclusions

In this study, we prepared PDRN from the sperm of *Apostichopus japonicus* for the first time and evaluated the antioxidant activity of AJS-PDRN through DPPH, ABTS, and hydroxyl radical scavenging assays. In subsequent in vitro antioxidant assays, we found that AJS-PDRN pretreatment significantly increased the survival of H_2O_2-induced RAW264.7 cells. The altered levels of oxidative stress biomarkers indicated that AJS-PDRN possesses significant antioxidant activity. Furthermore, iTRAQ proteomics analysis reveals that the protective effects of AJS-PDRN on the cell injury model are primarily achieved through the regulation of immune and inflammatory responses, modulation of the extracellular matrix and signal transduction pathways, promotion of membrane repair, and enhancement of cellular antioxidant capacity. The PPI network analysis indicated that AJS-PDRN pretreatment may mitigate oxidative damage by promoting the expression of multiple selenoproteins in cells. In summary, H_2O_2 can cause cytotoxicity in RAW264.7 cells, resulting in oxidative damage, whereas AJS-PDRN can inhibit this damage through multiple pathways and is not cytotoxic. This study demonstrated the excellent antioxidant activity of AJS-PDRN and revealed its protective effect on oxidatively damaged RAW264.7 cells. This suggests that AJS-PDRN has significant potential in preventing and treating diseases caused by oxidative stress, particularly neurodegenerative diseases, cardiovascular diseases, and skin aging.

Author Contributions: Conceptualization, Z.S. and G.W.; methodology, Z.S., Y.J. (Yizhi Ji) and G.W.; validation, Z.S., Y.J. (Yizhi Ji) and G.W.; data curation, Z.S., Y.J. (Yuexin Jing) and F.L.; writing—original draft preparation, Z.S. and Y.J. (Yizhi Ji); writing—review and editing, Z.S., Y.Z. and C.J.; visualization, Z.S.; supervision, J.Z. and Y.L.; funding acquisition, G.W. and J.Z. All authors have read and agreed to the published version of the manuscript.

Funding: This research was funded by the Shandong Modern Agricultural Industrial Technology System Sea Cucumber Industry Innovation Team Construction Project (SDAIT-22-07), the Yantai Science and Technology Innovation Development Program Policy Guidance Category (2023YD083), and the Key Project of Natural Science Foundation of Shandong Province (ZR2020KC034).

Institutional Review Board Statement: Not applicable.

Data Availability Statement: The data are available from the corresponding author upon reasonable request.

Conflicts of Interest: The authors declare no conflicts of interest.

References

1. Pangestuti, R.; Arifin, Z. Medicinal and health benefit effects of functional sea cucumbers. *J. Tradit. Complement. Med.* **2018**, *8*, 341–351. [CrossRef] [PubMed]
2. Zhao, Y.-C.; Xue, C.-H.; Zhang, T.-T.; Wang, Y.-M. Saponins from Sea Cucumber and Their Biological Activities. *J. Agric. Food Chem.* **2018**, *66*, 7222–7237. [CrossRef] [PubMed]
3. Khotimchenko, Y. Pharmacological Potential of Sea Cucumbers. *Int. J. Mol. Sci.* **2018**, *19*, 1342. [CrossRef] [PubMed]
4. Wang, J.; Shi, S.; Li, F.; Du, X.; Kong, B.; Wang, H.; Xia, X. Physicochemical properties and antioxidant activity of polysaccharides obtained from sea cucumber gonads via ultrasound-assisted enzymatic techniques. *LWT* **2022**, *160*, 113307. [CrossRef]
5. Luo, L.; Wu, M.; Xu, L.; Lian, W.; Xiang, J.; Lu, F.; Gao, N.; Xiao, C.; Wang, S.; Zhao, J. Comparison of Physicochemical Characteristics and Anticoagulant Activities of Polysaccharides from Three Sea Cucumbers. *Mar. Drugs* **2013**, *11*, 399–417. [CrossRef] [PubMed]
6. Gong, P.-X.; Wang, B.-K.; Wu, Y.-C.; Li, Q.-Y.; Qin, B.-W.; Li, H.-J. Release of antidiabetic peptides from *Stichopus japonicas* by simulated gastrointestinal digestion. *Food Chem.* **2020**, *315*, 126273. [CrossRef] [PubMed]
7. Cai, N.; Luo, W.; Yao, L.; Li, X.; Wang, Z.; Xu, H.; Li, H.; Hu, Z.; Bao, W.; Xu, X. Activation of murine RAW264.7 macrophages by oligopeptides from sea cucumber (*Apostichopus japonicus*) and its molecular mechanisms. *J. Funct. Foods* **2020**, *75*, 104229. [CrossRef]
8. Mao, J.; Zhang, Z.; Chen, Y.; Wu, T.; Fersht, V.; Jin, Y.; Meng, J.; Zhang, M. Sea cucumber peptides inhibit the malignancy of NSCLC by regulating miR-378a-5p targeted TUSC2. *Food Funct.* **2021**, *12*, 12362–12371. [CrossRef] [PubMed]
9. Cusimano, M.G.; Spinello, A.; Barone, G.; Schillaci, D.; Cascioferro, S.; Magistrato, A.; Parrino, B.; Arizza, V.; Vitale, M. A Synthetic Derivative of Antimicrobial Peptide Holothuroidin 2 from Mediterranean Sea Cucumber (*Holothuria tubulosa*) in the Control of Listeria monocytogenes. *Mar. Drugs* **2019**, *17*, 159. [CrossRef]
10. Hoang, L.; Le Thi, V.; Tran Thi Hong, H.; Nguyen Van, T.; Nguyen Xuan, C.; Nguyen Hoai, N.; Do Cong, T.; Ivanchina, N.V.; Do Thi, T.; Dmitrenok, P.S.; et al. Triterpene glycosides from the Vietnamese sea cucumber *Holothuria edulis*. *Nat. Prod. Res.* **2020**, *34*, 1061–1067. [CrossRef]
11. Malaiwong, N.; Chalorak, P.; Jattujan, P.; Manohong, P.; Niamnont, N.; Suphamungmee, W.; Sobhon, P.; Meemon, K. Anti-Parkinson activity of bioactive substances extracted from *Holothuria leucospilota*. *Biomed. Pharmacother.* **2019**, *109*, 1967–1977. [CrossRef] [PubMed]
12. Aminin, D.; Pislyagin, E.; Astashev, M.; Es'kov, A.; Kozhemyako, V.; Avilov, S.; Zelepuga, E.; Yurchenko, E.; Kaluzhskiy, L.; Kozlovskaya, E.; et al. Glycosides from edible sea cucumbers stimulate macrophages via purinergic receptors. *Sci. Rep.* **2016**, *6*, 39683. [CrossRef] [PubMed]
13. Lushchak, V.I. Free radicals, reactive oxygen species, oxidative stress and its classification. *Chem. Biol. Interact.* **2014**, *224*, 164–175. [CrossRef]
14. Zhao, X.-C.; Zhang, L.; Yu, H.-X.; Sun, Z.; Lin, X.-F.; Tan, C.; Lu, R.-R. Curcumin protects mouse neuroblastoma Neuro-2A cells against hydrogen-peroxide-induced oxidative stress. *Food Chem.* **2011**, *129*, 387–394. [CrossRef]
15. Casas, A.I.; Nogales, C.; Mucke, H.A.M.; Petraina, A.; Cuadrado, A.; Rojo, A.I.; Ghezzi, P.; Jaquet, V.; Augsburger, F.; Dufrasne, F.; et al. On the Clinical Pharmacology of Reactive Oxygen Species. *Pharmacol. Rev.* **2020**, *72*, 801. [CrossRef] [PubMed]
16. Siti, H.N.; Kamisah, Y.; Kamsiah, J. The role of oxidative stress, antioxidants and vascular inflammation in cardiovascular disease (a review). *Vasc. Pharmacol.* **2015**, *71*, 40–56. [CrossRef]
17. Xu, B.; Dong, Q.; Yu, C.; Chen, H.; Zhao, Y.; Zhang, B.; Yu, P.; Chen, M. Advances in Research on the Activity Evaluation, Mechanism and Structure-Activity Relationships of Natural Antioxidant Peptides. *Antioxidants* **2024**, *13*, 479. [CrossRef]

18. Zhou, H.; Li, X.; Shang, Y.; Chen, K. Radical Scavenging Activity of Puerarin: A Theoretical Study. *Antioxidants* **2019**, *8*, 590. [CrossRef]
19. Colangelo, M.T.; Galli, C.; Guizzardi, S. The effects of polydeoxyribonucleotide on wound healing and tissue regeneration: A systematic review of the literature. *Regener. Med.* **2020**, *15*, 1801–1821. [CrossRef]
20. Kim, S.-E.; Ko, I.-G.; Jin, J.-J.; Hwang, L.; Kim, C.-J.; Kim, S.-H.; Han, J.-H.; Jeon, J.W. Polydeoxyribonucleotide Exerts Therapeutic Effect by Increasing VEGF and Inhibiting Inflammatory Cytokines in Ischemic Colitis Rats. *BioMed Res. Int.* **2020**, *2020*, 2169083. [CrossRef]
21. Kim, H.M.; Byun, K.-A.; Oh, S.; Yang, J.Y.; Park, H.J.; Chung, M.S.; Son, K.H.; Byun, K. A Mixture of Topical Forms of Polydeoxyribonucleotide, Vitamin C, and Niacinamide Attenuated Skin Pigmentation and Increased Skin Elasticity by Modulating Nuclear Factor Erythroid 2-like 2. *Molecules* **2022**, *27*, 1276. [CrossRef] [PubMed]
22. Kim, T.-H.; Heo, S.-Y.; Oh, G.-W.; Heo, S.-J.; Jung, W.-K. Applications of Marine Organism-Derived Polydeoxyribonucleotide: Its Potential in Biomedical Engineering. *Mar. Drugs* **2021**, *19*, 296. [CrossRef] [PubMed]
23. Guan, W.; Liu, Y.; Liu, Y.; Wang, Q.; Ye, H.L.; Cheng, Y.G.; Kuang, H.X.; Jiang, X.C.; Yang, B.Y. Proteomics Research on the Protective Effect of Mangiferin on H9C2 Cell Injury Induced by H_2O_2. *Molecules* **2019**, *24*, 1911. [CrossRef] [PubMed]
24. Yang, Y.; Liu, M.-c.; Li, H.; Yang, Y.-g.; Su, N.; Wu, Y.-j.; Wang, H. Proteomics analysis of the protective effect of canola (*Brassica campestris* L.) bee pollen flavonoids on the tert butyl hydroperoxide-induced EA.hy926 cell injury model. *J. Funct. Foods* **2020**, *75*, 104223. [CrossRef]
25. Lai, C.; Liang, Y.; Zhang, L.; Huang, J.; Kaliaperumal, K.; Jiang, Y.; Zhang, J. Variations of Bioactive Phytochemicals and Antioxidant Capacity of Navel Orange Peel in Response to Different Drying Methods. *Antioxidants* **2022**, *11*, 1543. [CrossRef] [PubMed]
26. Kozlov, A.V.; Javadov, S.; Sommer, N. Cellular ROS and Antioxidants: Physiological and Pathological Role. *Antioxidants* **2024**, *13*, 602. [CrossRef]
27. Cui, Y.; Wang, R.; Cao, S.; Ismael, M.; Wang, X.; Lü, X. A galacturonic acid-rich polysaccharide from *Diospyros kaki* peel: Isolation, characterization, rheological properties and antioxidant activities in vitro. *Food Chem.* **2023**, *416*, 135781. [CrossRef]
28. Kim, Y.-J.; Kim, M.-J.; Kweon, D.-K.; Lim, S.-T.; Lee, S.-J. Polydeoxyribonucleotide Activates Mitochondrial Biogenesis but Reduces MMP-1 Activity and Melanin Biosynthesis in Cultured Skin Cells. *Appl. Biochem. Biotechnol.* **2020**, *191*, 540–554. [CrossRef] [PubMed]
29. Park, K.-J.; Kim, Y.-J.; Kim, J.; Kim, S.M.; Lee, S.Y.; Bae, J.-W.; Hwang, K.-K.; Kim, D.-W.; Cho, M.-C. Protective Effects of Peroxiredoxin on Hydrogen Peroxide Induced Oxidative Stress and Apoptosis in Cardiomyocytes. *Korean Circ. J.* **2012**, *42*, 23–32. [CrossRef]
30. Zhao, Y.; Jiang, Q.; Zhang, X.; Zhu, X.; Dong, X.; Shen, L.; Zhang, S.; Niu, L.; Chen, L.; Zhang, M.; et al. l-Arginine Alleviates LPS-Induced Oxidative Stress and Apoptosis via Activating SIRT1-AKT-Nrf2 and SIRT1-FOXO3a Signaling Pathways in C2C12 Myotube Cells. *Antioxidants* **2021**, *10*, 1957. [CrossRef]
31. Pan, Y.; Long, X.; Yi, R.; Zhao, X. Polyphenols in Liubao Tea Can Prevent CCl_4-Induced Hepatic Damage in Mice through Its Antioxidant Capacities. *Nutrients* **2018**, *10*, 1280. [CrossRef] [PubMed]
32. Petriccione, M.; Mastrobuoni, F.; Pasquariello, M.S.; Zampella, L.; Nobis, E.; Capriolo, G.; Scortichini, M. Effect of Chitosan Coating on the Postharvest Quality and Antioxidant Enzyme System Response of Strawberry Fruit during Cold Storage. *Foods* **2015**, *4*, 501–523. [CrossRef] [PubMed]
33. Li, Y.; Sun, M.; Cao, F.; Chen, Y.; Zhang, L.; Li, H.; Cao, J.; Song, J.; Ma, Y.; Mi, W.; et al. The Ferroptosis Inhibitor Liproxstatin-1 Ameliorates LPS-Induced Cognitive Impairment in Mice. *Nutrients* **2022**, *14*, 4599. [CrossRef] [PubMed]
34. Mendes, R.; Cardoso, C.; Pestana, C. Measurement of malondialdehyde in fish: A comparison study between HPLC methods and the traditional spectrophotometric test. *Food Chem.* **2009**, *112*, 1038–1045. [CrossRef]
35. Li, S.; Sampson, C.; Liu, C.; Piao, H.-l.; Liu, H.-X. Integrin signaling in cancer: Bidirectional mechanisms and therapeutic opportunities. *Cell Commun. Signal.* **2023**, *21*, 266. [CrossRef] [PubMed]
36. Liu, X.; Zhang, M.; Cheng, X.; Liu, X.; Sun, H.; Guo, Z.; Li, J.; Tang, X.; Wang, Z.; Sun, W.; et al. LC-MS-Based Plasma Metabolomics and Lipidomics Analyses for Differential Diagnosis of Bladder Cancer and Renal Cell Carcinoma. *Front. Oncol.* **2020**, *10*, 717. [CrossRef] [PubMed]
37. Arneth, B. Coevolution of the coagulation and immune systems. *Inflamm. Res.* **2019**, *68*, 117–123. [CrossRef] [PubMed]
38. Martinez-Val, A.; Bekker-Jensen, D.B.; Steigerwald, S.; Koenig, C.; Østergaard, O.; Mehta, A.; Tran, T.; Sikorski, K.; Torres-Vega, E.; Kwasniewicz, E.; et al. Spatial-proteomics reveals phospho-signaling dynamics at subcellular resolution. *Nat. Commun.* **2021**, *12*, 7113. [CrossRef] [PubMed]
39. Bader, G.D.; Hogue, C.W. An automated method for finding molecular complexes in large protein interaction networks. *BMC Bioinform.* **2003**, *4*, 2. [CrossRef]
40. Zhang, Z.-H.; Song, G.-L. Roles of Selenoproteins in Brain Function and the Potential Mechanism of Selenium in Alzheimer's Disease. *Front. Neurosci.* **2021**, *15*, 646518. [CrossRef]

41. Barrett, C.W.; Short, S.P.; Williams, C.S. Selenoproteins and oxidative stress-induced inflammatory tumorigenesis in the gut. *Cell. Mol. Life Sci.* **2017**, *74*, 607–616. [CrossRef] [PubMed]
42. Varone, E.; Pozzer, D.; Di Modica, S.; Chernorudskiy, A.; Nogara, L.; Baraldo, M.; Cinquanta, M.; Fumagalli, S.; Villar-Quiles, R.N.; De Simoni, M.-G.; et al. SELENON (SEPN1) protects skeletal muscle from saturated fatty acid-induced ER stress and insulin resistance. *Redox Biol.* **2019**, *24*, 101176. [CrossRef] [PubMed]
43. Wang, J.; Chang, Y.; Wu, F.; Xu, X.; Xue, C. Fucosylated chondroitin sulfate is covalently associated with collagen fibrils in sea cucumber *Apostichopus japonicus* body wall. *Carbohydr. Polym.* **2018**, *186*, 439–444. [CrossRef] [PubMed]
44. Liu, Y.; Dave, D.; Trenholm, S.; Ramakrishnan, V.V.; Murphy, W. Effect of Drying on Nutritional Composition of Atlantic Sea Cucumber (*Cucumaria frondosa*) Viscera Derived from Newfoundland Fisheries. *Processes* **2021**, *9*, 4. [CrossRef]
45. Mamelona, J.; Saint-Louis, R.; Pelletier, É. Proximate composition and nutritional profile of by-products from green urchin and Atlantic sea cucumber processing plants. *Int. J. Food Sci. Technol.* **2010**, *45*, 2119–2126. [CrossRef]
46. Hossain, A.; Yeo, J.; Dave, D.; Shahidi, F. Phenolic Compounds and Antioxidant Capacity of Sea Cucumber (*Cucumaria frondosa*) Processing Discards as Affected by High-Pressure Processing (HPP). *Antioxidants* **2022**, *11*, 337. [CrossRef] [PubMed]
47. Zhong, C.; Sun, L.-C.; Yan, L.-J.; Lin, Y.-C.; Liu, G.-M.; Cao, M.-J. Production, optimisation and characterisation of angiotensin converting enzyme inhibitory peptides from sea cucumber (*Stichopus japonicus*) gonad. *Food Funct.* **2018**, *9*, 594–603. [CrossRef] [PubMed]
48. Squadrito, F.; Bitto, A.; Irrera, N.; Pizzino, G.; Pallio, G.; Minutoli, L.; Altavilla, D. Pharmacological Activity and Clinical Use of PDRN. *Front. Pharmacol.* **2017**, *8*, 224. [CrossRef] [PubMed]
49. Hua, Z.; Zhang, J.; Cheng, W.; Wang, C.; Zhao, D. Ethanolic Extract from Seed Residues of Sea Buckthorn (*Hippophae rhamnoides* L.) Ameliorates Oxidative Stress Damage and Prevents Apoptosis in Murine Cell and Aging Animal Models. *Foods* **2023**, *12*, 3322. [CrossRef]
50. Čakar, U.; Čolović, M.; Milenković, D.; Medić, B.; Krstić, D.; Petrović, A.; Đorđević, B. Protective Effects of Fruit Wines against Hydrogen Peroxide—Induced Oxidative Stress in Rat Synaptosomes. *Agronomy* **2021**, *11*, 1414. [CrossRef]
51. Chiabrando, D.; Vinchi, F.; Fiorito, V.; Mercurio, S.; Tolosano, E. Heme in pathophysiology: A matter of scavenging, metabolism and trafficking across cell membranes. *Front. Pharmacol.* **2014**, *5*, 61. [CrossRef] [PubMed]
52. Ross, D.; Siegel, D. Functions of NQO1 in Cellular Protection and CoQ10 Metabolism and its Potential Role as a Redox Sensitive Molecular Switch. *Front. Physiol.* **2017**, *8*, 595. [CrossRef] [PubMed]
53. Yu, C.; Xiao, J.-H. The Keap1-Nrf2 System: A Mediator between Oxidative Stress and Aging. *Oxid. Med. Cell. Longev.* **2021**, *2021*, 6635460. [CrossRef] [PubMed]
54. Andrade, M.O.; Sforca, M.L.; Heleno Batista, F.A.; Migliorini Figueira, A.C.; Benedetti, C.E. The MAF1 Phosphoregulatory Region Controls MAF1 Interaction with the RNA Polymerase III C34 Subunit and Transcriptional Repression in Plants. *Plant Cell* **2020**, *32*, 3019–3035. [CrossRef] [PubMed]
55. Manivannan, S.N.; Darouich, S.; Masmoudi, A.; Gordon, D.; Zender, G.; Han, Z.; Fitzgerald-Butt, S.; White, P.; McBride, K.L.; Kharrat, M.; et al. Novel frameshift variant in MYL2 reveals molecular differences between dominant and recessive forms of hypertrophic cardiomyopathy. *PLoS Genet.* **2020**, *16*, e1008639. [CrossRef] [PubMed]
56. Hsia, D.A.; Tepper, C.G.; Pochampalli, M.R.; Hsia, E.Y.C.; Izumiya, C.; Huerta, S.B.; Wright, M.E.; Chen, H.-W.; Kung, H.-J.; Izumiya, Y. KDM8, a H3K36me2 histone demethylase that acts in the cyclin A1 coding region to regulate cancer cell proliferation. *Proc. Natl. Acad. Sci. USA* **2010**, *107*, 9671–9676. [CrossRef] [PubMed]
57. Anijs, M.; Devanna, P.; Vernes, S.C. *ARHGEF39*, a Gene Implicated in Developmental Language Disorder, Activates RHOA and Is Involved in Cell De-Adhesion and Neural Progenitor Cell Proliferation. *Front. Mol. Neurosci.* **2022**, *15*, 941494. [CrossRef] [PubMed]
58. Hallmann, K.; Kudin, A.P.; Zsurka, G.; Kornblum, C.; Reimann, J.; Stüve, B.; Waltz, S.; Hattingen, E.; Thiele, H.; Nürnberg, P.; et al. Loss of the smallest subunit of cytochrome c oxidase, COX8A, causes Leigh-like syndrome and epilepsy. *Brain* **2016**, *139*, 338–345. [CrossRef] [PubMed]
59. Cui, X.; Mi, T.; Xiao, X.; Zhang, H.; Dong, Y.; Huang, N.; Gao, P.; Lee, J.; Guelakis, M.; Gu, X. Topical glutathione amino acid precursors protect skin against environmental and oxidative stress. *J. Eur. Acad. Dermatol. Venereol.* **2024**, *38*, 3–11. [CrossRef]
60. Zhang, Y.; Roh, Y.J.; Han, S.-J.; Park, I.; Lee, H.M.; Ok, Y.S.; Lee, B.C.; Lee, S.-R. Role of Selenoproteins in Redox Regulation of Signaling and the Antioxidant System: A Review. *Antioxidants* **2020**, *9*, 383. [CrossRef]
61. Yu, M.; Yu, J.; Yi, Y.; Chen, T.; Yu, L.; Zeng, W.; Ouyang, X.-k.; Huang, C.; Sun, S.; Wang, Y.; et al. Oxidative stress-amplified nanomedicine for intensified ferroptosis-apoptosis combined tumor therapy. *J. Control. Release* **2022**, *347*, 104–114. [CrossRef] [PubMed]
62. Cawthorn, D.-M.; Steinman, H.A.; Witthuhn, R.C. Comparative study of different methods for the extraction of DNA from fish species commercially available in South Africa. *Food Control* **2011**, *22*, 231–244. [CrossRef]
63. Shao, P.; Chen, X.; Sun, P. Improvement of antioxidant and moisture-preserving activities of Sargassum horneri polysaccharide enzymatic hydrolyzates. *Int. J. Biol. Macromol.* **2015**, *74*, 420–427. [CrossRef] [PubMed]

64. Xu, B.; Zhang, A.; Zheng, Y.; Wang, H.; Zheng, X.; Jin, Z.; Liu, D.; Wang, N.; Kan, Y. Influences of superfine-grinding and enzymolysis separately assisted with carboxymethylation and acetylation on the in vitro hypoglycemic and antioxidant activities of oil palm kernel expeller fibre. *Food Chem.* **2024**, *449*, 139192. [CrossRef]
65. Souza, B.W.S.; Cerqueira, M.A.; Bourbon, A.I.; Pinheiro, A.C.; Martins, J.T.; Teixeira, J.A.; Coimbra, M.A.; Vicente, A.A. Chemical characterization and antioxidant activity of sulfated polysaccharide from the red seaweed *Gracilaria birdiae*. *Food Hydrocoll.* **2012**, *27*, 287–292. [CrossRef]

marine drugs

MDPI

Article

Influence of a Very High-Molecular Weight Fucoidan from *Laminaria hyperborea* on Age-Related Macular Degeneration-Relevant Pathomechanisms in Ocular Cell Models

Philipp Dörschmann [1,*], Georg Kopplin [2], Tabea Thalenhorst [1], Charlotte Seeba [1], Sadia Fida Ullah [3], Vaibhav Srivastava [3], Johann Roider [1] and Alexa Klettner [1]

1 Department of Ophthalmology, University Medical Center, University of Kiel, Arnold-Heller-Str. 3, Haus 25, 24105 Kiel, Germany; johann.roider@uksh.de (J.R.); alexa.klettner@uksh.de (A.K.)
2 Alginor ASA, Haraldsgata 162, 5525 Haugesund, Norway; georg@alginor.no
3 Division of Glycoscience, Department of Chemistry, School of Engineering Sciences in Chemistry, Biotechnology and Health, Royal Institute of Technology (KTH), AlbaNova University Centre, SE106 91 Stockholm, Sweden; ullahsf@kth.se (S.F.U.); vasri@kth.se (V.S.)
* Correspondence: philipp.doerschmann@uksh.de; Tel.: +49-431-500-13712

Abstract: Fucoidans from *Laminaria hyperborea* (LH) can be antioxidative, antiangiogenic, and anti-inflammatory. In this study, a very high-molecular weight (3700 kDa) fucoidan from LH, FucBB04, was tested regarding its bioactivity in age-related macular degeneration (AMD) models *in vitro*. Primary retinal pigment epithelium (RPE) from pig eyes, human uveal melanoma cell line OMM-1, and RPE cell line ARPE-19 were used. Substituents of the extract were determined with chemical analysis. Cell viability was tested with tetrazolium assay (MTT), oxidative stress was induced by H_2O_2 or erastin, respectively. Secreted vascular endothelial growth factor A (VEGF-A) was assessed with ELISA. Retinal pigment epithelium 65 kDa protein (RPE65) and protectin (CD59) protein expression were tested in Western blot. Cell barrier was assessed by measuring trans-epithelial electrical resistance (TEER), phagocytic ability by a fluorescence assay. Gene expression and secretion of interleukin 6 (IL-6) and interleukin 8 (IL-8) were tested in real-time PCR and ELISA. FucBB04 displayed no oxidative stress protective effects. Its effect on VEGF was inconsistent, with VEGF secretion reduced in primary RPE, but not in ARPE-19. On the other hand, Lipopolysaccharide (LPS) and polyinosinic/polycytidylic acid (PIC)-induced IL-6 or IL-8 secretion was reduced by FucBB04, while complement inhibiting protein CD59 was not affected. In addition, FucBB04 did not influence the gene expression of IL-6 or IL-8. Visual cycle protein RPE65 expression, phagocytic ability, and barrier function were reduced by FucBB04. Very high-molecular weight fucoidan from LH shows bioactivities against AMD-related pathological pathways, but adverse effects on RPE function may limit its suitability as a therapeutic compound. Smaller high-molecular weight fucoidans are recommended for further research.

Keywords: sulfated fucan; fucoidan; retinal pigment epithelium-specific 65 kDa protein (RPE65); vascular endothelial growth factor (VEGF); phagocytosis; gene expression; protectin (CD59); trans-epithelial electrical resistance (TEER); interleukin; toll-like receptor; polyinosinic/polycytidylic acid (PIC)

1. Introduction

Age-related macular degeneration (AMD) is the major cause for blindness and severe visual impairment in the elderly in the industrialized world [1]. The disease can be divided in an asymptomatic early and two vision threatening late forms. The late forms consist of the atrophic or "dry" form, in which degenerate changes in the retinal pigment epithelium (RPE) and the photoreceptors result in a slow progressive vision deterioration, and the neovascular exudative or "wet" form, in which vessels grow under or into the retina and visual acuity decreases rapidly. Currently, only the late wet form can be targeted by therapeutics (mainly intravitreal VEGF inhibitors), which may hold or reduce disease progression. New therapeutics targeting the early forms and slowing the progression are clearly warranted [2].

On a cellular level, the pathology of AMD occurs in the photoreceptor/RPE/choroid complex, with the RPE being the major player in AMD development [3]. The RPE exerts many functions in the retina, supporting the photoreceptors and upholding visual function. RPE cells protect the photoreceptors by scavenging stray light und protecting against oxidative stress [4]. They phagocytose shed photoreceptor outer segments and participate in recycling of the visual pigment [5]. Furthermore, they form the outer blood–retina barrier, thereby regulating transport from and to the photoreceptors and contributing to the retinal immune privilege [6]. On the other hand, they can contribute to inflammation, as they act as sentinels to danger signals, expressing toll-like receptors (TLR) 3 and 4, and secreting various pro-inflammatory stimuli upon activation [7,8].

On the cellular and tissue level, the pathomechanisms in AMD development include oxidative stress, lipid dysregulation, inflammation, complement activation, and, in the wet form, angiogenesis caused by increased VEGF secretion [8–11]. A compound that could target several of these mechanisms would be of high interest for treating early AMD development and slowing down or halting its progression.

Such a potential compound is fucoidan, a polysaccharide obtained from brown seaweed [12]. Our group has previously shown that fucoidans could exert antiangiogenic, antioxidative, and anti-inflammatory effects in retinal cells [13–15]. However, fucoidans are a heterogenic group and their bioactivity depends strongly on its species of origin and the extraction methods, as well as other factors [16]. In particular, the pro- and antiangiogenic properties of fucoidan have been linked to their molecular weight, with low-molecular weight fucoidans described as pro- and high-molecular weight fucoidans as antiangiogenic [17]. In addition, anti-inflammatory and complement-inhibiting properties of fucoidans have been related to their degree of sulfation and their fucose content [18,19]. Our own studies support these findings, as beneficial bioactivities of fucoidans regarding AMD-related pathways are connected to a higher molecular weight, a higher degree of sulfation, and a high content of fucose [13].

Previously, we could show that fucoidan from *Laminaria hyperborea* (LH) with a high-molecular weight (1549 kDa) showed promising characteristics compared to fucoidans of lower molecular weight from the same species [20]. Therefore, we wanted to investigate the effect of very high-molecular weight fucoidan (3700 kDa; FucBB04) from this species.

We investigated the bioactivity in regards to the important pathomechanisms of oxidative stress, inflammation, and angiogenesis (VEGF secretion) in ocular *in vitro* models, using the human RPE cell line ARPE-19 [21], primary porcine RPE cells [22], and the uveal melanoma cell line OMM-1 [23]. Primary porcine RPE cells are an excellent model for human RPE cells, displaying a highly differentiated phenotype (when used without further passaging) and a high barrier (as assessed in transepithelial electric resistance), exhibiting natural functions such as phagocytosis, sentinel functions, and cytokine secretion [24]. ARPE-19 cells are an RPE cell line with some similarities to RPE cells, such as a constitutive (albeit lesser) secretion of VEGF. Furthermore, concerning angiogenesis or cell death, they exhibit similar gene expression while being more susceptible to oxidative stress than fully differentiated RPE cells, rendering them a good model for testing oxidative stress protection [24,25]. OMM-1, an uveal melanoma cell line, was added as they are more susceptible to oxidative stress compared to primary RPE or ARPE-19 cells [26].

In addition to testing AMD-relevant bioactivity, we investigated the effect of this fucoidan on important functions of the RPE, assessing survival, phagocytosis, barrier properties, and the expression of a protein important for the visual cycle (retinal pigment epithelium 65 kDa protein, RPE65) [27] and complement inhibition (protectin, CD59) [28]. Furthermore, we present the highest molecular weight fucoidan reported so far.

2. Results

2.1. Chemical Characterization of Fucoidan

The applied extraction and purification methods omitted depolymerization and further removed lower molecular weight fractions (300 kDa molecular weight cut-off, MWCO) from the sample, aiming for high-molecular weight fucoidan from LH.

Monosaccharide analysis of FucBB04 revealed a fucose content of 91.59 ± 1.40%, classifying it as a fucan according to Deniaud-Bouët et al. (2017) [29]. Galactose (0.50 ± 0.42%), xylose (0.71 ± 0.05%), rhamnose (1.32 ± 0.26), mannose (0.44 ± 0.15), and three uronic acids, namely galacturonic acid (1.60 ± 0.12), mannuronic acid (1.95 ± 0.23), and guluronic acid (1.86 ± 0.08), were found (Table 1). Even though monosaccharide residues of xylose, rhamnose, and uronic are common in fucoidans from brown seaweed [30,31], this is, to our knowledge, the first time those are reported for fucoidan from LH [32,33].

Table 1. Monosaccharide composition of very high-molecular weight fucoidan from *Laminaria hyperborea*. Analysis performed in three replicates (molecular percentage and standard deviation are indicated). Fuc = fucose; Rha = rhamnose; Gal = galactose; Xyl = xylose; Man = mannose; GalA = galacturonic acid; ManA = mannuronic acid; GulA = guluronic acid; SD = standard deviation.

Sugar	Fuc	Rha	Gal	Xyl	Man	GalA	ManA	GulA	Other
Mol%	91.59	1.32	0.50	0.71	0.44	1.60	1.95	1.86	0.53
SD	1.40	0.26	0.42	0.05	0.15	0.12	0.23	0.08	–

Mass spectrometry of FucBB04 revealed a sulfur content (S) of 12.4%, corresponding to a sulfate content ($NaSO_3$) of 39.5% and a sulfation degree (DS) of approximately 0.95 [33] (Table 2). Raman spectra showed strong bands at 1063 cm^{-1} and 839 cm^{-1}, related to vibrations of the sulfate group, confirming sulfation in the C-4 position [34].

Table 2. Data overview of the sulfated fucan samples used in this study. Degree of sulfation (DS), weight average molar mass (Mw), number average molar mass (Mn), polydispersity index (PD), degree of polymerization (DP_n), Z-average radius of gyration (Rz), refractive index increment (dn/dc), slope of the RMS conformation plot (b = rms versus M), and the total phenolic content in the sample (TPC).

Fucoidan	DS	M_w [kDa]	M_n [kDa]	PD	DP_n	R_z [nm]	dn/dc	B	TPC [%]
FucBB04	0.95	3700	2500	1.48	10,300	249	0.115	0.44	0.0

SEC-MALS (Size-Exclusion Chromatography with Multi-Angle Light Scattering) revealed a very high-molecular weight average of M_w = 3700 kDa, resulting in an average degree of polymerization (DP_n) of 10,300, with an approximated average monosaccharide unit weight of 243 g/mol. To our knowledge, this is the highest molecular weight average for fucoidan yet reported [35,36]. The radius of gyration as the Z-average (R_z) was found to be 249.0 nm. The overall shape of the molecule was determined through an rms conformation plot (root mean square radius [nm] versus M [g/mol], Figure 1), displaying a slope

(b) of 0.44 and thus placing the overall shape of the molecule between random coil and sphere conformation (sphere b = 0.33; random coil b = 0.5; rigid rod b = 1) [37,38]. A high degree of branching for fucoidan from LH was previously reported [33]. However, light scattering experiments suggested an oligomeric branching 'short-chain branches', while a conformation towards a spherical shape is indicative of polymeric branching 'long-chain branches' or hyper-branching, respectively [39,40].

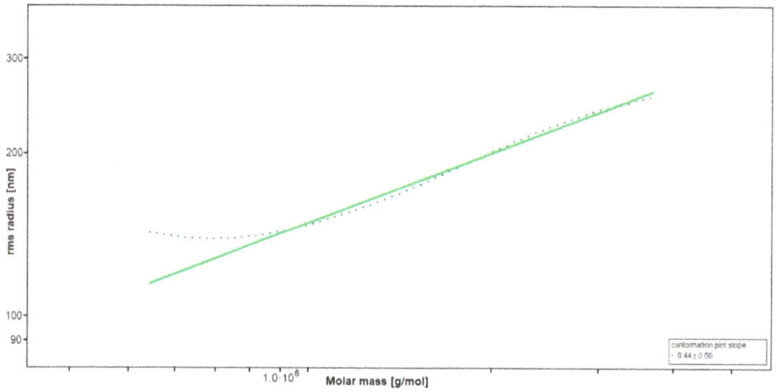

Figure 1. Rms conformation plot of the high-molecular weight fucoidan (FucBB04) giving the rms (root mean square) radius [nm] versus M [g/mol]. The slope (b) = 0.44 indicates a random coil with substantial branching.

Total phenolic content (TPC) analysis using the Folin–Ciocalteu TPC assay as well as Raman spectroscopy showed absence of any phenolic residues within the sample.

2.2. Oxidative Stress Assays

In the development of AMD, oxidative stress is a major factor [41]. The retina is burdened with a high life-long exposure to oxidative stress because of high oxygen pressure, constant light exposure, high mitochondrial metabolism, lipid peroxidation, and intracellular deposits such as lipofuscin [41].

Established oxidative stress models were utilized as previously described [26,42,43]. Human uveal melanoma cell line OMM-1 (Figure 2a) and human RPE cell line ARPE-19 (Figure 2b) were stimulated with 1, 10, 50, or 100 µg/mL LH fucoidan FucBB04, respectively, for 30 min. In addition, oxidative stress insult was applied by 500 µM H_2O_2 or 25 µM erastin for OMM-1 and 250 µM H_2O_2 or 20 µM erastin for ARPE-19 for 4 or 24 h, respectively. Tetrazolium bromide assay [3-(4,5-dimethylthiazol-2-yl)-2,5-diphenyltetrazolium bromide, MTT] was used to determine cell viability. Absorption was set into relation to the untreated control, set as 100%. Regarding short-term effects of fucoidan on cell viability, FucBB04 increased the viability signal to 111 ± 2% (p = 0.0001) in OMM-1 and decreased the viability slightly in all concentrations in ARPE-19. These small effects should be of little biological relevance. Concerning oxidative stress assays, in OMM-1, viability was reduced to 42 ± 11% with 500 µM H_2O_2 (p = 0.0005) and to 67 ± 6% with 25 µM erastin (p = 0.0001), after 4 h of stimulation. Cell viability was not relevantly influenced with co-treatment of the extract. In ARPE-19, cell viability was decreased by 250 µM H_2O_2 to 44 ± 22% (p = 0.0002) and by 20 µM erastin to 26 ± 16% (p = 0.0001) after 24 h of stimulation. Also, the extract did not show any relevant effects concerning oxidative stress protection. Taken together, these results indicate that FucBB04 lacked short-term antioxidative effects in the models tested.

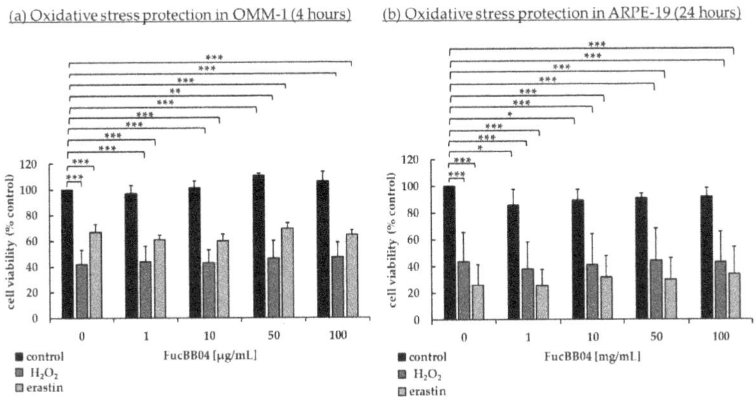

Figure 2. Oxidative stress assay. Human uveal melanoma cell line OMM-1 (**a**) and human retinal pigment epithelium cell line ARPE-19 (**b**) were treated with 1, 10, 50, or 100 µg/mL FucBB04 fucoidan. For oxidative stress insult, 500 µM H_2O_2 or 25 µM erastin for OMM-1 and 250 µM H_2O_2 or 20 µM erastin for ARPE-19 were applied for 4 h or 24 h, respectively. Cell survival was tested with tetrazolium bromide assay (MTT). Absorption was set into relation to the untreated control (100%). Data were normally distributed (Shapiro–Wilk test). One-sample *t*-test was conducted. * $p \leq 0.05$, ** $p \leq 0.01$, *** $p \leq 0.001$ (compared to control, 0 µg/mL FucBB04 = 100%), $n \geq 5$.

2.3. Vascular Endothelial Growth Factor Secretion

Increased VEGF secretion plays an important role in the development of wet AMD [44]. Fucoidans have been shown to decrease VEGF in the supernatant of ocular cells [13]. ARPE-19 (Figure 3) and primary porcine RPE (Figure 4) cells were stimulated with FucBB04 (1, 10, 50, and 100 µg/mL), with the former one for 3 days and the latter for 3, 7, and 28 days. As primary RPE resemble the in vivo situation more closely, more time points and long-term effects were examined. Also, they produce nearly four times more VEGF per hour than ARPE-19 (ARPE-19: 66 pg/h and RPE: 243 pg/h, [20]). Supernatants were harvested after 24 h collection time for ARPE-19 and 4 h collection time for RPE. Supernatants were applied in human VEGF-A DuoSet ELISA. MTT assay was conducted at the end of the experiments to control for potential toxic effects influencing VEGF secretion.

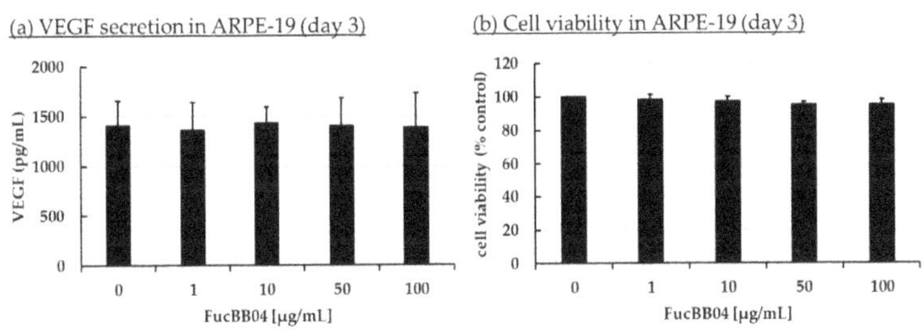

Figure 3. VEGF secretion and cell viability of ARPE-19. ARPE-19 cells were stimulated with 1, 10, 50, and 100 µg/mL FucBB04, respectively, for three days. Supernatant was collected for 24 h by renewing media with extracts on day 2. VEGF-A was determined in ELISA (**a**). MTT assay was performed at day 3 to measure cell viability (**b**). VEGF content in pg/mL of supernatants is shown. Data showed Gaussian distribution (Shapiro–Wilk test) and ANOVA by post hoc Dunnett's test was performed to calculate significances. No significant changes compared to 0 µg/mL FucBB04 were detected. $n = 4$.

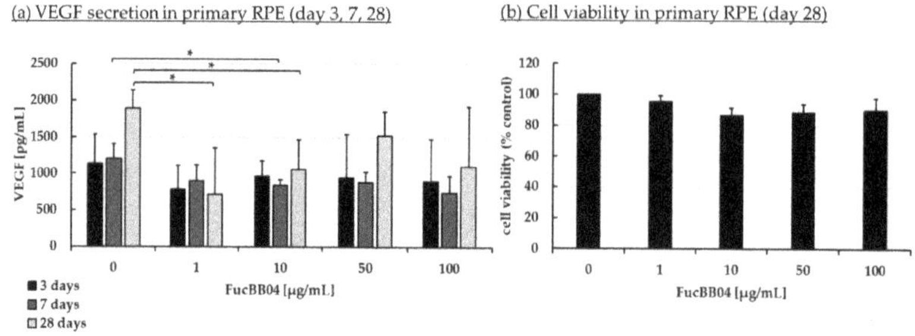

Figure 4. VEGF secretion and cell viability of primary RPE. Primary porcine RPE cells were stimulated with 1, 10, 50, and 100 µg/mL FucBB04 for 3, 7, and 28 days, respectively. Supernatant was collected on the individual days after changing media with extracts four hours before supernatant collection. VEGF-A was detected in ELISA (**a**). MTT assay was performed at day 28 to measure cell viability (**b**). VEGF content in pg/mL of supernatants is shown. Data showed Gaussian distribution (Shapiro–Wilk test) and ANOVA by post hoc Dunnett's test was performed to calculate significances. * $p \leq 0.05$ (compared to 0 µg/mL FucBB04 of the same day of treatment). $n = 3$.

In ARPE-19, no antiproliferative effects were found after three days (Figure 3b). VEGF secretion was also not significantly influenced (Figure 3a). In primary RPE cells, neither cell viability (Figure 4b) nor VEGF secretion (Figure 4a) was significantly altered by FucBB04 treatment after 28 days. Of note, a reduction is seen in VEGF content which does not reach statistical significance because of high standard deviation. After three days of treatment, all tested concentrations reduced VEGF slightly but not significantly. After seven days of stimulation, 10 µg/mL FucBB04 reduced VEGF content significantly from 1206 ± 202 pg/mL to 841 ± 73 ($p = 0.0422$). Here, 1, 50, and 100 µg/mL fucoidan reduced VEGF as well but reached no statistical significance. After 28 days of stimulation, secreted VEGF was significantly lowered by 1 and 10 µg/mL fucoidan from 1892 ± 248 pg/mL to 711 ± 640 pg/mL ($p = 0.0407$) and 1057 ± 411 pg/mL ($p = 0.0394$), respectively, while 50 and 100 µg/mL fucoidan also reduced it numerically without reaching significance.

2.4. Interleukin Secretion

Inflammation plays an important role in the development of AMD and we have previously shown fucoidans to exert anti-inflammatory effects on RPE cells [9,14]. Primary RPE were treated with FucBB04 for 30 min, followed by pro-inflammatory stimulation by applying 1 µg/mL lipopolysaccharide (LPS), 10 µg/mL polyinosinic/polycytidylic acid (PIC), 50 ng/mL tumor necrosis factor alpha (TNF), or 10 ng/mL Pam2CSK4 (Pam), respectively. These agents and concentrations are based on previous findings [7]. Appropriate controls with fucoidan or inflammatory stimuli were included. Cells were stimulated for 1, 3, 7, and 28 days and supernatant collected for 24 h. Supernatants were analyzed in ELISA for porcine IL-6 (Figure 5) and IL-8 (Figure 6). Also, MTT assays were performed to determine cell viability after 1, 3, 7, and 28 days of treatment. No significant or relevant antiproliferative effects regarding stressors or extracts were found (refer to Appendix A.1).

Regarding IL-6 secretion, significant secretion was induced by all agents, with LPS and PIC exhibiting significant secretion at any time point tested. Pam only exhibited a short time response, losing this effect from day 3 (Figure 5b), and TNF no longer displayed a significant increase at day 28 (Figure 5d). FucBB04 alone did not induce a significant IL-6 release, but it was nominally increased at day 1 (Figure 5a) to 1846 pg/mL ($p = 0.178$). In general, FucBB04 displayed little effect on the level of secreted IL-6, with the exception of IL-6 secretion at day 7 (Figure 5c) after stimulation with PIC. Here, FucBB04 significantly reduced the secretion from 958 ± 485 pg/mL to 194 ± 210 pg/mL IL-6 ($p = 0.001$). Of note, several pro-inflammatory activations by different stimuli lost their significance after treatment with FucBB04, and for PIC treatment it was also numerically decreased on day 3 and day 28.

Regarding IL-8 secretion, FucBB04 increased IL-8 release significantly on day 1 (Figure 6a) with 1396 ± 396 pg/mL ($p = 0.032$) compared to control with 135 ± 177 pg/mL. All pro-inflammatory stimuli significantly increased IL-8 secretion on all tested time points. FucBB04 reduced IL-8 in several stimulations: On day 1 and 28 (Figure 6d), LPS-induced IL-8 secretion was reduced by FucBB04 from 4475 ± 1924 pg/mL to 1809 ± 460 pg/mL ($p = 0.0009$), and from 1614 ± 813 pg/mL to 595 ± 381 pg/mL ($p = 0.023$), respectively. On day 3 (Figure 6b) and 7 (Figure 6c), PIC-induced IL-8 secretion was reduced from 1827 ± 920 pg/mL to 610 ± 335 pg/mL ($p = 0.016$), and from 1804 ± 656 pg/mL to 566 ± 345 pg/mL ($p = 0.009$), respectively. Taken together, FucBB04 seems to interact with LPS-induced TLR-4 activation at short-term and long-term conditions and on PIC-induced TLR-3 activation at mid-term conditions, indicating an anti-inflammatory potential. There are clear differences in the activity of fucoidan between IL-6 and IL-8 assays as well as for the inflammatory agents which excludes a mere scavenging effect.

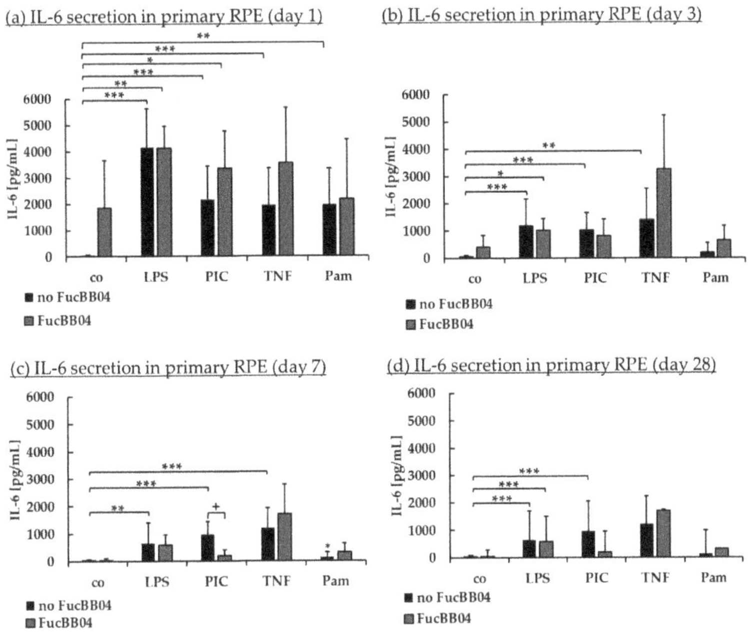

Figure 5. Interleukin 6 secretion. Primary porcine RPE cells were stimulated with 50 µg/mL FucBB04, and/or 1 µg/mL lipopolysaccharide (LPS), 10 µg/mL polyinosinic/polycytidylic acid (PIC), 50 ng/mL tumor necrosis factor alpha (TNF), or 10 ng/mL Pam2CSK4 (Pam) for 1 (**a**), 3 (**b**), 7 (**c**), and 28 days (**d**). Supernatants were collected and IL-6 was determined in ELISA. Data showed Gaussian distribution (Shapiro–Wilk test) and ANOVA by post hoc Dunnett's test was performed to calculate significances. * $p \leq 0.05$, ** $p \leq 0.01$, *** $p \leq 0.001$ (compared to co, no FucBB04); + $p \leq 0.05$ (compared to stress control LPS, PIC, TNF or Pam, no FucBB04); co = control, $n \geq 3$.

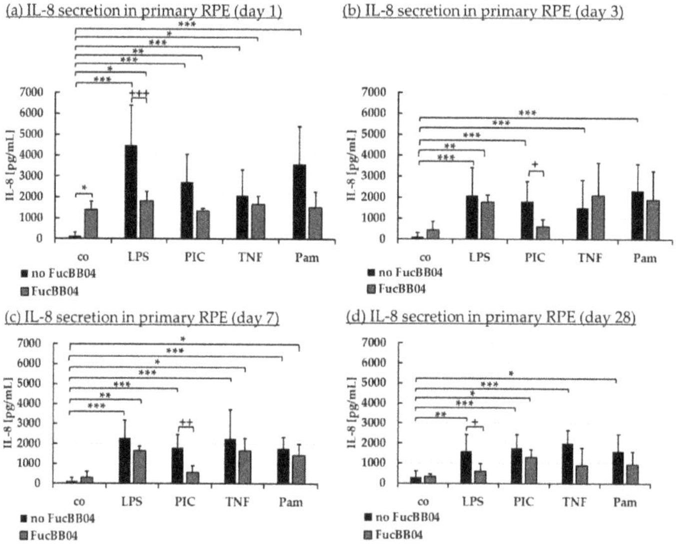

Figure 6. Interleukin 8 secretion. Porcine RPE cells were stimulated with 50 μg/mL FucBB04, and/or 1 μg/mL lipopolysaccharide (LPS), 10 μg/mL polyinosinic/polycytidylic acid (PIC), 50 ng/mL tumor necrosis factor alpha (TNF), or 10 ng/mL Pam2CSK4 (Pam) for 1 (**a**), 3 (**b**), 7 (**c**), and 28 days (**d**). Supernatants were collected and IL-8 was determined in ELISA. Data showed Gaussian distribution (Shapiro–Wilk test) and ANOVA by post hoc Dunnett's test was performed to calculate significances. * $p \leq 0.05$, ** $p \leq 0.01$, *** $p \leq 0.001$ (compared to co, no FucBB04); + $p \leq 0.05$, ++ $p \leq 0.01$, +++ $p \leq 0.001$ (compared to stress control LPS, PIC, TNF or Pam, no FucBB04); co = control, $n \geq 3$.

2.5. Interleukin Gene Expression

In addition to secreted proteins, we also investigated IL-6 and IL-8 gene expression. We focused on PIC-stimulated RPE cells (as they showed the most promising activities in Section 2.4) for three and seven days with 50 μg/mL FucBB04 and/or 10 μg/mL PIC. RNA was isolated, transcribed to cDNA, and real-time polymerase chain reaction was conducted to measure relative gene expression of IL-6 (*IL6*) and IL-8 (*CXCL8* or *IL8*). Glyceraldehyde-3-phosphate dehydrogenase (*GAPDH*) was used as endogenous control.

PIC stimulation did not significantly increase *IL6* or *IL8* gene expression after three days (Table 3), in contrast to the protein assays. *IL8* expression of control was more than two times lower the PIC (Rq = 0.434), but reached no significance. FucBB04 alone displayed no effect on *IL6* or *IL8* gene expression. *IL6* gene expression induced by PIC in the presence of fucoidan was numerically lower than PIC alone (Rq = 0.603), which, however, did not reach significance. Regarding seven days of gene expression, PIC stimulation led to an increased *IL6* and *IL8* gene expression (Table 4), which did not reach statistical significance. Additional treatment with FucBB04 did not display any significant influence on PIC-induced *IL6* or *IL8* gene expression.

Table 3. Inflammatory gene expression (three days). Real-time polymerase chain reaction (qPCR) was used to determine gene expression of *IL6* (interleukin 6) and *CXCL8/IL8* (interleukin 8) in primary porcine RPE. *GAPDH* was used as endogenous control. Cells were treated with 50 µg/mL FucBB04 and/or 10 µg/mL polyinosinic/polycytidylic acid (PIC) for three days. Thermo Fisher Connect was used to determine relative gene expression and significances (student's *t*-test). co = untreated control, Rq = relative fold gene expression level (= $2^{-\Delta\Delta CT}$), Rq Min = minimal Rq value, Rq Max = maximal Rq values. No significant findings, n = 3.

Bio Group Name	Target Name	Rq	Rq Min	Rq Max	*p*-Value
control	*IL6*	1.649	0.305	8.916	0.661
PIC	*IL6*	1.000	0.725	1.379	1.000
FucBB04	*IL6*	0.574	0.156	2.110	0.540
FucBB04+PIC	*IL6*	0.603	0.157	2.321	0.586
control	*CXCL8*	0.434	0.318	0.593	0.162
PIC	*CXCL8*	1.000	0.498	2.007	1.000
FucBB04	*CXCL8*	0.872	0.411	1.852	0.829
FucBB04+PIC	*CXCL8*	1.165	0.539	2.518	0.811

Table 4. Inflammatory gene expression (seven days). Real-time polymerase chain reaction (qPCR) was used to determine gene expression of *IL6* (interleukin 6) and *CXCL8/IL8* (interleukin 8) in primary porcine RPE. *GAPDH* was used as endogenous control. Cells were treated with 50 µg/mL FucBB04 and/or 10 µg/mL polyinosinic/polycytidylic acid (PIC) for three days. Thermo Fisher Connect was used to determine relative gene expression and significances (student's *t*-test). co = untreated control, Rq = relative fold gene expression level (= $2^{-\Delta\Delta CT}$), Rq Min = minimal Rq value, Rq Max = maximal Rq values. No significant findings, n = 3.

Bio Group Name	Target Name	Rq	Rq Min	Rq Max	*p*-Value
control	*IL6*	0.570	0.127	2.550	0.586
PIC	*IL6*	1.000	0.694	1.442	1.000
FucBB04	*IL6*	1.671	1.393	2.006	0.120
FucBB04+PIC	*IL6*	0.854	0.446	1.633	0.736
control	*CXCL8*	0.270	0.242	0.301	0.134
PIC	*CXCL8*	1.000	0.393	2.544	1.000
FucBB04	*CXCL8*	0.493	0.251	0.969	0.353
FucBB04+PIC	*CXCL8*	1.847	0.326	10.475	0.627

2.6. Barrier Measurement

The manifestation of a cell barrier is an important task of RPE, establishing the outer blood–retina barrier [45]. The influence of FucBB04 and pro-inflammatory agents on RPE barrier function was tested. Primary porcine RPE were cultivated on transwell plates. Immediately before treatment (day 0), transepithelial electrical resistance (TEER) was measured, and cells were treated with 50 µg/mL FucBB04 and/or 10 µg/mL PIC or 50 ng/mL tumor necrosis factor alpha (TNF). PIC was chosen regarding possible protective effects of fucoidans (Section 2.4 [43]) and TNF as a known barrier-reducing agent in the RPE [7,46]. After 1 and 3 days of stimulation, TEER was measured again and set in relation to day 0 values in percent (Figure 7). Significances were calculated compared to control with no FucBB04, to day 0 values of the same well, and to stress controls PIC or TNF with no FucBB04.

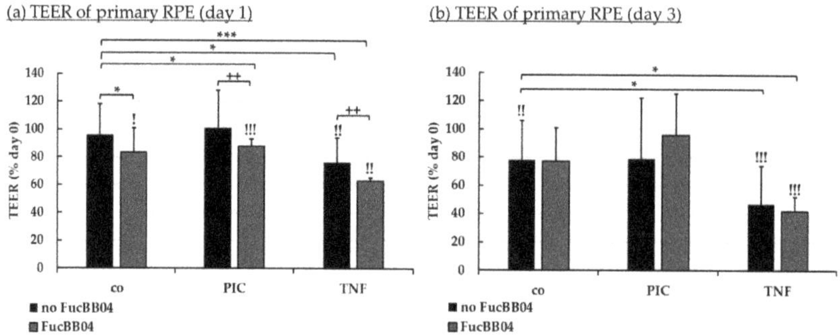

Figure 7. Barrier function of RPE. Porcine RPE cells cultured on transwell plates were treated with 50 µg/mL FucBB04 and/or 10 µg/mL polyinosinic/polycytidylic acid (PIC) or 50 ng/mL tumor necrosis factor α (TNF), respectively. Barrier function was determined by measuring the transepithelial electrical resistance (TEER) in $\Omega \cdot cm^2$. TEER was measured before stimulation (day 0), and after 1 (**a**) and 3 (**b**) days. TEER was calculated relatively to values of day 0 in percent. Data were normally distributed and one-sample *t*-test was conducted. * $p \leq 0.05$, *** $p \leq 0.001$ (compared to co, no FucBB04); ! $p \leq 0.05$, !! $p \leq 0.01$, !!! $p \leq 0.001$ (compared to initial measurement of the same well); ++ $p \leq 0.01$ (compared to stress control PIC or TNF, no FucBB04); co = control, $n = 4$.

After one day (Figure 7a), barrier function was reduced compared to control and to the day before treatment with FucBB04, FucBB04 plus PIC, TNF and FucBB04 plus TNF, but not PIC alone. Also, barrier function was significantly stronger decreased by FubBB04 treatment compared to stress control. Fucoidan reduced TEER after PIC treatment from 101% ± 21% to 88% ± 5% ($p = 0.0035$) when FucBB04 was co-applied, and after TNF treatment from 76% ± 18% to 63 ± 2% ($p = 0.0027$) when FucBB04 was co-applied. After three days (Figure 7b), the negative effects of fucoidan on the barrier are lost, while control and TNF-related treatments are reduced compared to TEER before treatment.

2.7. Protein Expression

Further tasks of RPE cells involve recycling of visual pigments with RPE65 as an important enzyme [47], and the regulation of the complement system on the basolateral site by expression of CD59 [48]. Protein expression of RPE65 (Figure 8) and CD59 (Figure 9) in primary RPE was tested by Western blotting. RPE were stimulated with 50 µg/mL FucBB04 and/or 10 µg/mL PIC for three days. Band volumes were evaluated and set into relation to control without PIC. Example blots are shown in Figures 8b and 9b.

PIC significantly reduced RPE65 expression (Figure 8a) to 0.6 ± 0.5 [arb. unit] ($p = 0.0002$). FucBB04 alone significantly reduced RPE65 to 0.5 ± 0.2 [arb. unit] ($p = 0.0033$) and to 0.3 ± 0.1 [arb. unit] ($p = 0.0003$) when co-applied with PIC. Regarding CD59 (Figure 9b), PIC significantly reduced its expression to 0.8 ± 0.3 [arb. unit] ($p = 0.0464$). FucBB04 displayed no significant influence on CD59 expression. Of note, the lowering effect of PIC on CD59 expression was lost under FucBB04 stimulation.

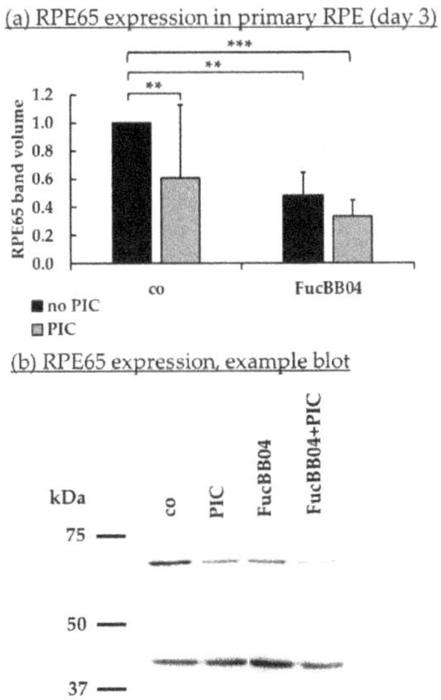

Figure 8. RPE65 protein expression. Primary porcine RPE cells were treated with 50 µg/mL FucBB04 and/or 10 µg/mL polyinosinic/polycytidylic acid (PIC) for three days. RPE65 expression was determined in Western blot (exemplary blot in (**b**)). β-actin (48 kDa) expression was used for normalization. Band volumes were calculated in TotalLab (**a**) in relation to untreated control. Data were normally distributed and one-sample *t*-test was conducted. ** $p \leq 0.01$, *** $p \leq 0.001$ (compared to co, no PIC); co = control, $n = 5$.

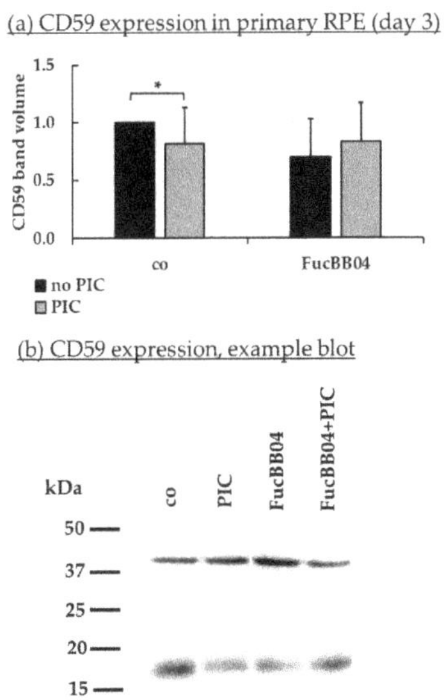

Figure 9. CD59 protein expression. Primary porcine RPE cells were treated with 50 µg/mL FucBB04 and/or 10 µg/mL polyinosinic/polycytidylic acid (PIC) for three days. Expression of CD59 was determined in Western blot (exemplary blot in (**b**)). β-actin (48 kDa) expression was used for normalization. Band volumes were calculated in TotalLab (**a**) in relation to the untreated control. Data were normally distributed and one-sample *t*-test was conducted. * $p \leq 0.05$ (compared to co, no PIC); co = control, $n = 5$.

2.8. Phagocytosis Assay

Phagocytosis is essential for photoreceptor outer segment renewal and visual pigment recycling [4]. Human RPE cell line ARPE-19 (Figure 10) and primary porcine RPE (Figure 11) were treated with 50 µg/mL FucBB04 and/or 10 µg/mL PIC for three days. Phagocytosis was assessed with fluorescent latex beads. Number of ingested beads were put in relation to cell nuclei. Exemplary photos are shown in Figures 10b and 11b. In ARPE-19, the co-stimulation with FucBB04 and PIC significantly reduced phagocytosis (Figure 10a) from 9 ± 5 beads/cell to 3 ± 2 beads/cell (p = 0.0002). Neither pro-inflammatory activation by PIC alone nor FucBB04 alone displayed a significant effect on phagocytosis. Concerning primary RPE, FucBB04 significantly reduced phagocytosis (Figure 11a) from 7 ± 3 beads/cell to 3 ± 1 beads/cell ($p < 0.0001$). Also, PIC and co-treatment with FucBB04 and PIC reduced RPE phagocytosis to 5 ± 1 beads/cell (p = 0.0268) and to 3 ± 1 beads/cell ($p < 0.0001$), respectively.

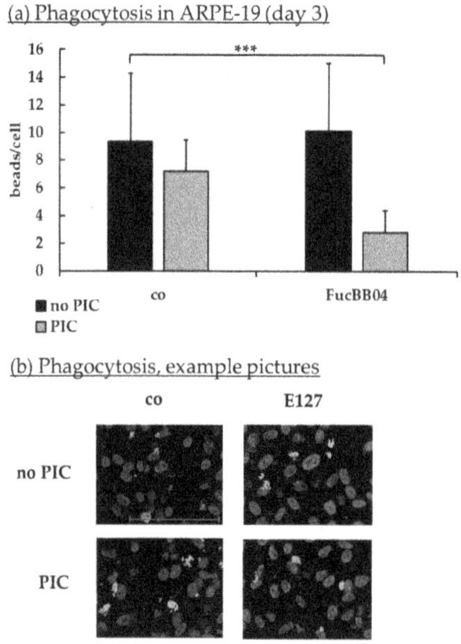

Figure 10. Phagocytosis of ARPE-19. ARPE-19 cells were stimulated with 50 µg/mL FucBB04 and/or 10 µg/mL polyinosinic/polycytidylic acid (PIC) for three days. Fluorescence-labeled beads opsonized with photoreceptor outer segments were applied to the cells (green dots, **b**). Fluoromount-G™ and 4′,6-diamidino-2-phenylindol (DAPI) was used to label cell nuclei (blue circles, **b**). Immunofluorescence photos were taken by Imager M2 (64× magnification, red scale bar = 100 µm). Nuclei number and beads were counted. Beads were calculated relatively to cell nuclei (**a**). Shapiro–Wilk test showed Gaussian distribution. Data were normally distributed and one-sample t-test was conducted. *** $p \leq 0.001$ (compared to control, no PIC), co = control, n = 15.

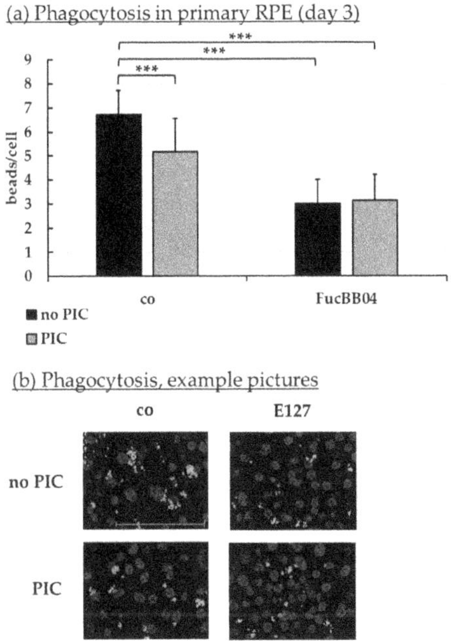

Figure 11. Phagocytosis of RPE. Primary porcine RPE cells were stimulated with 50 µg/mL FucBB04 and/or 10 µg/mL polyinosinic/polycytidylic acid (PIC) for three days. Fluorescence-labeled beads opsonized with photoreceptor outer segments were applied to the cells (green dots, **b**). Fluoromount-G™ and 4′,6-diamidino-2-phenylindol (DAPI) was used to label cell nuclei (blue circles, **b**). Immunofluorescence photos were taken by Imager M2 (64× magnification, red scale bar = 100 µm). Nuclei number and beads were counted. Beads were calculated relatively to cell nuclei (**a**). Shapiro–Wilk test showed Gaussian distribution. Data were normally distributed and one-sample *t*-test was conducted. *** $p \leq 0.001$ (compared to control, no PIC), co = control, $n = 15$.

3. Discussion

In our study, we purified a very high-molecular weight fucoidan (3700 kDa) from *Laminaria hyperborea* and tested its bioactivity in regard to a potential application for the treatment of AMD. While this fucoidan showed some interesting bioactivities, its influence on RPE cell function renders it not suitable for further development in AMD treatment.

The chemical characterization of fucoidan sample FucBB04 revealed the highest molecular weight average for fucoidan yet reported (3700 kDa), likely achieved through the mild extraction and purification methods as well as ultrafiltration applying 300 kDa MWCO filters, deliberately removing, beside other co-extracted seaweed polysaccharides such as laminarin or alginate, lower molecular weight fucoidan fractions [35]. The predominant sugar moiety is fucose with 91.59%. The rms conformation plot revealed a molecular shape indicative of polymeric branching or hyper-branching, respectively [39,40]. Considering previously reported structural elucidations [20,33], a fucoidan backbone structure remains likely, with polymeric side-chains containing sugar moieties such as rhamnose, xylose, and uronic acids, previously not detected in fucoidan from LH. However, the branching pattern and sugar moiety distribution is currently speculative and requires further experiments such as branching analysis via SEC-MALS, target-specific depolymerization using fucoidan degrading enzymes, selectively cleaving glycosidic linkages and sulfate groups [49,50], and/or mild hydrolysis followed by fractionation and subsequent analysis of the molecular segments.

The bioactivities of fucoidans are strongly related to their molecular properties, of which molecular weight is of high importance. For example, molecular weight can make the difference in pro- and antiangiogenic properties of fucoidan [17], can influence the antibacterial effect [51], the skin-whitening effect [52], or the anticoagulant effect of fucoidans [53].

Fucoidans have been described to exert antioxidative effects; however, the relation between structure and antioxidant activity is complex and some of their antioxidant behavior has been attributed to contaminant phenol contents [54,55]. FucBB04 did not exert any antioxidative protective effect in our tested cell culture models, which on the other hand was shown for a 1549 kDa LH fucoidan [20,42]. This LH fucoidan was slightly protective in OMM-1 against H_2O_2 [20], showed promising antiferroptotic activities, and increased GPX4 expression in both OMM-1 and ARPE-19 [42]. In our experience, the protective effect against oxidative stress of fucoidans is not very prominent in retinal pigment epithelial cell models, but is more easily determined in OMM-1 cells, as RPE cells are rather resistant to oxidative stress with a strong intrinsic protective response [56]. As FucBB04 did not exert any effect in OMM-1 cells, its oxidative stress protection can be considered negligible in the ocular context.

Fucoidans can exhibit antiangiogenic and VEGF-inhibiting effects which make them highly interesting for conditions such as AMD or diabetic retinopathy [12]. FucBB04 inhibited VEGF after seven days in primary porcine RPE cells at a similar concentration and time frame that has been shown to effectively reduce VEGF in other fucoidans [43]. Conversely, however, FucBB04 exhibited no VEGF-inhibiting effect in ARPE-19 cells. The lack of effect on ARPE-19 is surprising, as in our experience, VEGF inhibition is easier achieved in ARPE-19 than in primary porcine RPE cells, as RPE cells secrete much higher concentrations of VEGF than ARPE-19 per time unit [26]. Also, the VEGF inhibition in primary RPE cells did not reach the potency of the 1549 kDa LH fucoidan [20], rendering it inferior in VEGF inhibition compared to other tested fucoidans. Of note, the VEGF-reducing effects are only seen in lower concentrations of FucBB04. Similar results have been found in a different fucoidan regarding inflammation, with lower concentrations of fucoidan showing the strongest effect [57]. As fucoidans have been shown to bind simultaneously to VEGF and its receptor [58], inhibiting angiogenic signaling and potentially reducing VEGF expression this way [59,60], it is feasible that a higher concentration of fucoidan may sterically hinder this interaction or may reduce the probability of a fucoidan molecule binding VEGF and its receptor at the same time due to the abundance of the fucoidan-binding partner.

Inflammation is an important factor in the development of AMD [9], and RPE cells secrete pro-inflammatory cytokines after stimulation with a variety of pro-inflammatory insults [7]. Interestingly, the effect of fucoidans on cytokine secretion is dependent on the stimulus, indicating an interaction with the TLR-3 pathway [14,43]. FucBB04 displayed a similar influence, with reducing IL-6 and IL-8 after PIC treatment (3 and 7 days, respectively), with some effect on IL-8 secretion also seen after LPS stimulation (after 1 and 28 days). Taken together, the effect of FucBB04 on IL-6 and IL-8 secretion is comparable with that of other fucoidans, suggesting mainly an interaction with the TLR-3 pathway. RPE cells highly express TLR-3, and its activation does not only induce pro-inflammatory cytokine secretion, but also a reduction of RPE65 expression and phagocytosis, thereby reducing RPE function before inducing cell death [8,61]; however, the pathways leading to RPE65 and phagocytosis reduction are not elucidated so far. It would be feasible to suppose that the reduction of RPE65 and phagocytosis may be a consequence of a sub-lethal injury of the cell, rending them alive but no longer functional, as described by Spaide et al. [62].

The nature of this interaction between the TLR-3 pathway and fucoidans is not known so far, but could be mediated via a steric interaction with the TLR-3 pathway. As TLR-3 activation has been implicated to be involved in AMD-development [8,63–65], this stresses again the potential of fucoidans in preventive or early treatment of AMD. However, it should also be noted that FucBB04 significantly induced IL-8 after 1 day of stimulation in the absence of a pro-inflammatory stimulus, albeit to a lesser degree compared to pro-inflammatory stimuli. Indeed, fucoidans have been shown to induce cytokine release, thereby again stressing the importance of meticulous characterization of any fucoidan considered for potential therapeutic use [43].

The function of the RPE is vital for the survival of the photoreceptors and the maintenance of visual function. One important function is the phagocytosis of shed photoreceptor outer segments, which in vivo are shed every morning after the onset of light [4]. Indeed, impairment of RPE phagocytosis leads to blindness in animal models and patients [66,67]. In our study, FucBB04 significantly and relevantly reduced the phagocytic capabilities of RPE cells. Fucoidans have been shown before to be able to reduce phagocytosis of activated macrophages [68,69]. Indeed, we have recently shown that FucBB04 reduces the phagocytotic capabilities of retinal microglia [70]. However, the mechanisms of phagocytosis of macrophages differ from those of RPE cells [71]. In macrophages, fucoidan has been described to alter phagocytosis by modulating TNF production of peripheral blood mononuclear cells or by interfering with the scavenger receptor [68,69]. We have previously tested the effect of several fucoidans on phagocytotic activity. Commercially available fucoidan from *Fucus vesiculosus* (FV) did not impede phagocytic function in primary RPE cells [14,59]. On the other hand, fucoidan from a crude extract of *Fucus distichus* subspecies *evanescens* reduced phagocytosis in primary RPE cells [72]. Of interest, we have investigated the effect of a high-molecular weight fucoidan (1549 kDa) from LH which did not show a significant influence on phagocytosis in the same experimental setting [34], strongly indicating that the effect is molecular weight dependent. As the phagocytosis of photoreceptor outer segment fragments of the RPE is dependent on the interaction of $\alpha v\beta 5$ integrin with binding partners like lactadherin (MFGE8), the mechanism of inhibition could be a steric inhibition of this interaction by the large, negatively charged fucoidan [73].

Another vital function of the RPE is to contribute to the recycling of the visual pigment to uphold vision. An important enzyme in this process is the retinyl ester-binding protein RPE65. Lack of functional RPE65 can lead to blinding disease, such as retinitis pigmentosa or Leber's congenital amaurosis and has been successfully targeted in gene-therapy [74,75]. FucBB04 significantly and relevantly reduced the expression of RPE65 in primary RPE cells. We have previously tested the effect of LH fucoidan with a molecular weight of 1549 kDa on RPE65 expression, and no effect could be found [34]. This strongly suggests that the effect on RPE65 expression is molecular weight dependent. However, a study concerning different fucoidans from *Saccharina latissima* (SL) shows that a fucoidan from the Faeroe Islands with a molecular weight of 997 kDa does not influence RPE65 expression, while a Norwegian SL extract with a molecular weight of 312 kDa reduced RPE65 [43]. Of interest, commercially available fucoidan from FV did not influence RPE65 expression but protected RPE cells from RPE65 loss after pro-inflammatory stimulation [14] (this protection was not seen with SL fucoidans [43]). We do not know why and how some fucoidans reduce RPE65 expression, but this effect should be tested for fucoidans scheduled for further development as a potential AMD therapeutic in order to avoid any interaction with RPE65 expression.

Also of importance is the outer blood–retinal barrier, which contributes to the immune privilege of the retina [6]. FucBB04 transiently reduced the barrier properties of primary RPE cells one day after stimulation. In addition, it exacerbated the negative effect of TNF on the cell barrier. This effect was not found with FV fucoidan (which ameliorated

PIC-induced barrier reduction after 28 days) [14], but is similar to what is seen for two SL fucoidans, which also reduced barrier function after 1, but not after 3 days [43]. A transient reduction in the barrier function may not be of a high biological relevance. However, the exacerbation of pro-inflammatory effects would argue against an application in AMD, as inflammation is considered to be an important pathomechanism.

Our study has several limitations. It is an *in vitro* study using cell culture models. While this gives us valuable insight into cellular effects and mechanisms, it cannot reflect on the complex interactions that are seen in vivo. In particular, cancer cell lines like OMM-1 are highly abnormal compared to normal human tissue. In addition, ARPE-19 cells, while not derived from a tumor, only partially behave as RPE cells. Finally, while primary porcine RPE cells are an excellent model of adult human RPE cells, they lack the interaction with the adjacent cells and tissues of the eye and are of animal origin [24].

Taken together, our results show some protective bioactivities of FucBB04 such as a reduction of TLR-3-mediated cytokine release and VEGF inhibition, but also negative influences regarding RPE function such as a reduction of phagocytosis and RPE65 expression. As these negative effects are not found with a 1549 kDa LH fucoidan, we would advise against the use of very high-molecular weight fucoidan for further development of AMD therapeutics.

4. Materials and Methods

4.1. Algal Material, Fucoidan Extraction and Purification Method

Laminaria hyperborea (Laminariaceae, Phaeophyceae) were harvested on 6 April 2020 along the coast of Haugesund, Norway (Rogaland field 55E; N 59°11′ E 005°06′). A mild warm water extraction under stirring was performed for one hour at 60 °C, using freshly harvested, shredded LH leaves. The liquid phase was separated and $CaCl_2$ added. After one hour of settling, a centrifugation followed by microfiltration (at 100, 50, and 20 μm pore size, consecutively) was performed to remove remaining algae particles and precipitated alginate. Salt and smaller organic molecules were then removed through ultrafiltration using 300 kDa MWCO ceramic filters and 0.1 mol/L NaCl solution followed by distilled water. Fucoidan in the filtrate was precipitated using ethanol. Excess liquid was removed and the precipitated fucoidan vacuum dried.

4.2. Molecular Weight Determination

The molecular weight of FucBB04 was determined through size-exclusion chromatography (SEC) in the form of HPLC equipped with online multiangle static light scattering (MALS). The measurements were performed at ambient temperature using a Shodex LB-806 and LB-805, as well as a 2500 PWXL column as a separator. The measurement was executed with a Dawn HELEOS-8+ multiangle laser light scattering photometer (Wyatt, Santa Barbara, CA, USA) ($\lambda 0$ = 660 nm) and a subsequent Optilab T-rEX differential refractometer. The mobile phase was 0.15 mol/L CH_3COONH_4 (ammonium acetate at pH = 7) with 0.01 mol/L EDTA added. The flow rate was 0.5 mL/min. The injection volume was 5 μL, with a concentration of 5 g/L. The data were obtained and processed using Astra (v. 7) software (Wyatt, Santa Barbara, CA, USA).

4.3. Sulfate Content

The sulfur content was determined through an Agilent 7500 Series quadrupole ICP-MS. The fucoidan was dried at 70 °C for 90 min and 5.0 mg dissolved in 15.0 mL of 1 M HNO_3. The sulfation degree was calculated by using a mass balance equation, assuming that every sulfate group is associated with a sodium counterion. The sulfate position was verified via Raman micro-spectroscopy. Measurements were performed at room temperature using a

Bruker Senterra II Spectrometer equipped with a 785 nm laser and scanned from 100 to 4000 cm^{-1} (integration time 30 s, 3 accumulations). A sample size of <0.5 mg gave sufficient resolution due to the microscope array. No further sample preparation was necessary.

4.4. Total Phenolic Content

The total phenolic content (TPC) was determined using the Folin–Ciocalteu TPC assay applying a method optimized for seaweeds, as described in Wekre et al. (2022) [76,77]. Briefly, the method used 0.2 mL sample, blank, or standard, 1.59 mL undiluted Folin–Ciocalteu reagent, 4.0 mL 20% (w/v) Na_2CO_3 and yielded a total volume of 20 mL with water. The mixture was incubated for two hours in the dark, and absorbance was measured at 760 nm using a Hitachi Model U-5100 UV/Vis Spectrophotometer (Hitachi, Tokyo, Japan). Gallic acid and phloroglucinol calibration curves were used to validate the linearity, sensitivity, precision, and accuracy of the TPC method.

4.5. Monosaccharide Analysis

To analyze the monosaccharides composition, 1 mg of fucoidan was treated with 2 M trifluoroacetic acid (TFA) at 120 °C for three hours. After centrifugation at 10,000 rpm for ten minutes, 100 µL of supernatant was vacuum dried and resuspended in H_2O. Samples were then analyzed through high-performance anion-exchange chromatography with pulsed amperometric detection on an IC6000 system operated by Chromeleon software version 7.3 (Dionex, Sunnyvale, CA, USA). Analysis was conducted using Dionex CarboPac PA1 (4 × 250 mm) column at 20 °C and flow rate of 1 mL/min. Eluent A (water), B (300 mM NaOH), C (200 mM NaOH in 170 mM NaOAc), and D (1 M NaOAc) were prepared for the separation of uronic acids. All samples were prepared in triplicates. Monosaccharides were identified and quantified by comparing their retention times and peak areas to standards of known concentrations. The standards used were L-guluronic acid and D-mannuronic acid (purchased from Carbosynth, Berkshire, UK), while fucose, rhamnose, galactose, glucose, mannose, and xylose (purchased from Sigma-Aldrich, St. Louis, MO, USA) were dissolved in H_2O and run in different concentrations ranging from 0.005 g/L to 0.1 g/L. Water was used to elute natural sugars while a gradient was solely used to elute uronic acids.

4.6. Cell Culture

OMM-1 (RRID: CVCL_6939) cell line from human uveal melanoma [23] was kindly provided by Dr. Sarah Coupland. Hundred µL of cells at concentration of 200,000 cell per mL were seeded in 96-well plate (Sarstedt, Nümbrecht, Germany; #83.3924.005) and treated after 24 h of incubation at around 90% confluence, as media RPMI 1640 (Pan-Biotech, Aidenbach, Germany; #P04-18500) with 10% fetal bovine serum (Thermo Fisher Scientific, Waltham, MA, USA; #A5256701), and 1% penicillin/streptomycin (Sigma-Aldrich, St. Louis, MO, USA; #P0781) were used. Cells were split 1:4 after 3–4 days.

Immortal ARPE-19 cell line, originally from a 19-year-old human donor [21], was purchased from American Type Culture Collection (ATCC, Manassas, VA, USA; RRID: CVCL_0145; #CRL-2302). These cells were seeded in 12-well (1 mL per well, Sarstedt; #83.3921) or 96-well plates (100 µL per well) with 100,000 cells per mL and treated after one week in 12-well plates or after 24 h in 96-well plates (90% confluence), as media HyClone DMEM (Cytiva, Freiburg in Breisgau, Germany; #31053028) with 10% fetal bovine serum, 1% penicillin/streptomycin, 2.5% HEPES (Pan-Biotech; #P05-01100), and 1% non-essential amino acids (Pan-Biotech; #P08-32100) were used.

Primary RPE cells from pig eyes were isolated as described before [78]. Eyes were delivered from local slaughters as byproduct in food production. The use of these eyes was agreed to by animal welfare officer of University of Kiel. It is considered an active contribution to the reduction in animal experiments (German animal welfare act TierSchG) according to the 3R principle. The eyes were cleaned and cut open to remove retina and vitreous body. RPE cells were removed by incubation steps with trypsin (Pan-Biotech; #P10-021100) and trypsin/EDTA (Pan-Biotech; #P10-020100). After washing, cells were seeded into 12-well (1 mL per well) or 24-well (500 µL per well; #83.3922.005) plates with 100,000 cells per mL, as media HyClone DMEM with 10% fetal bovine serum, 1% penicillin/streptomycin, 2.5% HEPES, and 1% non-essential amino acids were used. Cells were always treated at 100% confluence (two weeks after seeding). To measure TEER, cells were seeded on 12-well plates containing a transwell insert (Sarstedt; #83.3931.041).

For phagocytosis assay, ARPE-19 and RPE cells were seeded on cover slips (Th. Geyer GmbH & Co. KG, Renningen, Germany; #9161050) which were coated with collagen I, also called collagen A (Pan-Biotech; #P06-20030), according to the manufacturer's instructions.

Cell cultures were incubated at 37 °C and 5% CO_2 in a humidified incubator. In general, cells were fed two times per week, also during long-term stimulation experiments for RPE (media were supplied with stimuli).

4.7. Stimulation

Cells were treated with 1–100 µg/mL FucBB04 depending on the experiment. For oxidative stress assays, ARPE-19 were treated first with FucBB04 for 30 min, followed by 250 µM H_2O_2 (Sigma-Aldrich; #H1009) and 20 µM erastin (Cayman Chemical, Ann Arbor, MI, USA; #CAY17754-5) for 24 h; OMM-1 were treated with 500 µM H_2O_2 or 25 µM erastin for 4 h after 30 min of fucoidan incubation, both applied in MTT assay (refer to Section 4.8). For VEGF assays, ARPE-19 were treated with FucBB04 for three days, followed by supernatant collection and MTT assay. Primary RPE were treated with fucoidan for 28 days, harvesting supernatants on day 3, 7, and 28 from the same well. The experiment was terminated by an MTT assay on day 28. For inflammation assays, cells were treated with FucBB04 for 30 min followed by a pro-inflammatory stimulus for 28 days with supernatant collection on day 1, 3, 7, and 28 days from the same well, finalizing with MTT assay on day 28 (1 µg/mL LPS (Merck, Darmstadt, Germany; #L4524), 10 µg/mL PIC (Tocris Bioscience, Bristol, UK; #4287/10), 50 ng/mL TNF (R&D System, Minneapolis, MN, USA; 210-TA-005/CF), or 10 ng/mL Pam2CSK4 (Pam, Tocris Biosciences; #4637)). For both VEGF and inflammation assays, RPE cells were re-stimulated after three to four days, as well as after supernatant harvest (refer to Section 4.10).

4.8. Cell Viability

MTT assay was used to assess cell viability and oxidative stress protection [79]. Wells were washed with phosphate-buffered saline (PBS, Pan-Biotech; #P04-53500) and then 0.5 mg/mL MTT solution (Sigma-Aldrich; #M2128) in HyClone DMEM without phenol red (Cytiva; #SH30284.01) was applied for two hours. MTT was discarded and cells lysed with dimethyl sulfoxide (Carl Roth, Karlsruhe, Germany; #11657618). Readout was performed at 550 nm by using the Elx800 (BioTek, Bad Friedrichshall, Germany).

4.9. Transepithelial Electrical Resistance (TEER)

For TEER measurements, primary porcine RPE were cultivated in 12-well plates with transwell inserts. TEER was measured with Epithelial Volt/Ohm (EVOM™) Meter 3 with STX4 electrodes (WPI, Sarasota, FL, USA). Between measurements, electrodes were washed in 70% ethanol (Th. Geyer GmbH & Co. KG; #11655285) and sterile distilled water (Fresenius Kabi AG, Bad Homburg, Germany; #1080224). TEER values were documented 7, 10, and 14 days after preparation. A well without cells and with media was used as blank. Only wells with a TEER of at least 150 Ohm·cm^2 were included in the study [80]. TEER was measured before stimulation (day 0) and after 1 and 3 days after stimulation.

4.10. Enzyme-Linked Immunosorbent Assay

ELISA was used to assess VEGF, IL-6, and IL-8 in supernatants. These were collected after indicated stimulation times. Supernatants were collected for 24 h (ARPE-19: VEGF, RPE: IL-6, IL-8) or 4 h (RPE: VEGF). ELISA DuoSet for human VEGF was used to determine VEGF-A of ARPE-19 and RPE samples. ELISA DuoSets for porcine IL-6 and IL-8 were used for RPE samples, all bought from R&D Systems (Minneapolis, MN, USA; # DY293B; #DY686; #DY535). All kits were used according to the manufacturer's instructions. Standard calibration curves for all ELISA are shown in Appendix A.2 (Figure A1).

4.11. Real-Time Polymerase Chain Reaction

RNA was isolated with NucleoSpin RNA Mini Kit (Macherey-Nagel, Düren, Germany; #11699517) according to the manual. Genomic DNA was digested with DNase, provided by the manufacturer. RNA was dissolved in 20 µL RNase-free water from the kit. NanoDrop™ One (Thermo Fisher Scientific) was used to analyze purity and concentration of the RNA samples. To transcribe RNA into cDNA, the High-Capacity cDNA Reverse Transcription Kit (Thermo Fisher Scientific; #4368814) was used according to the manual. Real-time PCR was conducted with TaqMan™ Fast Advanced Master Mix (Thermo Fisher Scientific; #4444557) and TaqMan™ gene expression assays (Thermo Fisher Scientific; #4331182) [dye label 5(6)-carboxyfluorescein-minor groove binder (FAM-MGB)]. The procedure was performed as described in the instructions of the TaqMan™ Fast Advanced Master Mix. Gene expression assays for *IL6* (interleukin 6, Ss03384604_u1), *CXCL8* (interleukin 8, Ss03392437_m1), and *GAPDH* (glyceraldehyde-3-phosphate dehydrogenase, Ss03375629_u1, endogenous control) were used. For evaluation, RQ module of Thermo Fisher Connect was used which is based on ΔΔCT method [81]. The ΔΔCT method calculated the relative normalized gene expression with ΔCT (=CT [gene of interest] − CT [housekeeping gene]), ΔΔCT (=ΔCT [sample of interest] − ΔCT [reference sample]), and relative fold gene expression level RQ (=$2^{-\Delta\Delta CT}$). Reference sample was PIC and set to RQ = 1.0.

4.12. Western Blotting

To assess RPE65 and CD59 protein expression, Western blots were conducted as previously described [43]. In brief, after treatment, cells were washed in PBS and lysed with Nonidet® P-40 containing lysis buffer (NP-40, nonylphenyl-polyethylene glycol, Sigma-Aldrich; #11332473001) for 45 min on ice. DC Protein Assay Kit II (Bio-Rad Laboratories, Munich, Germany; #5000112 and Genesys 10 Bio (Thermo Fisher) were used to determine protein concentrations as described by the manufacturer. SDS-PAGE was performed with 12% acrylamide gels and 15 µg sample. Wet tank Western blots were performed and membranes blocked with 4% skimming milk (Carl Roth GmbH + Co. KG, Karlsruhe, Germany; #T145.2). Membranes were incubated overnight at 4 °C with primary antibodies in 2% skimming milk (mouse anti-RPE65 Abcam, 65 kDa, 1:6000, Berlin, Germany; #ab235950; rabbit anti-CD59, 18 kDa, 1:3000, Proteintech Group, Inc., Rosemont, IL, USA; #10742-1-AP; rabbit anti-β-actin, 37 kDa, 1:1000, Cell Signaling Technologies, Denver, CO, USA; #4967). Conjugates with horseradish peroxidase (HRP) were applied for one hour (anti-mouse-HRP or anti-rabbit-HRP, Cell Signaling Technologies; #7076, #7074). For chemiluminescent signal, Amersham ECL Western Blotting Detection Reagent (GE Healthcare, Chicago, IL, USA; #12316992) was applied. Readout was performed with MF-ChemiBIS 1.6 (Biostep, Jahnsdorf, Germany). TotalLab TL100 (Biostep, version 1D v2008) software was used to generate quantitative values and β-actin was used for normalization

4.13. Phagocytosis Assay

Confluent RPE cells on collagen I-coated cover slips were treated and used for the phagocytosis assay (conducted as previously established [82]). Latex fluorescence beads (Sigma-Aldrich; #L4530) were incubated with photoreceptor outer segment fragments, prepared from porcine eyes' retinae as described previously [72]. The treated beads were applied to the respective cells for four hours. After washing cells with media and PBS, they were fixated in paraformaldehyde (Carl Roth GmbH + Co. KG; #0335.1) and mounted with Fluoromount-G™ with DAPI (Thermo Fisher Scientific; #00-4959-52). Images were taken with fluorescence microscope Axiovert Imager M.2 by using ZenBlue 2 Software (version) v2.0.0.0) (both Zeiss, Jena, Germany). Cell nuclei and beads were counted by self-programmed macro in Fiji (ImageJ2, https://imagej.net/software/fiji/downloads (accessed on 29 March 2021)). Counted beads were calculated in relation to the cell nuclei number.

4.14. Statistical Analysis

Microsoft Excel and PowerPoint (Microsoft Office 2010, Microsoft, Redmond, WA, USA) were used to generate diagrams depicting means and standard deviations. GraphPad Prism 9 (GraphPad Software, Inc., San Diego, CA, USA, version 9.1.1) was used for statistical evaluation. Normality was assessed with Shapiro–Wilk test. One-sample *t*-test was used for calculating significances between relative data and ANOVA (analysis of variance) followed by Dunnett's multiple comparison test was used for absolute data. PCR data were evaluated by Thermo Fisher Connect, which uses the student's *t*-test. Bio groups with p-values ≤ 0.5 were marked as significant.

5. Conclusions

The aim of this study was to assess the bioactivity of a very high-molecular weight (3700 kDa) fucoidan from *Laminaria hyperborea* from the coasts of Norway, concerning age-related macular degeneration-relevant pathomechanisms and their influence on retinal pigment epithelium cell functions. In former studies, another fucoidan from this species with a size of 1549 kDa showed antioxidative, antiangiogenic, and anti-inflammatory effects with no adverse effects on retinal pigment epithelium cell functions. With the bigger fucoidan from this study, we also determined vascular endothelial growth factor-inhibiting effects and a reduction in interleukin 6 and interleukin 8 secretion. Antioxidative effects were not found. Barrier function was transiently affected. Retinal pigment epithelium 65 kDa protein expression as well as phagocytic ability were reduced. Taken together, we determined antiangiogenic and anti-inflammatory effects in primary retinal pigment epithelium, but the effects on cellular functions advise against further development of this very high-molecular weight fucoidan from *Laminaria hyperborea* as a potential therapeutic in age-related macular degeneration.

Author Contributions: Conceptualization, A.K. and G.K.; Methodology, C.S., P.D. and T.T.; Validation, C.S., P.D. and T.T.; Formal Analysis, P.D., G.K., S.F.U. and V.S.; Investigation, C.S., P.D. and T.T.; Resources, A.K., G.K. and J.R.; Data Curation, C.S., P.D. and T.T.; Writing—Original Draft Preparation, A.K., G.K. and P.D.; Writing—Review and Editing, A.K., C.S., G.K., J.R., P.D., S.F.U., V.S. and T.T.; Visualization, G.K. and P.D.; Supervision, A.K. and J.R. All authors have read and agreed to the published version of the manuscript.

Funding: This study was supported by the Helmut–Ecker Foundation (grant number 01/20). This work was partially funded by the Research Council of Norway through the Fucomed project (NFR: 310167). We acknowledge financial support by Land Schleswig-Holstein within the funding programme Open Access Publikationsfonds.

Institutional Review Board Statement: Not applicable.

Informed Consent Statement: Not applicable.

Data Availability Statement: Data are available on request.

Conflicts of Interest: Georg Kopplin is employed by Alginor ASA, and the other authors declare that there are no potential conflicts of interest. Alginor ASA has no role in the study design, collection, analysis, interpretation of data, the writing of this article or the decision to submit it for publication.

Appendix A

Appendix A.1. Cell Viability Data for Section 2.5

In this section, supporting cell viability data determined by MTT assay for inflammation assays of Section 2.5 are listed (Table A1). Viability was determined 1, 3, 7, and 28 days after stimulation with FucBB04 and pro-inflammatory agents. There were no significant, relevant findings observed.

Table A1. Cell viability data with mean and standard deviation (SD). LPS = lipopolysaccharide, PIC = polyinosinic/polycytidylic acid, TNF = tumor necrosis factor alpha, Pam = Pam2CSK4 Pam.

Day 1	**co**	**LPS**	**PIC**	**TNF**	**Pam**	
no FucBB04	100	105	109	104	103	Mean
	0	11	14	32	9	SD
FucBB04	95	91	94	96	97	Mean
	3	7	7	5	1	SD
Day 3						
no FucBB04	100	94	96	105	99	Mean
	0	15	7	9	5	SD
FucBB04	98	87	77	95	96	Mean
	4	16	15	1	1	SD
Day 7						
no FucBB04	100	97	95	93	100	Mean
	0	13	14	18	12	SD
FucBB04	100	81	88	98	91	Mean
	6	9	5	15	9	SD
Day 28						
no FucBB04	100	90	98	99	81	Mean
	0	19	26	44	31	SD
FucBB04	75	64	78	90	63	Mean
	16	16	16	13	15	SD

Appendix A.2. Standard Calibration Curves for ELISA

In this section, standard calibration curves for Section 2.3 (VEGF-ELISA ARPE-19 and RPE) and Section 2.4 (IL-6-ELISA and IL-8-ELISA) are shown (Figure A1).

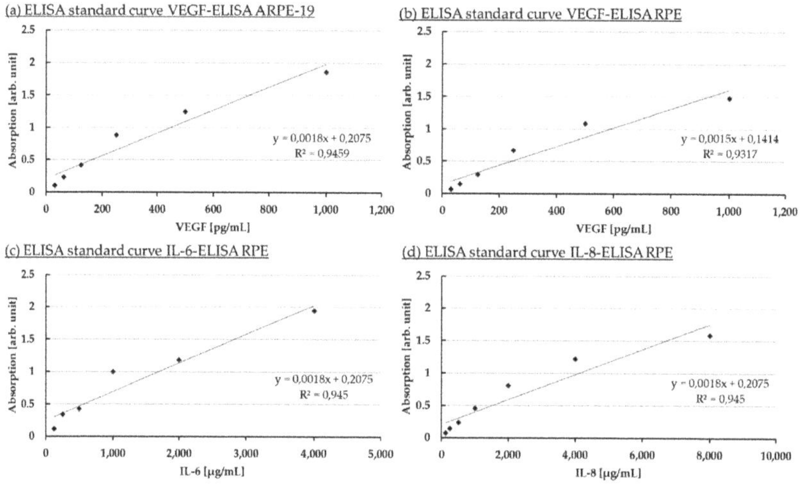

Figure A1. Standard calibration curves. Standard curves for Section 2.3 (VEGF-ELISA ARPE-19 and RPE) and Section 2.4 (IL-6-ELISA and IL-8-ELISA) are shown.

References

1. Bourne, R.R.A.; Jonas, J.B.; Bron, A.M.; Cicinelli, M.V.; Das, A.; Flaxman, S.R.; Friedman, D.S.; Keeffe, J.E.; Kempen, J.H.; Leasher, J.; et al. Prevalence and causes of vision loss in high-income countries and in Eastern and Central Europe in 2015: Magnitude, temporal trends and projections. *Br. J. Ophthalmol.* **2018**, *102*, 575–585. [CrossRef] [PubMed]
2. Guymer, R.H.; Campbell, T.G. Age-related macular degeneration. *Lancet* **2023**, *401*, 1459–1472. [CrossRef] [PubMed]
3. Bhutto, I.; Lutty, G. Understanding age-related macular degeneration (AMD): Relationships between the photoreceptor/retinal pigment epithelium/Bruch's membrane/choriocapillaris complex. *Mol. Aspects Med.* **2012**, *33*, 295–317. [CrossRef] [PubMed]
4. Strauss, O. The retinal pigment epithelium in visual function. *Physiol. Rev.* **2005**, *85*, 845–881. [CrossRef] [PubMed]
5. Mazzoni, F.; Safa, H.; Finnemann, S.C. Understanding photoreceptor outer segment phagocytosis: Use and utility of RPE cells in culture. *Exp. Eye Res.* **2014**, *126*, 51–60. [CrossRef]
6. Du, Y.; Yan, B. Ocular immune privilege and retinal pigment epithelial cells. *J. Leukoc. Biol.* **2023**, *113*, 288–304. [CrossRef]
7. Dietrich, L.; Lucius, R.; Roider, J.; Klettner, A. Interaction of inflammatorily activated retinal pigment epithelium with retinal microglia and neuronal cells. *Exp. Eye Res.* **2020**, *199*, 108167. [CrossRef] [PubMed]
8. Klettner, A.; Roider, J. Retinal Pigment Epithelium Expressed Toll-like Receptors and Their Potential Role in Age-Related Macular Degeneration. *Int. J. Mol. Sci.* **2021**, *22*, 8387. [CrossRef] [PubMed]
9. Datta, S.; Cano, M.; Ebrahimi, K.; Wang, L.; Handa, J.T. The impact of oxidative stress and inflammation on RPE degeneration in non-neovascular AMD. *Prog. Retin. Eye Res.* **2017**, *60*, 201–218. [CrossRef]
10. Lin, J.B.; Halawa, O.A.; Husain, D.; Miller, J.W.; Vavvas, D.G. Dyslipidemia in age-related macular degeneration. *Eye* **2022**, *36*, 312–318. [CrossRef] [PubMed]
11. Miller, J.W. Beyond VEGF-The Weisenfeld Lecture. *Investig. Ophthalmol. Vis. Sci.* **2016**, *57*, 6911–6918. [CrossRef]
12. Klettner, A. Fucoidan as a Potential Therapeutic for Major Blinding Diseases--A Hypothesis. *Mar. Drugs* **2016**, *14*, 31. [CrossRef]
13. Dörschmann, P.; Klettner, A. Fucoidans as Potential Therapeutics for Age-Related Macular Degeneration-Current Evidence from In Vitro Research. *Int. J. Mol. Sci.* **2020**, *21*, 9272. [CrossRef] [PubMed]
14. Dörschmann, P.; Seeba, C.; Thalenhorst, T.; Roider, J.; Klettner, A. Anti-inflammatory properties of antiangiogenic fucoidan in retinal pigment epithelium cells. *Heliyon* **2023**, *9*, e15202. [CrossRef]
15. Dörschmann, P.; Akkurt, H.; Kopplin, G.; Mikkelsen, M.D.; Meyer, A.S.; Roider, J.; Klettner, A. Establishment of specific age-related macular degeneration relevant gene expression panels using porcine retinal pigment epithelium for assessing fucoidan bioactivity. *Exp. Eye Res.* **2023**, *231*, 109469. [CrossRef] [PubMed]
16. Pomin, V.H.; Mourão, P.A.S. Structure, biology, evolution, and medical importance of sulfated fucans and galactans. *Glycobiology* **2008**, *18*, 1016–1027. [CrossRef] [PubMed]
17. Ustyuzhanina, N.E.; Bilan, M.I.; Ushakova, N.A.; Usov, A.I.; Kiselevskiy, M.V.; Nifantiev, N.E. Fucoidans: Pro- or antiangiogenic agents? *Glycobiology* **2014**, *24*, 1265–1274. [CrossRef] [PubMed]

18. Birgersson, P.S.; Chahal, A.S.; Klau, L.J.; Holte, H.B.; Arlov, Ø.; Aachmann, F.L. Structural characterization and immunomodulating assessment of ultra-purified water extracted fucoidans from *Saccharina latissima*, *Alaria esculenta* and *Laminaria hyperborea*. *Carbohydr. Polym.* **2024**, *343*, 122448. [CrossRef] [PubMed]
19. Ersoydan, S.; Rustemeyer, T. Investigating the Anti-Inflammatory Activity of Various Brown Algae Species. *Mar. Drugs* **2024**, *22*, 457. [CrossRef] [PubMed]
20. Dörschmann, P.; Kopplin, G.; Roider, J.; Klettner, A. Effects of Sulfated Fucans from Laminaria hyperborea Regarding VEGF Secretion, Cell Viability, and Oxidative Stress and Correlation with Molecular Weight. *Mar. Drugs* **2019**, *17*, 548. [CrossRef]
21. Dunn, K.C.; Aotaki-Keen, A.E.; Putkey, F.R.; Hjelmeland, L.M. ARPE-19, a human retinal pigment epithelial cell line with differentiated properties. *Exp. Eye Res.* **1996**, *62*, 155–169. [CrossRef] [PubMed]
22. Wiencke, A.K.; Kiilgaard, J.F.; Nicolini, J.; Bundgaard, M.; Röpke, C.; La Cour, M. Growth of cultured porcine retinal pigment epithelial cells. *Acta Ophthalmol. Scand.* **2003**, *81*, 170–176. [CrossRef]
23. Luyten, G.P.M.; Naus, N.C.; Mooy, C.M.; Hagemeijer, A.; Kan-Mitchell, J.; van Drunen, E.; Vuzevski, V.; de Jong, P.T.V.M.; Luider, T.M. Establishment and characterization of primary and metastatic uveal melanoma cell lines. *Int. J. Cancer* **1996**, *66*, 380–387. [CrossRef]
24. Schnichels, S.; Paquet-Durand, F.; Löscher, M.; Tsai, T.; Hurst, J.; Joachim, S.C.; Klettner, A. Retina in a dish: Cell cultures, retinal explants and animal models for common diseases of the retina. *Prog. Retin. Eye Res.* **2021**, *81*, 100880. [CrossRef]
25. Strunnikova, N.V.; Maminishkis, A.; Barb, J.J.; Wang, F.; Zhi, C.; Sergeev, Y.; Chen, W.; Edwards, A.O.; Stambolian, D.; Abecasis, G.; et al. Transcriptome analysis and molecular signature of human retinal pigment epithelium. *Hum. Mol. Genet.* **2010**, *19*, 2468–2486. [CrossRef]
26. Dörschmann, P.; Bittkau, K.S.; Neupane, S.; Roider, J.; Alban, S.; Klettner, A. Effects of Fucoidans from Five Different Brown Algae on Oxidative Stress and VEGF Interference in Ocular Cells. *Mar. Drugs* **2019**, *17*, 258. [CrossRef]
27. Kiser, P.D. Retinal pigment epithelium 65 kDa protein (RPE65): An update. *Prog. Retin. Eye Res.* **2022**, *88*, 101013. [CrossRef] [PubMed]
28. Schnabolk, G.; Tomlinson, S.; Rohrer, B. The complement regulatory protein CD59: Insights into attenuation of choroidal neovascularization. *Adv. Exp. Med. Biol.* **2014**, *801*, 435–440. [CrossRef] [PubMed]
29. Deniaud-Bouët, E.; Hardouin, K.; Potin, P.; Kloareg, B.; Hervé, C. A review about brown algal cell walls and fucose-containing sulfated polysaccharides: Cell wall context, biomedical properties and key research challenges. *Carbohydr. Polym.* **2017**, *175*, 395–408. [CrossRef] [PubMed]
30. Cumashi, A.; Ushakova, N.A.; Preobrazhenskaya, M.E.; D'Incecco, A.; Piccoli, A.; Totani, L.; Tinari, N.; Morozevich, G.E.; Berman, A.E.; Bilan, M.I.; et al. A comparative study of the anti-inflammatory, anticoagulant, antiangiogenic, and antiadhesive activities of nine different fucoidans from brown seaweeds. *Glycobiology* **2007**, *17*, 541–552. [CrossRef]
31. Sellimi, S.; Kadri, N.; Barragan-Montero, V.; Laouer, H.; Hajji, M.; Nasri, M. Fucans from a Tunisian brown seaweed *Cystoseira barbata*: Structural characteristics and antioxidant activity. *Int. J. Biol. Macromol.* **2014**, *66*, 281–288. [CrossRef]
32. Halling, B.P.; Vetvicka, V.; Blakemore, W.R. Evaluation of The Immunomodulatory in vivo Activity of *Laminaria hyperborea* Fucoidan Relative to Commercial (1,3/1,6)-B-D-Glucans from Yeast and Mushrooms. *J. Nutr. Health Sci.* **2015**, *2*, 1–13. [CrossRef]
33. Kopplin, G.; Rokstad, A.M.; Mélida, H.; Bulone, V.; Skjåk-Bræk, G.; Aachmann, F.L. Structural Characterization of Fucoidan from *Laminaria hyperborea*: Assessment of Coagulation and Inflammatory Properties and Their Structure-Function Relationship. *ACS Appl. Bio Mater.* **2018**, *1*, 1880–1892. [CrossRef] [PubMed]
34. Dörschmann, P.; Kopplin, G.; Roider, J.; Klettner, A. Interaction of High-Molecular Weight Fucoidan from *Laminaria hyperborea* with Natural Functions of the Retinal Pigment Epithelium. *Int. J. Mol. Sci.* **2023**, *24*, 2232. [CrossRef]
35. Gómez-Ordóñez, E.; Jiménez-Escrig, A.; Rupérez, P. Molecular weight distribution of polysaccharides from edible seaweeds by high-performance size-exclusion chromatography (HPSEC). *Talanta* **2012**, *93*, 153–159. [CrossRef] [PubMed]
36. Fletcher, H.R.; Biller, P.; Ross, A.B.; Adams, J. The seasonal variation of fucoidan within three species of brown macroalgae. *Algal Res.* **2017**, *22*, 79–86. [CrossRef]
37. Smidsrød, O.; Moe, S.T. *Biopolymer Chemistry*; Tapir: Trondheim, Norway, 2008; ISBN 978-82-519-2384-2.
38. Chang, Y.; Hu, Y.; Yu, L.; McClements, D.J.; Xu, X.; Liu, G.; Xue, C. Primary structure and chain conformation of fucoidan extracted from sea cucumber *Holothuria tubulosa*. *Carbohydr. Polym.* **2016**, *136*, 1091–1097. [CrossRef] [PubMed]
39. Podzimek, S. *Light Scattering, Size Exclusion Chromatography and Asymmetric Flow Field Flow Fractionation*; John Wiley & Sons, Inc.: Hoboken, NJ, USA, 2011. [CrossRef]
40. Hoai, N.T.; Sasaki, A.; Sasaki, M.; Kaga, H.; Kakuchi, T.; Satoh, T. Synthesis, characterization, and lectin recognition of hyperbranched polysaccharide obtained from 1,6-anhydro-D-hexofuranose. *Biomacromolecules* **2011**, *12*, 1891–1899. [CrossRef] [PubMed]
41. Klettner, A.; Kauppinen, A.; Blasiak, J.; Roider, J.; Salminen, A.; Kaarniranta, K. Cellular and molecular mechanisms of age-related macular degeneration: From impaired autophagy to neovascularization. *Int. J. Biochem. Cell Biol.* **2013**, *45*, 1457–1467. [CrossRef] [PubMed]

42. Dörschmann, P.; Apitz, S.; Hellige, I.; Neupane, S.; Alban, S.; Kopplin, G.; Ptak, S.; Fretté, X.; Roider, J.; Zille, M.; et al. Evaluation of the Effects of Fucoidans from Fucus Species and *Laminaria hyperborea* against Oxidative Stress and Iron-Dependent Cell Death. *Mar. Drugs* **2021**, *19*, 557. [CrossRef] [PubMed]
43. Dörschmann, P.; Thalenhorst, T.; Seeba, C.; Tischhöfer, M.-T.; Neupane, S.; Roider, J.; Alban, S.; Klettner, A. Comparison of Fucoidans from *Saccharina latissima* Regarding Age-Related Macular Degeneration Relevant Pathomechanisms in Retinal Pigment Epithelium. *Int. J. Mol. Sci.* **2023**, *24*, 7939. [CrossRef]
44. Mitchell, P.; Liew, G.; Gopinath, B.; Wong, T.Y. Age-related macular degeneration. *Lancet* **2018**, *392*, 1147–1159. [CrossRef] [PubMed]
45. Wang, M.; Li, H.; Wang, F. Roles of Transepithelial Electrical Resistance in Mechanisms of Retinal Pigment Epithelial Barrier and Retinal Disorders. *Discov. Med.* **2022**, *34*, 19–24. [PubMed]
46. Shirasawa, M.; Sonoda, S.; Terasaki, H.; Arimura, N.; Otsuka, H.; Yamashita, T.; Uchino, E.; Hisatomi, T.; Ishibashi, T.; Sakamoto T. TNF-α disrupts morphologic and functional barrier properties of polarized retinal pigment epithelium. *Exp. Eye Res.* **2013**, *110* 59–69. [CrossRef] [PubMed]
47. Cai, X.; Conley, S.M.; Naash, M.I. RPE65: Role in the visual cycle, human retinal disease, and gene therapy. *Ophthalmic Genet* **2009**, *30*, 57–62. [CrossRef] [PubMed]
48. Yang, P.; Tyrrell, J.; Han, I.; Jaffe, G.J. Expression and modulation of RPE cell membrane complement regulatory proteins. *Investig Ophthalmol. Vis. Sci.* **2009**, *50*, 3473–3481. [CrossRef] [PubMed]
49. Silchenko, A.S.; Rasin, A.B.; Zueva, A.O.; Kusaykin, M.I.; Zvyagintseva, T.N.; Rubtsov, N.K.; Ermakova, S.P. Discovery of a fucoidan endo-4O-sulfatase: Regioselective 4O-desulfation of fucoidans and its effect on anticancer activity in vitro. *Carbohydr. Polym.* **2021**, *271*, 118449. [CrossRef] [PubMed]
50. Sichert, A.; Corzett, C.H.; Schechter, M.S.; Unfried, F.; Markert, S.; Becher, D.; Fernandez-Guerra, A.; Liebeke, M.; Schweder, T.; Polz, M.F.; et al. Verrucomicrobia use hundreds of enzymes to digest the algal polysaccharide fucoidan. *Nat. Microbiol.* **2020**, *5*, 1026–1039. [CrossRef] [PubMed]
51. Sun, X.; Ai, C.; Wen, C.; Peng, H.; Yang, J.; Cui, Y.; Song, S. Inhibitory effects of fucoidan from *Laminaria japonica* against some pathogenic bacteria and SARS-CoV-2 depend on its large molecular weight. *Int. J. Biol. Macromol.* **2023**, *229*, 413–421. [CrossRef] [PubMed]
52. Chen, Q.; Kou, L.; Wang, F.; Wang, Y. Size-dependent whitening activity of enzyme-degraded fucoidan from *Laminaria japonica*. *Carbohydr. Polym.* **2019**, *225*, 115211. [CrossRef]
53. Lakshmana Senthil, S. A comprehensive review to assess the potential, health benefits and complications of fucoidan for developing as functional ingredient and nutraceutical. *Int. J. Biol. Macromol.* **2024**, *277*, 134226. [CrossRef] [PubMed]
54. Lahrsen, E.; Schoenfeld, A.-K.; Alban, S. Size-dependent pharmacological activities of differently degraded fucoidan fractions from Fucus vesiculosus. *Carbohydr. Polym.* **2018**, *189*, 162–168. [CrossRef] [PubMed]
55. Fernandes, P.A.R.; Coimbra, M.A. The antioxidant activity of polysaccharides: A structure-function relationship overview. *Carbohydr. Polym.* **2023**, *314*, 120965. [CrossRef]
56. Klettner, A. Oxidative stress induced cellular signaling in RPE cells. *Front. Biosci.* **2012**, *4*, 392. [CrossRef]
57. Ahmad, T.; Eapen, M.S.; Ishaq, M.; Park, A.Y.; Karpiniec, S.S.; Stringer, D.N.; Sohal, S.S.; Fitton, J.H.; Guven, N.; Caruso, V.; et al. Anti-Inflammatory Activity of Fucoidan Extracts In Vitro. *Mar. Drugs* **2021**, *19*, 702. [CrossRef] [PubMed]
58. Chen, H.; Cong, Q.; Du, Z.; Liao, W.; Zhang, L.; Yao, Y.; Ding, K. Sulfated fucoidan FP08S2 inhibits lung cancer cell growth in vivo by disrupting angiogenesis via targeting VEGFR2/VEGF and blocking VEGFR2/Erk/VEGF signaling. *Cancer Lett.* **2016**, *382*, 44–52. [CrossRef] [PubMed]
59. Dithmer, M.; Fuchs, S.; Shi, Y.; Schmidt, H.; Richert, E.; Roider, J.; Klettner, A. Fucoidan reduces secretion and expression of vascular endothelial growth factor in the retinal pigment epithelium and reduces angiogenesis in vitro. *PLoS ONE* **2014**, *9*, e89150. [CrossRef]
60. Klettner, A.; Westhues, D.; Lassen, J.; Bartsch, S.; Roider, J. Regulation of constitutive vascular endothelial growth factor secretion in retinal pigment epithelium/choroid organ cultures: P38, nuclear factor κB, and the vascular endothelial growth factor receptor-2/phosphatidylinositol 3 kinase pathway. *Mol. Vis.* **2013**, *19*, 281–291. [PubMed]
61. Klettner, A.; Koinzer, S.; Meyer, T.; Roider, J. Toll-like receptor 3 activation in retinal pigment epithelium cells—Mitogen-activated protein kinase pathways of cell death and vascular endothelial growth factor secretion. *Acta Ophthalmol.* **2013**, *91*, e211–e218. [CrossRef]
62. Spaide, R.F.; Vavvas, D.G. Complement Inhibition for Geographic Atrophy: Review of Salient Functional Outcomes and Perspective. *Retina* **2023**, *43*, 1064–1069. [CrossRef]
63. Ma, L.; Tang, F.Y.; Chu, W.K.; Young, A.L.; Brelen, M.E.; Pang, C.P.; Chen, L.J. Association of toll-like receptor 3 polymorphism rs3775291 with age-related macular degeneration: A systematic review and meta-analysis. *Sci. Rep.* **2016**, *6*, 19718. [CrossRef] [PubMed]

54. Gao, M.-L.; Wu, K.-C.; Deng, W.-L.; Lei, X.-L.; Xiang, L.; Zhou, G.-H.; Feng, C.-Y.; Cheng, X.-W.; Zhang, C.-J.; Gu, F.; et al. Toll-Like Receptor 3 Activation Initiates Photoreceptor Cell Death In Vivo and In Vitro. *Investig. Ophthalmol. Vis. Sci.* **2017**, *58*, 801–811. [CrossRef] [PubMed]
55. Kleinman, M.E.; Kaneko, H.; Cho, W.G.; Dridi, S.; Fowler, B.J.; Blandford, A.D.; Albuquerque, R.J.C.; Hirano, Y.; Terasaki, H.; Kondo, M.; et al. Short-interfering RNAs induce retinal degeneration via TLR3 and IRF3. *Mol. Ther.* **2012**, *20*, 101–108. [CrossRef] [PubMed]
56. D'Cruz, P.M.; Yasumura, D.; Weir, J.; Matthes, M.T.; Abderrahim, H.; LaVail, M.M.; Vollrath, D. Mutation of the receptor tyrosine kinase gene Mertk in the retinal dystrophic RCS rat. *Hum. Mol. Genet.* **2000**, *9*, 645–651. [CrossRef] [PubMed]
57. Audo, I.; Mohand-Said, S.; Boulanger-Scemama, E.; Zanlonghi, X.; Condroyer, C.; Démontant, V.; Boyard, F.; Antonio, A.; Méjécase, C.; El Shamieh, S.; et al. MERTK mutation update in inherited retinal diseases. *Hum. Mutat.* **2018**, *39*, 887–913. [CrossRef] [PubMed]
58. Kim, H.-M.; Ahn, C.; Kang, B.-T.; Kang, J.-H.; Jeung, E.-B.; Yang, M.-P. Fucoidan suppresses excessive phagocytic capacity of porcine peripheral blood polymorphonuclear cells by modulating production of tumor necrosis factor-alpha by lipopolysaccharide-stimulated peripheral blood mononuclear cells. *Res. Vet. Sci.* **2018**, *118*, 413–418. [CrossRef]
59. Hult, A.; Toss, F.; Malm, C.; Oldenborg, P.-A. In vitro phagocytosis of liquid-stored red blood cells requires serum and can be inhibited with fucoidan and dextran sulphate. *Vox Sang.* **2020**, *115*, 647–654. [CrossRef] [PubMed]
70. Dörschmann, P.; Hunger, F.; Schroth, H.; Chen, S.; Kopplin, G.; Roider, J.; Klettner, A. Effects of Fucoidans on Activated Retinal Microglia. *Int. J. Mol. Sci.* **2024**, *25*, 6018. [CrossRef] [PubMed]
71. Irschick, E.U.; Sgonc, R.; Böck, G.; Wolf, H.; Fuchs, D.; Nussbaumer, W.; Göttinger, W.; Huemer, H.P. Retinal pigment epithelial phagocytosis and metabolism differ from those of macrophages. *Ophthalmic Res.* **2004**, *36*, 200–210. [CrossRef]
72. Rohwer, K.; Neupane, S.; Bittkau, K.S.; Galarza Pérez, M.; Dörschmann, P.; Roider, J.; Alban, S.; Klettner, A. Effects of Crude Fucus distichus Subspecies evanescens Fucoidan Extract on Retinal Pigment Epithelium Cells-Implications for Use in Age-Related Macular Degeneration. *Mar. Drugs* **2019**, *17*, 538. [CrossRef] [PubMed]
73. Lieffrig, S.A.; Gyimesi, G.; Mao, Y.; Finnemann, S.C. Clearance phagocytosis by the retinal pigment epithelial during photoreceptor outer segment renewal: Molecular mechanisms and relation to retinal inflammation. *Immunol. Rev.* **2023**, *319*, 81–99. [CrossRef] [PubMed]
74. Wolf, G. Function of the protein RPE65 in the visual cycle. *Nutr. Rev.* **2005**, *63*, 97–100. [CrossRef] [PubMed]
75. Miraldi Utz, V.; Coussa, R.G.; Antaki, F.; Traboulsi, E.I. Gene therapy for RPE65-related retinal disease. *Ophthalmic Genet.* **2018**, *39*, 671–677. [CrossRef]
76. Wekre, M.E.; Holmelid, B.; Underhaug, J.; Pedersen, B.; Kopplin, G.; Jordheim, M. Characterization of high value products in the side-stream of *Laminaria hyperborea* alginate production—Targeting the phenolic content. *Algal Res.* **2023**, *72*, 103109. [CrossRef]
77. Wekre, M.E.; Hellesen Brunvoll, S.; Jordheim, M. Advancing quantification methods for polyphenols in brown seaweeds-applying a selective qNMR method compared with the TPC assay. *Phytochem. Anal.* **2022**, *33*, 1099–1110. [CrossRef] [PubMed]
78. Klettner, A.; Roider, J. Comparison of bevacizumab, ranibizumab, and pegaptanib in vitro: Efficiency and possible additional pathways. *Investig. Ophthalmol. Vis. Sci.* **2008**, *49*, 4523–4527. [CrossRef] [PubMed]
79. Riss, T.L.; Moravec, R.A.; Niles, A.L.; Duellman, S.; Benink, H.A.; Worzella, T.J.; Minor, L. *Assay Guidance Manual: Cell Viability Assays*; Eli Lilly & Co.: Bethesda, ML, USA, 2004.
80. Rizzolo, L.J. Barrier properties of cultured retinal pigment epithelium. *Exp. Eye Res.* **2014**, *126*, 16–26. [CrossRef] [PubMed]
81. Livak, K.J.; Schmittgen, T.D. Analysis of relative gene expression data using real-time quantitative PCR and the 2(-Delta Delta C(T)) Method. *Methods* **2001**, *25*, 402–408. [CrossRef]
82. Klettner, A.; Möhle, F.; Lucius, R.; Roider, J. Quantifying FITC-labeled latex beads opsonized with photoreceptor outer segment fragments: An easy and inexpensive method of investigating phagocytosis in retinal pigment epithelium cells. *Ophthalmic Res.* **2011**, *46*, 88–91. [CrossRef] [PubMed]

marine drugs

MDPI

Article

Alginate from *Ericaria crinita* Possesses Antioxidant Activity and Attenuates Systemic Inflammation via Downregulation of Pro-Inflammatory Cytokines

Paolina Lukova [1], Vesela Kokova [2], Alexandra Baldzhieva [3,4], Marianna Murdjeva [3,4], Plamen Katsarov [4,5], Cédric Delattre [6,7] and Elisaveta Apostolova [2,4,*]

[1] Department of Pharmacognosy and Pharmaceutical Chemistry, Faculty of Pharmacy, Medical University-Plovdiv, Vasil Aprilov Str. 15A, 4002 Plovdiv, Bulgaria

[2] Department of Pharmacology, Toxicology, and Pharmacotherapy, Faculty of Pharmacy, Medical University-Plovdiv, Vasil Aprilov Str. 15A, 4002 Plovdiv, Bulgaria

[3] Department of Medical Microbiology and Immunology "Prof. Dr. Elissay Yanev", Faculty of Medicine, Medical University-Plovdiv, Vasil Aprilov Str. 15A, 4002 Plovdiv, Bulgaria

[4] Research Institute at Medical University-Plovdiv, Vasil Aprilov Str. 15A, 4002 Plovdiv, Bulgaria

[5] Department of Pharmaceutical Sciences, Faculty of Pharmacy, Medical University-Plovdiv, Vasil Aprilov Str. 15A, 4002 Plovdiv, Bulgaria

[6] Clermont Auvergne INP, CNRS, Institut Pascal, Université Clermont Auvergne, 63000 Clermont-Ferrand, France

[7] Institut Universitaire de France (IUF), 1 rue Descartes, 75005 Paris, France

* Correspondence: elisaveta.apostolova@mu-plovdiv.bg; Tel.: +359-886-056557

Abstract: Alginates are anionic polysaccharides present in the cell walls of brown seaweeds. Various biological activities of alginate and its derivatives have been described. In this study, we assessed the potential of alginate obtained from *Ericaria crinita* (formerly *Cystoseira crinita*) to scavenge free radicals and function as a ferric ion reductor. The anti-inflammatory effect on the serum levels of TNF-α, IL-1β, IL-6, and IL-10 of rats with LPS-induced systemic inflammation after 14 days of treatment was also examined. *Ericaria crinita* alginate showed antioxidant activities of IC_{50} = 505 μg/mL (DPPH) and OD_{700} > 2 (ferric reducing power). A significant decrease in serum levels of IL-1β was observed only in animals treated with the polysaccharide at a dose of 100 mg/kg bw. Both doses of *E. crinita* alginate (25 and 100 mg/kg bw) significantly reduced the serum concentrations of pro-inflammatory cytokines TNF-α and IL-6, but no statistical significance was observed in the levels of the anti-inflammatory cytokine IL-10. Our findings show the potential of *E. crinita* alginate to act as an antioxidant and anti-inflammatory agent. It is likely that the exhibited antioxidant ability of the polysaccharide contributes to its antiphlogistic effects. More in-depth studies are needed to fully understand the specific mechanisms and the molecular pathways involved in these activities.

Keywords: alginate; *Cystoseira crinita*; *Ericaria crinita*; antioxidant effect; anti-inflammatory effect; cytokines; IL-1β; TNF-α; Il-6

1. Introduction

Inflammation is a key component of the immune system of the body and an essential mechanism to survive against pathogens and chemical or mechanical stress. While normally a tightly controlled response, inflammation must be monitored to prevent its spreading and the cause of irreparable damage. Excessive production of pro-inflammatory cytokines, chemokines, and reactive oxygen species, primarily secreted by macrophages and other immune cells as lymphocytes, can cause severe impairment and contribute to the pathogenesis of different inflammatory diseases [1].

Lipopolysaccharide (LPS) is a potent endotoxin that is a component of the outer membrane of Gram-negative bacteria, which plays a major role in the pathogenesis of inflammatory diseases [2,3]. LPS stimulates the activity of immune cells and in macrophages causes excessive release of pro-inflammatory mediators through activation of nuclear factor-kappa B (NF-κB) and mitogen-activated protein kinase (MAPK) signaling pathways [4]. Such critical mediators produced by LPS-stimulated macrophages are prostaglandins and NO, which are generated following the activation of cyclooxygenase-2 (COX-2) and nitric oxide synthases (NOS), respectively [5]. Many inflammatory cytokines, including tumor necrosis factor (TNF)-α, interleukin (IL)-6, and IL-1β, can be secreted by LPS-activated mononuclear phagocytes (monocytes and macrophages) and other types of cells [6]. The increase of these inflammatory mediators levels is closely associated with the development of inflammation-related diseases [7]. Therefore, inhibition of these inflammatory cytokines is considered to be an effective strategy for anti-inflammatory therapy.

Reactive oxygen species (ROS) are a group of short-lived, highly reactive molecules that are involved in numerous physiological processes like cell maturation, signaling, immune defense, and cytotoxicity against pathogens [8,9]. However, the overproduction of ROS is recognized as causing cellular abnormalities such as DNA alteration, lipid peroxidation, protein damage, and enzyme deactivation, which contribute to pathological conditions such as autoimmune disorders, cardiovascular diseases, atherosclerosis, rheumatoid arthritis, diabetes, and tumorigenesis [10,11]. Generally, antioxidants are defined as synthetic or natural substances that at low concentrations can prevent, inhibit, or delay the deterioration of oxidizable substrates [12]. The European Food Safety Authority (EFSA) assesses the scientific evidence regarding the use, benefits, and safety of antioxidants in food products and supplements [13].

While numerous synthesized chemicals effectively scavenge free radicals, they often have significant side effects. Moreover, available anti-inflammatory agents, such as nonsteroidal anti-inflammatory drugs and steroids, cause serious adverse effects with long-term use. Therefore, developing alternative treatments against inflammation and oxidative stress that are effective and less toxic remains an ongoing challenge. Natural products play an essential role in the process of new drug discovery and development. Nowadays, significant focus has been placed on the preparation and modification of polysaccharides, especially marine-derived polysaccharides such as fucoidans, alginates, laminarins, ulvans, agar, and chitosan [14–16].

Alginates are biopolymers commercially produced from brown marine algae; however, bacterial alginates from some *Pseudomonas* sp. and *Azotobacter* sp. are also used. Structurally alginates are composed of β-D-mannuronic acid (M) and its C-5 epimer, α-L-guluronic acid (G), linked by β-(1,4) bonds. The mannuronic and guluronic residues are arranged in homopolymeric (MM, GG) or heteropolymeric block structures (MG, GM) [17,18]. Alginates' MG block ratio, molecular weight, and molecular conformations block structure significantly influence their biological and physicochemical properties. Alginates have numerous proven properties, such as being non-toxic, water-soluble, biodegradable, biocompatible, film-forming, gelling, thickening, and anti-allergic [19,20]. Moreover, alginates are also known for their anti-inflammatory, antibacterial, antioxidant, prebiotic, mucoprotective, antidiabetic, and anti-obesity properties [17–19].

In this study, we aimed to achieve the following: (a) to examine the anti-inflammatory effect of the previously extracted and characterized alginate derived from the brown algae *Ericaria crinita* (*E. crinita*) (formerly *Cystoseira crinita*) [17] on the serum levels of TNF-α, IL-1β, IL-6, and IL-10 of rats with LPS-induced systemic inflammation after 14 days of treatment, (b) to evaluate the antioxidant capacity of *E. crinita* alginate to scavenge free radicals and to reduce ferric ions by donating an electron, and (c) to compare the obtained results with the activities of alginate structures isolated from other marine algae. Therefore, the performed analyses will highlight the importance of utilizing natural antioxidants and anti-inflammatory substances of marine origin, with a particular emphasis on alginate derived from *E. crinita*. By advancing the understanding of marine polysaccharides' therapeutic potential, this research will contribute to the development of safer, more sustainable, and effective alternatives to synthetic compounds in treating oxidative stress and inflammation, improving health outcomes.

2. Results

2.1. Changes in Serum Levels of Pro-Inflammatory Cytokines (IL-1β, TNF-α, and IL-6)

A significant decrease in serum levels of IL-1β was observed only in animals treated with the higher dose of alginate from *E. crinita* (100 mg/kg bw) in comparison to controls (835.13 ± 70.22 vs. 1318.97 ± 171.14; $p < 0.05$; Figure 1A). The reducing effect was also observed in TNF-α serum levels of rats treated with alginate isolated from *E. crinita* at a dose of 25 mg/kg bw (83.31.48 ± 8.37 vs. 129.33 ± 13.81; $p < 0.05$) and 100 mg/kg bw (79.67 ± 7.36 vs. 129.33 ± 13.81; $p < 0.05$) when compared with the control group (Figure 1B). As shown in Figure 1C, the levels of IL-6 in the serum of rats treated with both doses of *E. crinita* alginate were significantly decreased (80.29 ± 7.25 for the lower dose and 86.89 ± 7.82 for the higher dose vs. 121.08 ± 11.16; $p < 0.05$) in comparison to controls.

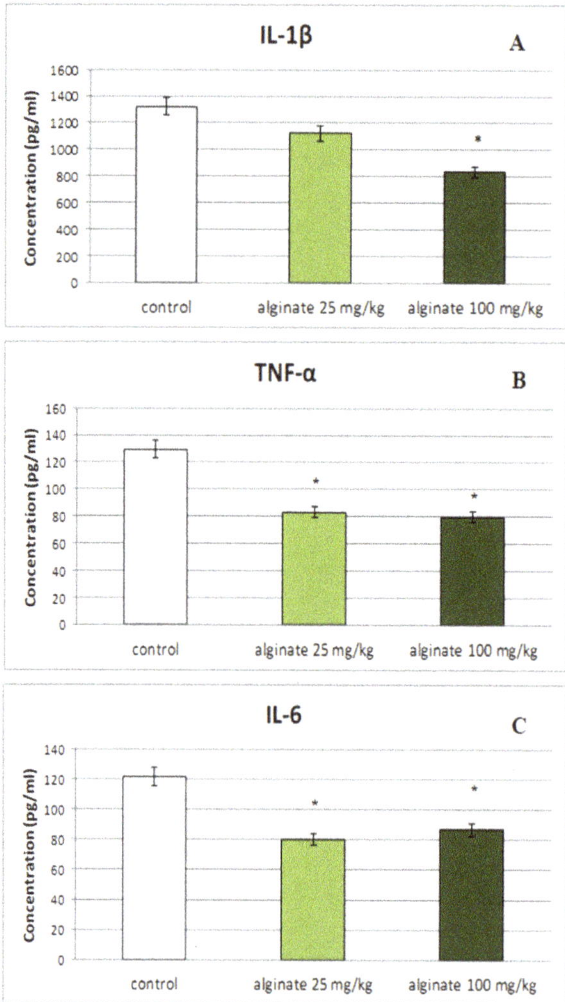

Figure 1. Effect of subchronic treatment with alginate from *E. crinita* (25 and 100 mg/kg bw) on serum levels of the pro-inflammatory cytokines IL-1β (panel (**A**)), TNF-α (panel (**B**)), and IL-6 (panel (**C**)) in LPS-induced systemic inflammation in rats. * $p < 0.05$ vs. same cytokine controls.

2.2. Changes in Serum Levels of Anti-Inflammatory Cytokine IL-10

Subchronic treatment of rats with *E. crinita* alginate at doses of 25 mg/kg and 100 mg/kg bw did not significantly change serum levels of the anti-inflammatory cytokine IL-10 in a model of LPS-induced systemic inflammation in comparison to controls (Figure 2).

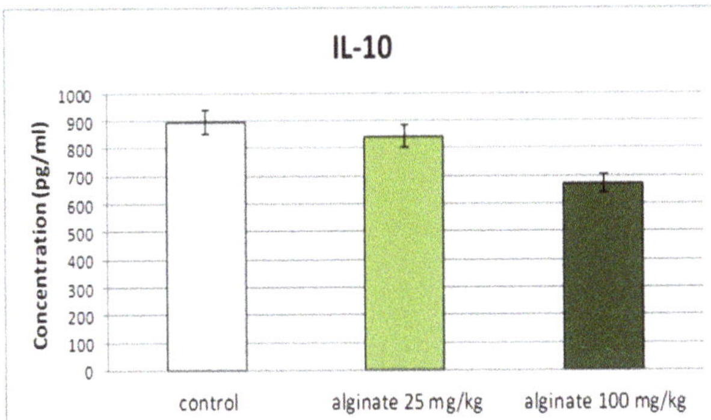

Figure 2. Effect of subchronic treatment with alginate from *E. crinita* (25 and 100 mg/kg bw) on serum levels of the anti-inflammatory cytokine IL-10 in rats with LPS-induced systemic inflammation.

2.3. 2,2-Diphenyl-1-Picryl-Hydrazyl-Hydrate (DPPH) Radical Scavenging Effect

As shown in Figure 3, the sample of *Ericaria crinita* alginate (ECA) was able to produce a stable form of DPPH in a dose-dependent manner. The inhibitory effect of ECA varied from 12.45% to 72.36% at concentrations of 0.05–2.5 mg/mL. Furthermore, in the range from 1.75 to 2.5 mg/mL, no remarkable augmentation of the antioxidant activity of ECA (from 71.78% to 72.36%) was established. An IC_{50} value of 505 μg/mL was calculated for ECA, which was lower than those of the two commercial antioxidants butylated hydroxytoluene (BHT) (IC_{50} = 5.5 μg/mL) and ascorbic acid (AA) (IC_{50} = 4.1 μg/mL).

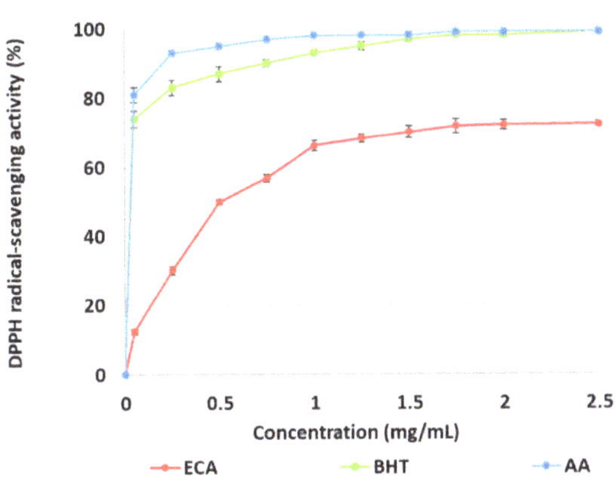

Figure 3. DPPH radical scavenging activity of *E. crinita* alginate (ECA), butylated hydroxytoluene (BHT), and ascorbic acid (AA).

2.4. Ferric Reducing Power

Figure 4 illustrates the capacity of ECA to facilitate the reduction of ferric to ferrous ions in a redox-linked colorimetric reaction. The OD_{700} of ECA exhibited a considerable range, from 0.37 to 2.02, across a concentration spectrum of 0.05 to 1.25 mg/mL. Hence, the most pronounced rise in activity, almost 50%, was noted between 0.5–0.75 mg/mL, respectively from 0.98 to 1.45. However, BHT and AA demonstrated higher reducing capacity in the tested concentrations (Figure 4).

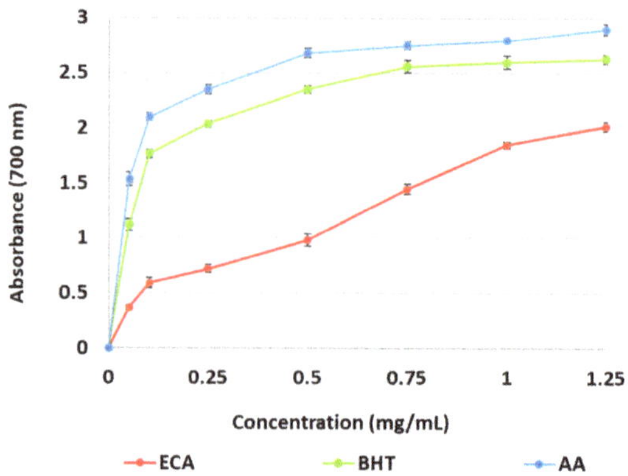

Figure 4. Ferric reducing power of *E. crinita* alginate (ECA), butylated hydroxytoluene (BHT), and ascorbic acid (AA).

3. Discussion

Alginates and their oligosaccharides have attractive pharmaceutical properties that exert many beneficial biological activities [19,21]. However, little is known about the anti-inflammatory effect of alginate isolated from *E. crinita*. Previously, we reported decreased levels of TNF-α, IL-6, and IL-1β after a single dose of *E. crinita* alginate [17]. In the current study, we found that *E. crinita* alginate at a dose of 25 and 100 mg/kg bw could ameliorate LPS-induced systemic inflammation after 14 days of treatment. We discovered that alginate from *E. crinita* could reduce serum levels of the pro-inflammatory cytokines IL-1β, TNF-α, and IL-6. These data confirm that alginate protects and possesses anti-inflammatory activity.

Our results are supported by the in vivo and in vitro findings of many other authors. Alginate isolated from *E. maxima* stipes attenuates particulate matter-induced inflammation in lung macrophages and downregulated the production of pro-inflammatory cytokines TNF-α, IL-6, and IL-1β [22]. The anti-inflammatory effects of oral and intraperitoneal administrated alginate gels in experimental models of ulcerative colitis and glomerulonephritis have been reported [23]. Low-viscosity sodium alginate (LVA), purified from *Macrocystis pyrifera* (concentration of 0.5% (*w*/*v*), administrated orally in drinking water for 1 week) suppressed the progression of colonic inflammatory lesions and decreased the serum and colonic mucosal levels of IL-6, TNF-α, leukotriene B4 (LTB4), and prostaglandin E2 (PGE2), in a model of acute colitis in rats [24]. Furthermore, its 6-week application reduced these serum levels, as well as colonic mucosal secretion of IL-6, TNF-α, LTB4, and the colonic damage score, in a model of chronic ulcerative colitis in rats [25]. The same LVA (dose 50 mg/kg bw, administrated i.p.) decreased proteinuria and serum creatinine, and inhibited antibody production and the glomerular deposition of immune complexes, as well as the development of glomerular lesions, in a model of immune complex glomerulonephritis in rats [26]. In another in vitro study, alginic acid from *Macrocystis pyrifera* with an approximate composition of 61% mannuronic and 39% guluronic acid, inhibited IL-1β and TNF-α production and mRNA expression but not IL-6 and IL-8 secretion. The authors suggested that alginic acid has different regulatory effects, including mast cell stabilization and inhibition of NF-kB, which might explain its anti-inflammatory properties [27]. Evidence of a local anti-inflammatory effect of sodium alginate and its compounds has been found in several studies [28–31].

Nevertheless, some research data indicate that alginate may have pro-inflammatory properties. For instance, sodium alginate with a molecular weight of 9500 kDa and an M/G ratio of 1.96 activated RAW264.7 macrophages, leading to increased levels of the pro-inflammatory cytokines TNF-α, IL-1β, IL-6, and IL-12 and triggered innate immunity via NF-κB activation [32]. Another study reported that high mannuronic acid-containing alginate (HMA) derived from *Macrocystis pyrifera* has an immunostimulatory effect, increases the number of peritoneal macrophages in mice, and promotes phagocytosis, secretion, and tumoricidal activity of macrophages through the production of cytokines and cytotoxic molecules such as TNF-α, NO, and H_2O_2 [33]. Additionally, alginate from *Ascophyllum nodosum* with high M- and MG-blocks was significantly more effective in inducing TNF-α IL-1, and IL-6 production than alginate with high G-blocks from *Laminaria digitata* [34]. Mannoglucan was also shown to have TNF-α-like antitumor activity [35]. These findings contrast with the anti-inflammatory effects of alginate observed in our studies. The first reason may be that these experiments were conducted in vitro whereas ours were performed in vivo. Secondly, different factors may influence the biological activities of alginates and alginate oligosaccharides (AOS), including their structure, molecular weight, M and G content (M/G ratio), and spatial conformation of molecules. Other factors, such as molecular weight, algal source, and extraction methods, should also be considered. This also applies to the immunogenicity of alginate, which can vary depending on its chemical composition. A higher proportion of mannuronic acid in alginate, such as the structure in the last cited studies, could enhance its immunostimulatory effects. For example, the M/G ratio of the examined alginate in Yang and Jones' research [32] was 1.96. The content of β-D-mannuronic acid in our *E. crinita* alginate was lower (M/G ratio 1.018). Likewise, the anti-inflammatory properties of AOS are dependent on the M and G monomer content. M−block AOS were found to increase the production of TNF-α, RANTES, and granulocyte-colony stimulating factor (G-CSF) from RAW macrophages as compared to G-block AOS [36]. Thus, alginates rich in mannuronic acid appear to stimulate pro-inflammatory cytokine production and activate the innate immune response via the NF-κB pathway. On the other hand, G-block AOS were reported to reduce the secretion of ROS, NO, PGE2, IL-1β, TNF-α and IL-6, and the expression of COX-2 after LPS activation [37]. It was proposed that G-block AOS can prevent the binding of LPS to Toll-like receptor 4 (TLR4), averting downstream NF-κB signaling [38].

Monocytes and macrophages respond to bacterial LPS and activate several host defense functions through the secretion of many inflammatory mediators. When activated with a specific source of LPS, monocytes exhibit rapid expression of mRNA for TNF-a, IL-1β, and IL-8, which is followed by IL-6 [39]. TNF-α can cause inflammation and apoptosis and can mediate the release of other cytokines, such as IL-6 and IL-8 by stimulating macrophages [40]. It is known that IL-1β is a potent pro-inflammatory cytokine that leads to vasodilatation, promotes the attraction of granulocytes to the site of inflammation, and induces prostaglandin production during an acute inflammation [41]. IL-1β also participates in chronic inflammation and stimulates other cytokine secretion by Th17 cells, promoting the development of chronic inflammatory diseases [42]. Furthermore, sensitive to IL-1β is a subtype of Th1 cells that express CD161, functionally related to Th17 cells [43]. Besides the pro-inflammatory activity, IL-1β plays a key role in the innate immune response. IL-1β has been suggested to link innate and acquired immunity through its additional effects on T cells [44]. IL-6 is a pleiotropic pro-inflammatory cytokine that participates actively in inflammatory and immunomodulatory mechanisms. Its production is mainly activated by IL-1β and TNFα, although there are also other ways to promote its secretion such as Toll-like receptor activation (TLRs), stress response, prostaglandins, adipokines, and other cytokines [45]. IL-6 induces an increase in the concentrations of various acute phase proteins such as C-reactive protein (CRP), serum amyloid A, fibrinogen, haptoglobin, and α1-antichymotrypsin, whereas it inhibits the production of albumin. These changes in acute-phase protein levels are used to evaluate the severity of inflammation in routine clinical laboratory tests. IL-6 not only evokes acute phase reactions but also leads to the development of specific cellular and humoral immune responses and plays an important role in acquired immunity by end-stage B-cell differentiation, stimulation of antibody secretion, and T-cell activation. Thus, IL-6 is an important mediator for the transition from acute to chronic stage of inflammation and performs an important function in the linking of innate to acquired immune response. Dysregulated continual synthesis of IL-6 is associated with the development of autoimmune and chronic inflammatory diseases [46–48]. Our data suggest that alginate could reduce inflammation induced by LPS. Our study found that TNF-α, IL-6, and IL-1β levels were decreased by *E. crinita* alginate. Alginate could ameliorate LPS-induced systemic inflammation by modulating serum levels of cytokines related to inflammation.

Cytokines and reactive oxygen species are closely interconnected [49]. Free radicals play a crucial role in triggering and maintaining inflammatory processes, so neutralizing them with antioxidants and radical scavengers can help reduce inflammation [50]. One study reported that alginic acid, derived from the brown algae *Sargassum wightii*, showed anti-inflammatory and antioxidant effects in rats with arthritis induced by complete Freund's adjuvant when administered orally at a dose of 100 mg/kg. The treatment led to a reduction in paw edema, decreased COX-2 and 5-LOX activities, and less neutrophil infiltration. Additionally, alginic acid decreased lipid peroxidation by enhancing the cellular antioxidant defense system, increasing the activity of antioxidant enzymes, and boosting reduced glutathione levels [51]. Furthermore, alginate inhibited TNF-α-induced intercellular adhesion molecule-1 expression, nitric oxide production, and hydrogen peroxide levels [52], suggesting that the antioxidant properties of alginate contribute to its anti-inflammatory effects.

Studies on the antioxidant activity of alginates demonstrated their in vitro ability to scavenge free hydroxyl and superoxide radicals, along with acting as a chelator/reductor of Fe ions and bleaching of β-carotene [53]. Several factors influence the antioxidant properties of alginates, including molecular weight, concentration, pretreatment techniques, period of collection, and in the case of alginate oligosaccharides, the method of depolymerization. Generally, the reported antioxidant effect was concentration- and time-dependent, and inversely proportional to alginate molecular weight [15,54]. Low molecular weight (LWM) alginates have better antioxidant ability compared to high molecular weight ones. It is supposed that this could be due to the presence of additional functional groups in the LWM alginates [53]. Moreover, polysaccharides with higher molecular weight exhibit a denser structure, leading to stronger intramolecular hydrogen linkages, which limit the accessibility of hydrogen groups [54]. This claim has been proven by several authors [18,54], including the results from our study for *E. crinita* alginate. Benslima et al. [54] isolated four alginate polymers from *Cystoseira schiffneri* collected in different months of the year with Mw ranging from 1.23×10^6 to 4.49×10^3 g/mol. The alginates with higher Mw (up to 2.33×10^5 g/mol) exhibited a lower DPPH radical scavenging effect ($IC_{50} > 1500$ µg/mL), while the alginate with Mw = 4.49×10^3 g/mol had an IC_{50} value of 190 µg/mL. Similarly, Borazjani et al. [55] reported the DPPH scavenging activity of four alginates obtained from the brown algae *Sargassum angustifolium* using different pretreatment agents. The enzyme-treated alginates resulted in the lowest Mw (357×10^3 g/mol) and, respectively, the highest antioxidant properties (more than 66% of inhibition) (Table 1). The same inversely proportional relationship between molecular weight and DPPH antioxidant activity was observed when comparing the scavenging effect of the obtained alginate from *E. crinita* with those of other brown species: *Cystoseira compressa* [18], *Cystoseira schiffneri* [54], and *Sargassum angustifolium* [55] (Table 1). Contrary to the above-mentioned comparisons, Sellimi et al. [56] reported the highest value for the DPPH scavenging effect (IC_{50}~150 µg/mL) of *Cystoseira barbata* alginate, which had a higher value of Mw (2.99×10^5 g/mol). Nonetheless, Mw appears to be the major factor in the control of alginates' DPPH antioxidant effect.

Table 1. Compositional data of alginates extracted from different species of brown algae.

DPPH		OD_{700} (0.5 mg/mL)	Uronic Acids (%, *w*/*w*)	Mw (g/mol)	Period of Collection	Pretreatment	Algal Source	Ref.
IC_{50} (μg/mL)	% Inh. (1 mg/mL)							
505	66.2	0.98	50.14	7.31×10^4	July	0.1 M HCl	*Ericaria cirnita* (*Cystoseira crinita*)	Current study
560	~70	~1.0	46.48	1×10^5	February	0.1 M HCl	*Cystoseira compressa*	[18]
~150	~73	~0.7	58.1	2.99×10^5	November	0.1 M HCl	*Cystoseira barbata*	[56]
>1500 >1500 >1500 190	~15 ~23 ~17 ~80	~2.0 ~0.3 ~1.0 ~2.8	47 53 66 62	1.23×10^6 1.16×10^5 2.33×10^5 4.49×10^3	December April July September	0.1 M HCl	*Cystoseira schiffneri*	[54]
-	39.9 ~43 66.5 66.7	0.25 0.28 0.38 0.37	-	480.3×10^3 557.1×10^3 $\sim 357 \times 10^3$ $\sim 357 \times 10^3$	-	Water 0.1 M HCl 5% Alcalase 5% Cellulase	*Sargassum angustifolium*	[55]
-	74.7 86.8 61.1	-	-	A-1.10×10^5 PolyG-7.5×10^2 PolyM-6.9×10^2	May	0.1 M H_2SO_4	*Sargassum vulgare*	[57]

A—Alginate; PolyG—homopolymeric polyguluronate; PolyM—homopolymeric polymannuronate.

Moreover, some authors claim that the antioxidant activity of alginates is independent of the relative content of mannuronate and guluronate, considering that the only distinction between pM and pG is the orientation of the C5 carboxyl groups [21]. However, the study of Nouha Sari-Chmayssem et al. [57] demonstrated 25% higher hydroxyl radical scavenging activity for the homopolymeric polyguluronate fraction compared to the homopolymeric polymanuronate fraction with slightly similar molecular weight (Table 1). These observations could be attributed to the diaxial linkage in guluronate blocks, which may result in a restricted rotation around the glycosidic linkage. The enhanced flexibility of guluronate blocks may be responsible for the rigid and extended configuration of the alginate chains, which could affect the accessibility of the sodium alginate hydroxyl groups [57].

Allegedly, the ferric reducing power of polysaccharides was found to be related to their molecular weight and the number of hydroxyl and carboxyl groups present in the uronic acids [18,54]. *E. crinita* alginate at a concentration of 0.5 mg/mL showed values for ferric reducing antioxidant activity (OD_{700} = 0.98) comparable to those reported for alginate extracted from *Cystoseira compressa* (OD_{700}~1) with similar uronic acid content but higher Mw [18]. Moreover, alginate from *C. barbata* with higher Mw and higher uronic acid exhibited lower ferric-reducing capacity (OD_{700}~0.7) [56] (Table 1). Similarly to the DPPH results, Borazjani et al. [55] reported the highest reducing ability for *Sargassum angustifolium* alginate fraction, which had the lowest Mw. Nevertheless, contrary findings have also been reported by other researchers. Regarding the results from Benslima et al. [54], the reducing capacity of *Cystoseira schiffneri* alginate was not found to be correlated with either their uronic acid amount or their molecular weight. It may be necessary to consider additional factors, such as the polyphenol content retained in alginates or other structural characteristics [54,58].

The antioxidant and anti-inflammatory activities of alginate have significant implications for health, industry, and the environment. By further unveiling its mechanisms and applications, alginate could play a significant role in various health fields. The current study, for example, suggests the potential use of polysaccharides for the treatment and prevention of inflammatory diseases. Moreover, by neutralizing free radicals, alginate can reduce cellular damage and potentially lower the risk of chronic disorders. The ability of alginate to modulate inflammatory pathways can help manage these conditions, offering therapeutic approaches for reducing severe symptoms and improving quality of life. Furthermore, alginate's antioxidant properties can be utilized in food preservation, extending food product shelf life by preventing oxidation and improving its chemical stability. Due to their unique properties and valuable therapeutic effects, alginates are also widely exploited in pharmaceutical technology. As natural biodegradable materials, these polysaccharides are preferred excipients and drug carriers, whose antioxidant and anti-inflammatory properties can enhance the efficacy of certain active substances, particularly in treating diseases characterized by oxidative stress and inflammation.

4. Materials and Methods

4.1. Algae Material and Chemicals

Talluses of the brown algae *Ericaria crinita* (Duby) Molinari & Guiry were gathered from the Black Sea coast, Bulgaria, in July 2019. The taxonomy, species identification, and pretreatment of the algae were detailed in our earlier research [17]. Test substances used in the experiments were alginic acid sodium salt (Product No. 180947), lipopolysaccharides from *E. coli* O55:B5 (LPS), butylated hydroxytoluene, ascorbic acid, and 2 and 2,2-diphenyl-1-picryl-hydrazyl-hydrate. All the reagents were purchased from Sigma Aldrich. The tested alginates and LPS were dissolved in saline.

4.2. Animals

Male Wistar 4-month-old rats weighing 160–205 g were used. The animals were housed in standard laboratory conditions: temperature 22 °C ± 1 °C, humidity 45%, light/dark cycle of 12/12 h, with access to food and water ad libitum.

4.3. Extraction and Structural Characterization of Ericaria crinita Alginate

The procedure of the alginate extraction and its structural analysis were outlined in our prior study [17]. *E. crinita* sodium alginate was extracted using an alkaline solvent (3% Na_2CO_3, pH 11) for 2 h, at a temperature of 60 °C. The extraction yield was determined to be 20.18% based on the dry weight of the algae. The uronic acid and neutral sugar contents were estimated to be 50.14% and 19.66%, respectively. The purity of *E. crinita* alginate was evaluated based on the low percentage of sulfate groups (0.63%), proteins (less than 0.04%), and total polyphenols (less than 0.10%). The average molecular weight in mass (Mw) and average molecular weight in number (Mn) of *E. crinita* alginate were estimated using size-exclusion chromatography–multi-angle light scattering (SEC/MALS). The calculated Mn and Mw were found to be 5.29×10^4 g/mol and 7.31×10^4 g/mol, respectively. The polydispersity index of 1.38 indicated a narrow mass distribution, confirming the polymer's homogeneity. The Fourier-transform infrared (FTIR) spectroscopy showed two characteristic peaks at 1090 and 1035 cm^{-1} corresponding to the mannuronic and guluronic acid. Further analysis of the chemical structure and block distribution of the alginate polymer was accomplished using proton nuclear magnetic resonance (^{1}H NMR) spectroscopy. The results revealed typical 500 MHz-^{1}H NMR signals attributed to repeating guluronic and mannuronic acid units. M/G ratio of 1.018 was estimated, indicating relatively equal levels of β-D-mannuronic and α-L-guluronic acids. Moreover, the homopolymorphic MM or GG regions were almost equivalent to the alternating blocks. The FTIR and ^{1}H NMR spectra of the *E. crinita* alginate revealed no traces of fucoidan, as confirmed by the absence of characteristic signals from the methyl groups in the fucose and sulfate ester groups.

4.4. Detection of Pro-Inflammatory and Anti-Inflammatory Cytokines

The effect of multiple applications of alginate from *E. crinita* on serum cytokine levels was studied. Twenty-four male Wistar rats were randomly divided into three experimental groups, each consisting of eight animals, and treated intraperitoneally for 14 days as follows: 1st group (control)—treated with saline (0.1 mL/100 g bw); 2nd group (alginate 25 mg/kg)—treated with 25 mg/kg bw alginate from *E. crinita*; and 3rd group (alginate 100 mg/kg)—treated with 100 mg/kg bw alginate from *E. crinita*. Thirty minutes after the last application of the substances, a solution of LPS at a dose of 0.25 mg/kg was injected intraperitoneally. Four hours after the LPS challenge, blood samples were collected in test tubes for serum yield. They were transported immediately to the Department of Medical Microbiology and Immunology "Prof. Dr. Elissay Yanev" in an ice container.

The collected rat blood samples were promptly processed through centrifugation at 1000× *g* for 10 min at room temperature, using a Hermle Z36-HK centrifuge (HERMLE Labortechnik GmbH, Wehingen, Germany), situated in the Department of Medical Microbiology and Immunology "Prof. Dr. Elissay Yanev". The centrifugation process separated the serum, which was then carefully removed from the monovettes using sterile techniques in order to avoid contamination. This serum was divided into smaller portions (aliquots), each ranging from 250 to 500 µL depending on the initial volume of the collected blood. This division was conducted to minimize the need for multiple freeze-thaw cycles, which could deteriorate the samples' and the cytokines' quality and stability. These aliquots were then placed in labeled cryovials and stored at −80 °C to preserve them for further examination.

The study focused on measuring the concentrations of four specific cytokines: Rat IL-1β, Rat IL-6, Rat IL-10, and Rat TNF-α in the serum samples. This was achieved using an enzyme-linked immunosorbent assay (ELISA) with pre-coated strip plates provided by Diaclone (CEDEX—Besançon, Franche-Comté, France). Those kits were selected due to their well-documented sensitivity, specificity, and compatibility with rat serum samples. The entire procedure was performed strictly following the manufacturer's instructions to ensure accuracy and reliability.

Optical density measurements based on the linear relationship between light absorbance and particle concentration were taken at a wavelength of 450 nm, with an optional reference filter at 620 nm, using a Tecan Sunrise Microplate Reader (Tecan Austria GmbH, Salzburg, Austria) paired with the Magellan™ Data Analysis Standard v7.2 Software. To quantify the cytokine levels, a standard curve was generated using known concentrations of cytokine standards included in the ELISA kits. The concentrations of cytokines in the samples were then calculated using the linear equation derived from this standard curve. The results were expressed in picograms per milliliter (pg/mL), providing a precise measure of the cytokine levels in each serum sample.

4.5. DPPH Radical Scavenging Activity

The DPPH free radical scavenging activity of *E. crinita* alginate was conducted as per the method outlined by Kao and Chen [59], with slight modifications. Specifically, 0.5 mM DPPH in methanol (0.2 mL) was mixed with the alginate solution (1 mL) at concentrations ranging from 0.05 to 2.5 mg/mL. These mixtures were incubated at room temperature in darkness for 15 min. Subsequently, the reduction in absorbance at 517 nm was estimated using a UV-VIS spectrophotometer Evolution 300 (Thermo Fisher Scientific, Waltham, MA, USA). A blend of the polysaccharide solution and methanol served as a blank. The antioxidant efficacy was quantified as a percentage of inhibition, calculated using the equation:

$$\%\ \text{Inhibition} = \frac{A_0 - A_{15}}{A_0} \times 100$$

where A_0 denoted the blank sample absorbance at 0 min and A_{15} designated the polysaccharide solution absorbance after 15 min. Results were presented based on triplicate measurements with standard deviation (±SD), and the IC_{50} values were deduced from linear regression plots.

4.6. Ferric Reducing Power

The ferric reducing power was assessed using the method of Yildirim et al. [60]. A 0.3 mL volume of polysaccharide solution at different concentrations (0.05–1.25 mg/mL) was mixed with 1.25 mL phosphate buffer (0.2 M, pH 6.6) and 1.25 mL of 1% potassium ferricyanide. Following a 30 min incubation period at 50 °C, the mixture was treated with 10% 1.25 mL of trichloroacetic acid and subsequently subjected to centrifugation for 10 min at 3500 rpm. Then, 1.25 mL of the supernatant, 1.25 mL of distilled water, and 0.25 mL of 0.1% ferric chloride solution were mixed in a test tube. The ferric reducing power was estimated by measuring the increase in absorbance after 10 min at a wavelength of 700 nm. Blanks lacking ferric chloride were prepared for each concentration and BHA and AA were employed as standards. The values were determined through triplicate measurements with ±SD.

4.7. Statistical Analysis

Statistical evaluation was executed with SPSS 17.0 employing one-way ANOVA and Bonferroni post hoc tests. The normality of distribution was determined with the one-sample Kolmogorov–Smirnov test. The number of tested animals is given as n. Results are presented as arithmetic mean ± standard error of the mean (± SEM). p-value ≤ 0.05 was considered statistically significant.

5. Conclusions

Our study demonstrated that subchronic treatment with alginate isolated from *E. crinita* in doses of 25 mg/kg and 100 mg/kg bw could ameliorate LPS-induced systemic inflammation by reducing serum levels of pro-inflammatory cytokines IL-1β, TNF-α, and IL-6 in rats. The antioxidant activity of *E. crinita* alginate, as evidenced by DPPH radical scavenging and reducing power assays, showed a concentration-dependent increase. Although the obtained data on *E. crinita* alginate's antioxidant and anti-inflammatory activities are encouraging, more in-depth studies are needed to fully understand the specific mechanisms and the molecular pathways involved in these processes. Future research may also focus on their multifunctional applications offering benefits beyond antioxidant and anti-inflammatory effects. The full potential of marine alginates can be harnessed to provide novel, effective, and sustainable therapeutic options for the treatment and prevention of various acute and chronic diseases.

The study has the following limitations: (1) the rats received intraperitoneal injections of alginate once a day for 14 days, so different treatment periods or application routes could result in different outcomes; (2) the results were obtained in rats and could not be extrapolated to humans without additional experiments; (3) the cytokines were evaluated 4 h after the LPS challenge, so changes in the time point of evaluation could have influenced the results; (4) the antioxidant properties of the compound were studied in vitro; however, there is no guarantee that the same activity will occur in vivo.

Author Contributions: Conceptualization, V.K., P.L. and E.A.; writing—original draft preparation, V.K., P.L. and A.B.; writing—critical review and editing, C.D., E.A., P.K. and M.M. All authors have read and agreed to the published version of the manuscript.

Funding: This research was financially supported by Medical University-Plovdiv through Doctoral (PhD) and Postdoctoral Project number DPDP-02/2019.

Institutional Review Board Statement: Approvals from the Bulgarian Food Safety Agency (permit number: 252/22 November 2019) and the Ethics Committee of the Medical University-Plovdiv, Bulgaria (protocol number: 1/13 February 2020), were obtained before the beginning of the experiments. The study was performed according to the following guidelines: ARRIVE, the EU Directive 2010/63/EU for animal experiments, and the relevant national and institutional rules and regulations.

Data Availability Statement: The data presented in this study are available on request from the corresponding author.

Conflicts of Interest: The authors declare no conflicts of interest.

References

1. Afonina, I.S.; Zhong, Z.; Karin, M.; Beyaert, R. Limiting Inflammation—The Negative Regulation of NF-KB and the NLRP3 Inflammasome. *Nat. Immunol.* **2017**, *18*, 861–869. [CrossRef] [PubMed]
2. Maldonado, R.F.; Sá-Correia, I.; Valvano, M.A. Lipopolysaccharide modification in Gram-negative bacteria during chronic infection. *FEMS Microbiol. Rev.* **2016**, *40*, 480–493. [CrossRef] [PubMed]
3. Hamesch, K.; Borkham-Kamphorst, E.; Strnad, P.; Weiskirchen, R. Lipopolysaccharide-induced inflammatory liver injury in mice. *Lab. Anim.* **2015**, *49*, 37–46. [CrossRef] [PubMed]
4. Jeong, Y.H.; Oh, Y.C.; Cho, W.K.; Yim, N.H.; Ma, J.Y. Anti-Inflammatory effect of rhapontici radix ethanol extract via inhibition of NF-κB and MAPK and induction of HO-1 in macrophages. *Mediat. Inflamm.* **2016**, *2016*, 7216912. [CrossRef] [PubMed]
5. Zhao, F.; Chen, L.; Bi, C.; Zhang, M.; Jiao, W.; Yao, X. In vitro anti-inflammatory effect of picrasmalignan A by the inhibition of iNOS and COX2 expression in LPS activated macrophage RAW264.7 cells. *Mol. Med. Rep.* **2013**, *8*, 1575–1579. [CrossRef]
6. An, S.J.; Pae, H.O.; Oh, G.S.; Choi, B.M.; Jeong, S.; Jang, S.I.; Oh, H.; Kwon, T.O.; Song, C.E.; Chung, H.T. Inhibition of TNF-α, IL-1β, and IL-6 productions and NF-κB activation in lipopolysaccharide-activated RAW 264.7 macrophages by catalposide, an iridoid glycoside isolated from *Catalpa ovata* G. Don (Bignoniaceae). *Int. Immunopharmacol.* **2002**, *2*, 1173–1181. [CrossRef]
7. Kany, S.; Vollrath, J.T.; Relja, B. Cytokines in Inflammatory Disease. *Int. J. Mol. Sci.* **2019**, *20*, 6008. [CrossRef]
8. Parcheta, M.; Świsłocka, R.; Orzechowska, S.; Akimowicz, M.; Choińska, R.; Lewandowski, W. Recent Developments in Effective Antioxidants: The Structure and Antioxidant Properties. *Materials* **2021**, *14*, 1984. [CrossRef]
9. Srinivas, U.S.; Tan, B.W.Q.; Vellayappan, B.A.; Jeyasekharan, A.D. ROS and the DNA Damage Response in Cancer. *Redox Biol.* **2019**, *25*, 101084. [CrossRef]
10. Zhao, X.; Li, B.; Xue, C.; Sun, L. Effect of Molecular Weight on the Antioxidant Property of Low Molecular Weight Alginate from Laminaria Japonica. *J. Appl. Phycol.* **2012**, *24*, 295–300. [CrossRef]
11. Alfadda, A.A.; Sallam, R.M. Reactive Oxygen Species in Health and Disease. *J. Biomed. Biotechnol.* **2012**, *2012*, 936486. [CrossRef] [PubMed]
12. Fernandes, R.D.P.P.; Trindade, M.A.; De Melo, M.P. Natural Antioxidants and Food Applications: Healthy Perspectives. In *Alternative and Replacement Foods*; Elsevier: Amsterdam, The Netherlands, 2018; pp. 31–64, ISBN 978-0-12-811446-9.
13. EFSA Panel on Dietetic Products, Nutrition and Allergies (NDA). Scientific Opinion on the Substantiation of Health Claims Related to Various Food(s)/Food Constituent(s) and Protection of Cells from Premature Aging, Antioxidant Activity, Antioxidant Content and Antioxidant Properties, and Protection of DNA, Proteins and Lipids from Oxidative Damage Pursuant to Article 13(1) of Regulation (EC) No 1924/2006. *EFSA J.* **2010**, *8*, 1489. [CrossRef]
14. Zhong, Q.; Wei, B.; Wang, S.; Ke, S.; Chen, J.; Zhang, H.; Wang, H. The Antioxidant Activity of Polysaccharides Derived from Marine Organisms: An Overview. *Mar. Drugs* **2019**, *17*, 674. [CrossRef] [PubMed]
15. Kelishomi, Z.H.; Goliaei, B.; Mahdavi, H.; Nikoofar, A.; Rahimi, M.; Moosavi-Movahedi, A.A.; Mamashli, F.; Bigdeli, B. Antioxidant Activity of Low Molecular Weight Alginate Produced by Thermal Treatment. *Food Chem.* **2016**, *196*, 897–902. [CrossRef]
16. Sindhi, V.; Gupta, V.; Sharma, K.; Bhatnagar, S.; Kumari, R.; Dhaka, N. Potential Applications of Antioxidants—A Review. *J. Pharm. Res.* **2013**, *7*, 828–835. [CrossRef]
17. Kokova, V.; Lukova, P.; Baldzhieva, A.; Katsarov, P.; Delattre, C.; Molinié, R.; Petit, E.; Elboutachfaiti, R.; Murdjeva, M.; Apostolova, E. Extraction, structural characterization, and in vivo anti-inflammatory effect of alginate from *Cystoseira crinita* (Desf.) Borry harvested in the Bulgarian Black Sea. *Mar. Drugs* **2023**, *21*, 245. [CrossRef]
18. Hentati, F.; Delattre, C.; Ursu, A.V.; Desbrières, J.; Le Cerf, D.; Gardarin, C.; Abdelkafi, S.; Michaud, P.; Pierre, G. Structural Characterization and Antioxidant Activity of Water-Soluble Polysaccharides from the Tunisian Brown Seaweed Cystoseira Compressa. *Carbohydr. Polym.* **2018**, *198*, 589–600. [CrossRef]
19. Szekalska, M.; Puciłowska, A.; Szymańska, E.; Ciosek, P.; Winnicka, K. Alginate: Current use and future perspectives in pharmaceutical and biomedical applications. *Int. J. Polym. Sci.* **2016**, *2016*, 7697031. [CrossRef]
20. Giridhar Reddy, S. Alginates—A Seaweed Product: Its Properties and Applications. In *Properties and Applications of Alginates*; Deniz, I., Imamoglu, E., Keskin-Gundogdu, T., Eds.; IntechOpen: London, UK, 2022; ISBN 978-1-83969-499-8.
21. Xing, M.; Cao, Q.; Wang, Y.; Xiao, H.; Zhao, J.; Zhang, Q.; Ji, A.; Song, S. Advances in research on the bioactivity of alginate oligosaccharides. *Mar. Drugs* **2020**, *18*, 144. [CrossRef]
22. Nagahawatta, D.P.; Lee, H.G.; Liyanage, N.M.; Jayawardhana, H.H.A.C.K.; Wang, L.; Kim, H.S.; Jeon, Y.J. Alginic acid, a functional dietary ingredient derived from Ecklonia maxima stipe, attenuates the pro-inflammatory responses on particulate matter-induced lung macrophages. *J. Funct. Foods* **2023**, *104*, 105539. [CrossRef]
23. Mirshafiey, A.; Rehm, B.H. Alginate and its comonomer mannuronic acid: Medical relevance as drugs. In *Alginates: Biology and Applications*, 1st ed.; Rehm, B.H., Ed.; Springer: Berlin/Heidelberg, Germany, 2009; pp. 229–260.
24. Mirshafiey, A.; Khodadadi, A.; Rehm, B.H.; Khorramizadeh, M.R.; Eslami, M.B.; Razavi, A.; Saadat, F. Sodium alginate as a novel therapeutic option in experimental colitis. *Scand. J. Immunol.* **2005**, *64*, 316–321. [CrossRef] [PubMed]
25. Razavi, A.; Khodadadi, A.; Eslami, M.B.; Eshraghi, S.; Mirshafiey, A. Therapeutic effect of sodium alginate in experimental chronic ulcerative colitis. *Iran J. Allergy Asthma Immunol.* **2008**, *7*, 13–18. [PubMed]

26. Mirshafiey, A.; Borzooy, Z.; Abhari, R.S.; Razavi, A.; Tavangar, M.; Rehm, B.H. Treatment of experimental immune complex glomerulonephritis by sodium alginate. *Vascul. Pharmacol.* **2005**, *43*, 30–35. [CrossRef] [PubMed]
27. Jeong, H.J.; Lee, S.A.; Moon, P.D.; Na, H.J.; Park, R.K.; Um, J.Y.; Kim, H.M.; Hong, S.H. Alginic acid has anti-anaphylactic effects and inhibits inflammatory cytokine expression via suppression of nuclear factor-κB activation. *Clin. Exp. Allergy* **2006**, *36*, 785–794. [CrossRef] [PubMed]
28. Abramowitz, L.; Weyandt, G.H.; Havlickova, B.; Matsuda, Y.; Didelot, J.M.; Rothhaar, A.; Sobrado, C.; Szabadi, A.; Vitalyos, T.; Wiesel, P. The diagnosis and management of haemorrhoidal disease from a global perspective. *Aliment. Pharmacol. Ther.* **2010**, *31*, 1–58. [CrossRef]
29. Slezka, I.E.; Miroshichenko, V.A.; Vostrikova, O.G.; Ziganshina, O.A. Applications of bioactive compounds from marine organisms in atherosclerosis prophylaxis in children, new biomedical technologies using bioactive additives. In *Proceedings of the All Russian Conference*; IMKVL Siberian Branch, Ross Akad Med Nauk: Vladivostok, Russia, 1998; pp. 90–94.
30. Hasegawa, T.; Takahashi, T.; Inada, Y.; Yamada, C.; Tanaka, Y. Reparative effects of sodium alginate (Alloid G) on radiation stomatitis. *Nihon Igaku Hoshasen Gakkai Zasshi. Nippon Acta Radiol.* **1989**, *49*, 1047–1051.
31. Katayama, S.; Ohshita, J.; Sugaya, K.; Hirano, M.; Momose, Y.; Yamamura, S. New medicinal treatment for severe gingivostomatitis. *Int. J. Mol. Med.* **1998**, *2*, 675–684. [CrossRef]
32. Yang, D.; Jones, K.S. Effect of alginate on innate immune activation of macrophages. *J. Biomed. Mater. Res. A* **2009**, *90*, 411–418. [CrossRef]
33. Son, E.H.; Moon, E.Y.; Rhee, D.K.; Pyo, S. Stimulation of various functions in murine peritoneal macrophages by high mannuronic acid-containing alginate (HMA) exposure in vivo. *Int. Immunopharmacol.* **2001**, *1*, 147–154. [CrossRef]
34. Otterlei, M.; Ostgaard, K.; Skjåk-Braek, G.; Smidsrød, O.; Soon-Shiong, P.; Espevik, T. Induction of cytokine production from human monocytes stimulated with alginate. *J. Immunother.* **1991**, *10*, 286–291. [CrossRef]
35. Takahashi, K.; Watanuki, Y.; Yamazaki, M.; Abe, S. Local induction of a cytotoxic factor in a murine tumor by systemic administration of an antitumor polysaccharide, MGA. *Br. J. Cancer* **1988**, *57*, 170–173. [CrossRef] [PubMed]
36. Wang, M.; Chen, L.; Zhang, Z. Potential applications of alginate oligosaccharides for biomedicine—A mini review. *Carbohydr. Polym.* **2021**, *271*, 118408. [CrossRef] [PubMed]
37. Yamamoto, Y.; Kurachi, M.; Yamaguchi, K.; Oda, T. Induction of multiple cytokine secretion from RAW264. 7 cells by alginate oligosaccharides. *Biosci. Biotechnol. Biochem.* **2007**, *71*, 238–241. [CrossRef]
38. Zhou, R.; Shi, X.; Gao, Y.; Cai, N.; Jiang, Z.; Xu, X. Anti-inflammatory activity of guluronate oligosaccharides obtained by oxidative degradation from alginate in lipopolysaccharide-activated murine macrophage RAW 264.7 cells. *J. Agric. Food Chem.* **2015**, *63*, 160–168. [CrossRef] [PubMed]
39. Agarwal, S.; Piesco, N.P.; Johns, L.P.; Riccelli, A.E. Differential Expression of IL-1β, TNF-α, IL-6, and IL-8 in Human Monocytes in Response to Lipopolysaccharides from Different Microbes. *J. Dent. Res.* **1995**, *74*, 1057–1065. [CrossRef] [PubMed]
40. Yamagishi, S.; Ohnishi, M.; Pawankar, R. IL-1 and TNF-α-mediated regulation of IL-6, IL-8, and GM-CSF release from cultured nasal epithelial cells. *Nihon Jibiinkoka Gakkai Kaiho* **2000**, *103*, 829–835. [CrossRef]
41. Galozzi, P.; Bindoli, S.; Doria, A.; Sfriso, P. The revisited role of interleukin-1 alpha and beta in autoimmune and inflammatory disorders and in comorbidities. *Autoimmun. Rev.* **2021**, *20*, 102785. [CrossRef]
42. Sutton, C.E.; Lalor, S.J.; Sweeney, C.M.; Brereton, C.F.; Lavelle, E.C.; Mills, K.H. Interleukin-1 and IL-23 induce innate IL-17 production from gammadelta T cells, amplifying Th17 responses and autoimmunity. *Immunity* **2009**, *31*, 331–341. [CrossRef]
43. Chung, Y.; Chang, S.H.; Martinez, G.J.; Yang, X.O.; Nurieva, R.; Kang, H.S.; Ma, L.; Watowich, S.S.; Jetten, A.M.; Tian, Q.; et al. Critical regulation of early Th17 cell differentiation by interleukin-1 signaling. *Immunity* **2009**, *30*, 576–587. [CrossRef]
44. Ben-Sasson, S.Z.; Hu-Li, J.; Quiel, J.; Cauchetaux, S.; Ratner, M.; Shapira, I.; Dinarello, C.A.; Paul, W.E. IL-1 acts directly on CD4 T cells to enhance their antigen-driven expansion and differentiation. *Proc. Natl. Acad. Sci. USA* **2009**, *106*, 7119–7124. [CrossRef]
45. Hunter, C.A.; Jones, S.A. IL-6 as a keystone cytokine in health and disease. *Nat. Immunol.* **2015**, *16*, 448–457. [CrossRef] [PubMed]
46. Tanaka, T.; Narazaki, M.; Kishimoto, T. IL-6 in inflammation, immunity, and disease. *Cold Spring Harb. Perspect. Biol.* **2014**, *6*, a016295. [CrossRef] [PubMed]
47. Kaplanski, G.; Marin, V.; Montero-Julian, F.; Mantovani, A.; Farnarier, C. IL-6: A regulator of the transition from neutrophil to monocyte recruitment during inflammation. *Trends Immunol.* **2003**, *24*, 25–29. [CrossRef] [PubMed]
48. Kaur, S.; Bansal, Y.; Kumar, R.; Bansal, G. A panoramic review of IL-6: Structure, pathophysiological roles and inhibitors. *Bioorganic Med. Chem.* **2020**, *28*, 115327. [CrossRef] [PubMed]
49. Bhol, N.K.; Bhanjadeo, M.M.; Singh, A.K.; Dash, U.C.; Ojha, R.R.; Majhi, S.; Duttaroy, A.K.; Jena, A.B. The interplay between cytokines, inflammation, and antioxidants: Mechanistic insights and therapeutic potentials of various antioxidants and anti-cytokine compounds. *Biomed. Pharmacother.* **2024**, *178*, 117177. [CrossRef]
50. De la Coba, F.; Aguilera, J.; Figueroa, F.L.; De Gálvez, M.V.; Herrera, E. Antioxidant activity of mycosporine-like amino acids isolated from three red macroalgae and one marine lichen. *J. Appl. Phycol.* **2009**, *21*, 161–169. [CrossRef]
51. Sarithakumari, C.H.; Renju, G.L.; Kurup, G.M. Anti-inflammatory and antioxidant potential of alginic acid isolated from the marine algae, *Sargassum wightii* on adjuvant-induced arthritic rats. *Inflammopharmacology* **2013**, *21*, 261–268. [CrossRef]
52. Mo, S.J.; Son, E.W.; Rhee, D.K.; Pyo, S. Modulation of tnf-α-induced icam-1 expression, no and h 2 0 2 production by alginate, allicin and ascorbic acid in human endothelial cells. *Arch. Pharm. Res.* **2003**, *26*, 244–251. [CrossRef]

53. Ye, S.; Xie, C.; Agar, O.T.; Barrow, C.J.; Dunshea, F.R.; Suleria, H.A.R. Alginates from Brown Seaweeds as a Promising Natural Source: A Review of Its Properties and Health Benefits. *Food Rev. Int.* **2024**, 1–29. [CrossRef]
54. Benslima, A.; Sellimi, S.; Hamdi, M.; Nasri, R.; Jridi, M.; Cot, D.; Li, S.; Nasri, M.; Zouari, N. The Brown Seaweed Cystoseira Schiffneri as a Source of Sodium Alginate: Chemical and Structural Characterization, and Antioxidant Activities. *Food Biosci.* **2021**, *40*, 100873. [CrossRef]
55. Borazjani, N.J.; Tabarsa, M.; You, S.; Rezaei, M. Effects of Extraction Methods on Molecular Characteristics, Antioxidant Properties and Immunomodulation of Alginates from Sargassum Angustifolium. *Int. J. Biol. Macromol.* **2017**, *101*, 703–711. [CrossRef] [PubMed]
56. Sellimi, S.; Younes, I.; Ayed, H.B.; Maalej, H.; Montero, V.; Rinaudo, M.; Dahia, M.; Mechichi, T.; Hajji, M.; Nasri, M. Structural, Physicochemical and Antioxidant Properties of Sodium Alginate Isolated from a Tunisian Brown Seaweed. *Int. J. Biol. Macromol.* **2015**, *72*, 1358–1367. [CrossRef] [PubMed]
57. Sari-Chmayssem, N.; Taha, S.; Mawlawi, H.; Guégan, J.-P.; Jeftić, J.; Benvegnu, T. Extracted and Depolymerized Alginates from Brown Algae Sargassum Vulgare of Lebanese Origin: Chemical, Rheological, and Antioxidant Properties. *J. Appl. Phycol.* **2016**, *28*, 1915–1929. [CrossRef]
58. Wang, J.; Hu, S.; Nie, S.; Yu, Q.; Xie, M. Reviews on Mechanisms of In Vitro Antioxidant Activity of Polysaccharides. *Oxidative Med. Cell. Longev.* **2016**, *2016*, 5692852. [CrossRef]
59. Kao, T.-H.; Chen, B.-H. Functional Components in Soybean Cake and Their Effects on Antioxidant Activity. *J. Agric. Food Chem.* **2006**, *54*, 7544–7555. [CrossRef]
60. Yıldırım, A.; Mavi, A.; Kara, A.A. Determination of Antioxidant and Antimicrobial Activities of *Rumex Crispus* L. Extracts. *J. Agric. Food Chem.* **2001**, *49*, 4083–4089. [CrossRef]

marine drugs

MDPI

Article

Codium fragile Extract Ameliorates Respiratory Function by Controlling Allergic Inflammation in Ovalbumin-Induced Bronchial Disorders in Mice

Hyo Lim Lee, Yeong Hyeon Ju, In Young Kim, Hye Ji Choi, Yu Mi Heo, Hwa Rang Na and Ho Jin Heo *

Division of Applied Life Science (BK21), Institute of Agriculture and Life Science, Gyeongsang National University, Jinju 52828, Republic of Korea; gyfla059@gnu.ac.kr (H.L.L.); ju8172001@gnu.ac.kr (Y.H.J.); inzero331@gnu.ac.kr (I.Y.K.); hjchoi0820@gnu.ac.kr (H.J.C.); yumi@gnu.ac.kr (Y.M.H.); hrna@gnu.ac.kr (H.R.N.)
* Correspondence: hjher@gnu.ac.kr; Tel.: +82-55-772-1907; Fax: +82-55-772-1909

Abstract: This study investigated the effect of *Codium fragile* (WCF) water extract in reducing allergic inflammation in ovalbumin (OVA)-induced mice. Mice were sensitized to OVA + aluminum hydroxide, administered WCF for one week, and exposed to 1% aerosolized OVA. As a result, WCF intake reduced the OVA-induced increase in $CD4^+$ T cells, $CD8^+$ T cells, the T helper type 2 (Th2)/T helper type 1 (Th1) cell ratio, and inflammatory cells such as eosinophils and lymphocytes. Furthermore, WCF reduced Th2 cytokines such as interleukin (IL)-5, IL-13, and IL-33 and inflammatory cytokines such as tumor necrosis factor α (TNF-α) and IL-1β in lung tissues. A histological analysis showed that WCF intake decreases OVA-induced pulmonary inflammation, bronchial wall thickness, and mucus score and increases pulmonary alveolar area. Moreover, WCF inhibited the nuclear factor κB (NF-κB) pathway, the transforming growth factor β (TGF-β)/Smad pathway, and apoptosis-related proteins in lung tissues that OVA excessively activated. The oleamide (9-octadecenamide) content, representing a physiologically active component of WCF, was analyzed and validated using a high-performance liquid chromatography-photodiode array (HPLC-PDA) system. These results demonstrate that WCF may serve as a potential preventive agent for respiratory dysfunction such as allergic asthma by suppressing NF-κB and TGF-β/Smad pathways.

Keywords: *Codium fragile*; oleamide; allergic inflammation; Th2 cytokine; fibrosis; pulmonary function

1. Introduction

A recent chronic respiratory disease (CRD) morbidity and mortality study reported that non-communicable diseases, such as respiratory diseases, cardiovascular diseases, and neurological diseases, accounted for 73.4% of total deaths [1]. Respiratory diseases, including asthma and chronic obstructive pulmonary disease (COPD), affect several pulmonary components, including the airways and lungs, thus resulting in abnormal physiological function [2]. Globally, asthma is one of the most common chronic diseases in which airway inflammation, the hypersecretion of mucus, airway remodeling, and leukocyte infiltration are observed, which are related to a decline in lung function [3]. Used as representative clinical indicators, T helper type 2 (Th2) cytokines such as interleukin (IL)-4, IL-5, and IL-13 secreted by Th2 cells play an important role in the pathogenesis of eosinophilic asthma [4]. Th2 immune hyperactivation is a distinct characteristic of asthma and promotes eosinophil activation, increased immunoglobulin (Ig)E-mediated allergic responses, and fibrosis [4,5]. Various treatment approaches are available to alleviate complications associated with respiratory inflammation, including oxygen therapy, steam inhalation, mucus drainage, and the use of antihistamines [6]. Pharmacological agents commonly prescribed to manage asthma symptoms include β_2-adrenoceptor agonists, inhaled corticosteroids, leukotriene receptor antagonists such as montelukast, muscarinic antagonists (M-cholinolytics), phosphodiesterase inhibitors, lipoxygenase (LOX) inhibitors, and mast cell stabilizers. However, long-term use of these agents has been associated with adverse effects [7]. In addition, biologics targeting IgE and interleukins, such as omalizumab, mepolizumab, benralizumab, and dupilumab, have emerged as effective therapies for allergic diseases, including asthma [8]. Despite the clinical efficacy of these biologics, their high cost and the risk of symptom recurrence after discontinuation highlight the need for alternative strategies to ensure sustained asthma control [9]. Therefore, it is necessary to research phytochemicals as anti-inflammatory agents to discover safe and effective treatments for asthma. The use of plant products in the treatment of asthma has been reported in traditional medicine for over 5000 years [10]. The most studied plant-derived compounds are alkaloids, stilbenes, flavonoids, glycosides, and saponins, which have been shown to have activity against anti-inflammatory properties with respiratory diseases [6].

The marine environment, with its vast biodiversity, is a rich source of natural compounds. For this reason, numerous studies have investigated the antimicrobial, antioxidant, anti-inflammatory, and anti-asthmatic properties of various algae and marine natural products [11]. *Codium fragile* (*C. fragile*) is a type of seaweed commonly consumed in Korea belonging to the *Codiaceae* family. It is found in many countries around the world, including Korea, Japan, and North America [12]. Several in vitro and in vivo studies reported that *C. fragile* has antioxidant and anti-inflammatory effects [13,14]. Moreover, it has been reported by previous studies that oleamide (9-octadecenamide), known as an indicator component and effective ingredient of *C. fragile*, has strong anti-allergic, anti-inflammatory, and antioxidant effects [15–17]. Utilizing this knowledge as a foundation, we preliminarily confirmed through a preliminary study that water extract of *C. fragile* improves particulate matter-induced pulmonary dysfunction [12]. However, the improvement effect of *C. fragile* on ovalbumin (OVA)-induced allergy inflammation and lung damage has not yet been elucidated. Therefore, this study was conducted to investigate the effects of the hot water extract of *C. fragile* (WCF) on respiratory function in mice with OVA-induced allergic bronchial disorders. Furthermore, a method was developed for analyzing the indicator component, oleamide, in WCF for industrial applications. The reliability of this analytical method was confirmed through validation.

2. Results

2.1. High-Performance Liquid Chromatography with Photodiode Array Detection (HPLC-PDA) Analysis

2.1.1. Quantitative Analysis of Oleamide in WCF

WCF and oleamide HPLC chromatograms are presented in Figure 1. The oleamide standard compound was identified at 15.930 min. The peak at 15.943 min in the chromatogram of WCF showed a similarity index of 0.999 with oleamide. A calibration curve was created using the linear relationships between the peak area and concentration of the standard solution. Based on this, the concentration of oleamide in WCF was calculated as 3.85 ± 0.06 μg/mg of dried weight.

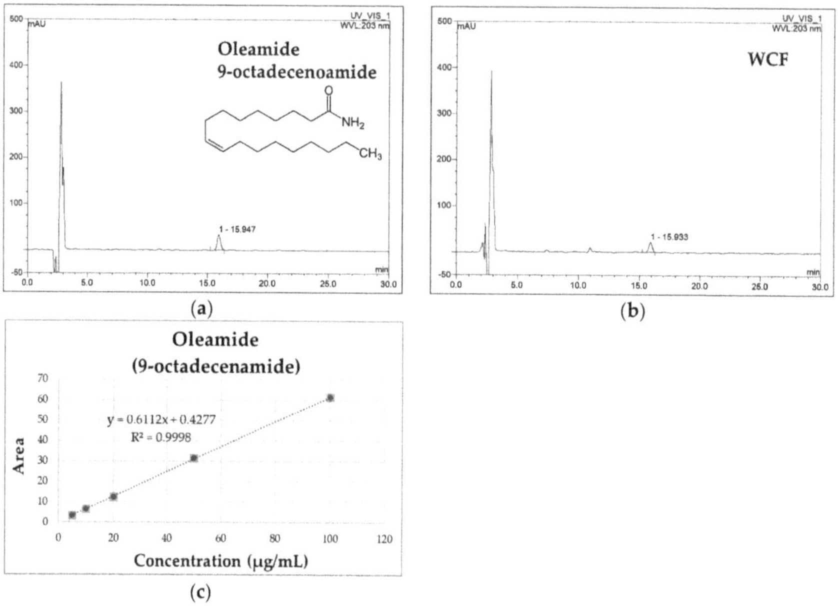

Figure 1. The HPLC chromatograms of oleamide standard (**a**) and water extract of *Codium fragile* (WCF) (**b**). The calibration curve of oleamide (**c**).

2.1.2. Method Validation

Table 1 shows the HPLC-PDA method validation for oleamide detection. The chromatograms of the standard solution and the WCF test solution were compared to verify the separation of the peak corresponding to the standard compound. The results show that the peak was separated as a single peak without interference from other substances, and the retention times of the standard solution and the test solution peaks were identical (Figure 1). In addition, the ultraviolet (UV) spectra of the standard solution and the WCF test solution were measured. The results demonstrate identical spectra with a similarity index of 999, confirming the specificity of the analytical method. The coefficient of determination (R^2) of the calibration curve, fit by analyzing three times in the measured concentration range of 5–100 μg/mL, showed a high linearity of 0.999. The detection limit was calculated using the slope and standard deviation (y-intercept) of the calibration curve obtained through linearity verification. The limit of detection (LOD) was 0.37 ± 0.00 μg/mL, and the limit of quantitation (LOQ) was 1.12 ± 0.00 μg/mL. The coefficient of variability (CV%) of the measurement value was analyzed three times with a standard solution prepared at a concentration of 20 μg/mL, and it was calculated to be below 2.5%. It is below the limit as per the recommendations of the Association of Official Analytical Chemists (AOAC) guidelines [18]. To evaluate the recovery of oleamide, it was used in test solutions according to concentration, mixed with WCF, and analyzed three times each. As a result, the recovery of the oleamide standard compounds at concentrations of 5, 10, and 20 μg/mL was 100 ± 5%. These results suggest that the recovery rates are high, falling within the AOAC recovery guidelines of 90–107% [18].

Table 1. Validation parameters of high-performance liquid chromatography with photodiode array detection (HPLC-PDA) analysis for oleamide.

Parameters	Oleamide (9-octadecenamide)		
Linearity range (μg/mL)	5–100		
Regression equation	y = 0.6112x + 0.4277		
Correlation coefficient (R^2)	0.9998		
Intra-day precision (%) [1]	0.14		
Inter-day precision (%) [1]	0.84		
LOD (μg/mL) [2]	0.37 ± 0.00		
LOQ (μg/mL) [2]	1.12 ± 0.00		
Recovery rate (%) [3]	Concentration (μg/mL)		
	5	10	20
	96.64 ± 1.10	99.62 ± 0.91	100.72 ± 1.10

The results are expressed as the mean ± SD (n = 3). [1] Oleamide precision was assessed via three replicates on one day and over three days. Intra- and inter-day variability are expressed as %CV, calculated by (SD/mean) × 100. [2] The LOD and LOQ were calculated by using the equations LOD = 3.3 × δ/S and LOQ = 10 × δ/S. 'δ' is the standard deviation of the peak areas of the oleamide, and 'S' is the slope of the corresponding calibration curve. [3] Accuracy was assessed through a recovery evaluation performed via the standard addition approach.

2.2. Effect of WCF on Activation of T Cells in Whole Blood of OVA-Induced Mice

The numbers of helper T (Th), cytotoxicity T (Tc), and Th1/Th2 cells in the whole blood were detected to evaluate respiratory damage caused by inflammation (Figure 2). Th and Tc cells were detected by analyzing CD4 and CD8 positive cells, respectively. They are considered markers of increased inflammation and tissue damage in asthma models. Both $CD3^+CD4^+$ and $CD3^+CD8^+$ T cells were significantly elevated in the OVA group compared with the control group ($p < 0.001$). However, their numbers were decreased in the WCF200 group compared with the OVA group ($p < 0.001$). Th1 and Th2 cells were assessed by measuring $CD3^+CD4^+IFN\text{-}\gamma^+$ and $CD3^+CD4^+IL\text{-}4^+$ cells, respectively (Figure 2d,e). As a result, $CD3^+CD4^+IFN\text{-}\gamma^+$ cells decreased ($p < 0.05$) in the OVA group compared to the control group, while $CD3^+CD4^+IL\text{-}4^+$ cells increased ($p < 0.01$). In contrast, WCF200 treatment increased $CD3^+CD4^+IFN\text{-}\gamma^+$ cells ($p < 0.01$) and reduced $CD3^+CD4^+IL\text{-}4^+$ cells ($p < 0.05$) compared with the OVA group. Based on this, the Th2/Th1 ratio was analyzed by calculating the ratio of $CD3^+CD4^+IFN\text{-}\gamma^+$ cells and $CD3^+CD4^+IL\text{-}4^+$ cells (Figure 2f). As a result, it was confirmed that it increased in the OVA group ($p < 0.01$) compared with the control group and decreased in the WCF200 group ($p < 0.01$) compared with the OVA group.

2.3. Effect of WCF on Allergic Inflammatory Cytokines in Lung Tissues of OVA-Induced Mice

The expression levels of Th2 and pro-inflammatory cytokines in lung tissues were detected to evaluate the effects of WCF on lung allergic inflammation (Figure 3). Asthma is characterized by a Th2-mediated immune response, which plays a key role in the pathogenesis of allergic airway inflammation by secreting Th2 cytokines such as IL-33, IL-5, and IL-13. IL-1β and tumor necrosis factor (TNF)-α are pro-inflammatory cytokines secreted primarily by macrophages and activate T cells and inflammatory responses. OVA stimulation significantly increased ($p < 0.05$ or less) the expression levels of the Th2 and pro-inflammatory cytokines in lung tissues compared with the control group. However, the expression levels of IL-33, IL-5, IL-13, and IL-1β decreased in the WCF200 group ($p < 0.05$ or less) compared with the OVA group. The WCF200 group did not significantly reduce OVA-induced TNF-α elevation.

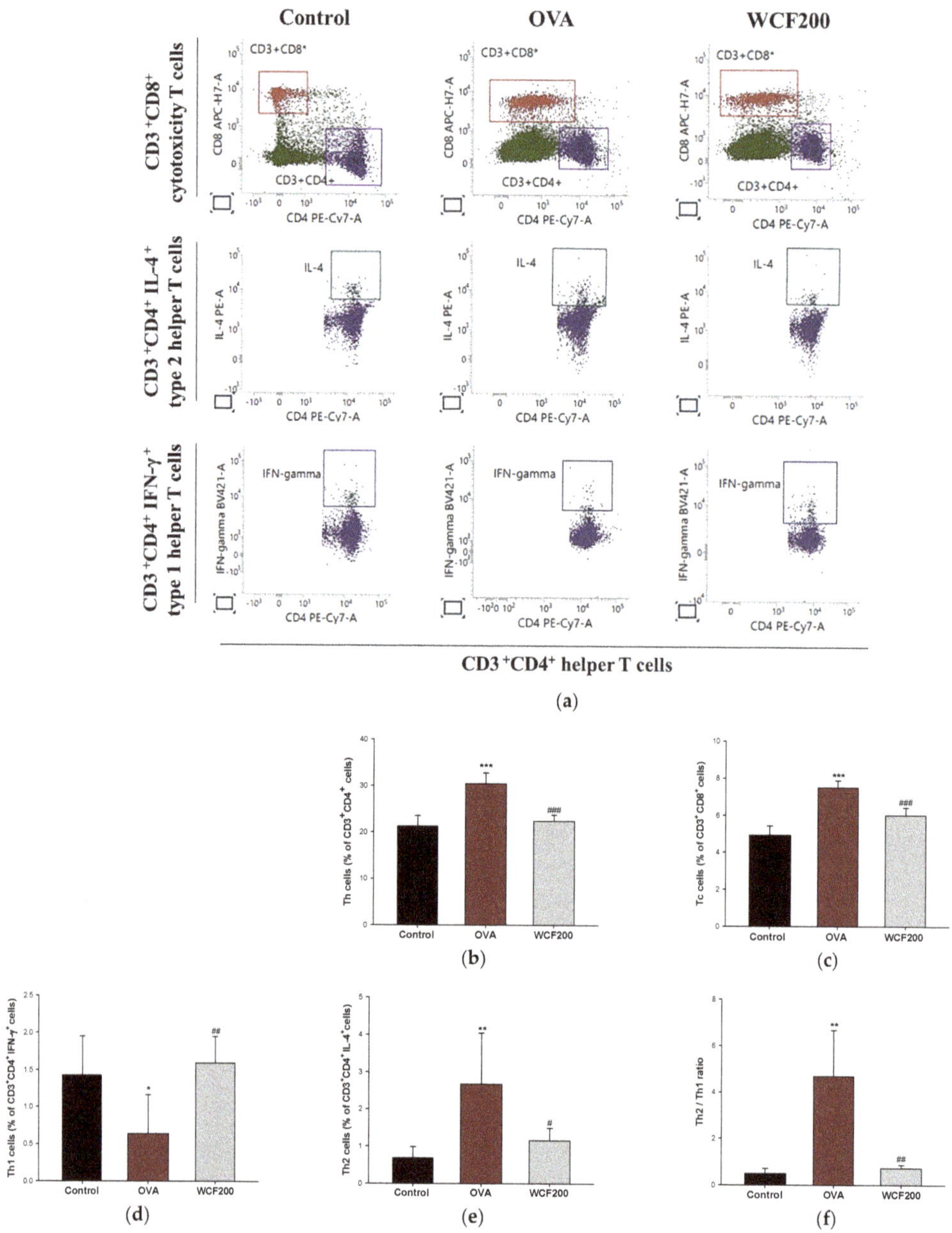

Figure 2. Effect of water extract of *Codium fragile* (WCF) on activation of T cells in whole blood of ovalbumin (OVA)-induced mice. Representative FACS plots (**a**), proportion of $CD3^+CD4^+$ as Th cells (**b**), and $CD3^+CD8^+$ as Tc cells (**c**). Th cell identification was performed by detecting intracellular cytokines IFN-γ and IL-4. Proportion of $CD3^+CD4^+$ IFN-γ^+ as Th1 cells (**d**) and $CD3^+CD4^+$ IL-4^+ as Th2 cells (**e**), and Th2/Th1 ratio (**f**). Data are presented as mean ± SD (n = 5). * $p < 0.05$, ** $p < 0.01$, and *** $p < 0.001$: OVA group vs. control group; # $p < 0.05$, ## $p < 0.01$, and ### $p < 0.001$: WCF groups vs. OVA group.

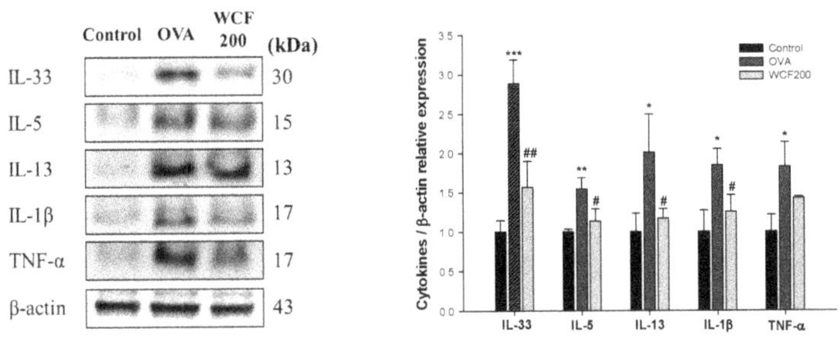

(a) (b)

Figure 3. Effect of water extract of *Codium fragile* (WCF) on allergic inflammatory cytokines in lung tissues of ovalbumin (OVA)-induced mice. Western blot images (**a**) and relative expression levels of IL-33, IL-5, IL-13, IL-1β, and TNF-α (**b**). Data are presented as mean ± SD (n = 3). * $p < 0.05$, ** $p < 0.01$, and *** $p < 0.001$: OVA group vs. control group; # $p < 0.05$ and ## $p < 0.01$: WCF groups vs. OVA group.

2.4. Effect of WCF on Number of Leukocytes in Bronchoalveolar Lavage Fluid (BALF) of OVA-Induced Mice

The number of leukocytes in BALF were analyzed to confirm the intensity and nature of lung inflammation (Table 2). In asthma models, leukocytes are an important indicator of the intensity and type of inflammatory response. The leukocytes were classified into eosinophils, lymphocytes, neutrophils, and monocytes. The total leukocyte counts were significantly higher in the OVA group compared to the control group, especially eosinophils, lymphocytes, and neutrophils ($p < 0.001$). In contrast, WCF treatment reduced eosinophils, lymphocytes, and neutrophils as well as total leukocytes ($p < 0.05$ or less). In particular, neutrophils showed a significant difference only in the WCF200 group ($p < 0.05$). There was no significant difference in monocyte counts between all groups.

Table 2. The number of leukocytes in the bronchoalveolar lavage fluid (BALF) of ovalbumin (OVA)-induced mice.

Groups	Total Leukocytes	Leukocyte Classification Unit: 10^5/mL			
		Eosinophils	Lymphocytes	Neutrophils	Monocytes
Control	2.70 ± 0.41	N.D.	N.D.	N.D.	2.67 ± 0.38
OVA	7.64 ± 0.43 ***	3.31 ± 0.88 ***	1.15 ± 0.19 ***	0.86 ± 0.31 ***	2.30 ± 0.43
WCF50	5.26 ± 0.56 ##	1.62 ± 0.23 ##	0.68 ± 0.19 ##	0.68 ± 0.22	2.29 ± 0.25
WCF100	5.16 ± 1.94 #	1.96 ± 0.84 #	0.64 ± 0.20 ##	0.56 ± 0.22	2.13 ± 1.00
WCF200	5.30 ± 0.82 #	1.76 ± 0.25 ##	0.63 ± 0.12 ###	0.42 ± 0.09 #	2.50 ± 0.46

N.D. means not detected. The results are expressed as the mean ± SD (n = 5). *** $p < 0.001$: OVA group vs. control group; # $p < 0.05$, ## $p < 0.01$, and ### $p < 0.001$: WCF groups vs. OVA group.

2.5. Effect of WCF on OVA-Specific IgE Levels in BALF and Serum of OVA-Induced Mice

OVA-specific IgE levels in BALF and serum were measured to confirm the induction of an allergic reaction (Figure 4). IgE is a protein that plays an important role in allergic reactions and is a key indicator of OVA sensitization and the challenge model's success. The OVA-specific IgE level was significantly higher in the OVA group ($p < 0.001$) than in the control group, but WCF groups ($p < 0.01$ or less) down-regulated this level in BALF (Figure 4a). In serum, the OVA-specific IgE level was not detected in the control group, but it was raised in the OVA group (Figure 4b). However, the WCF100 and WCF200 groups were significantly reduced ($p < 0.05$) compared with the OVA group.

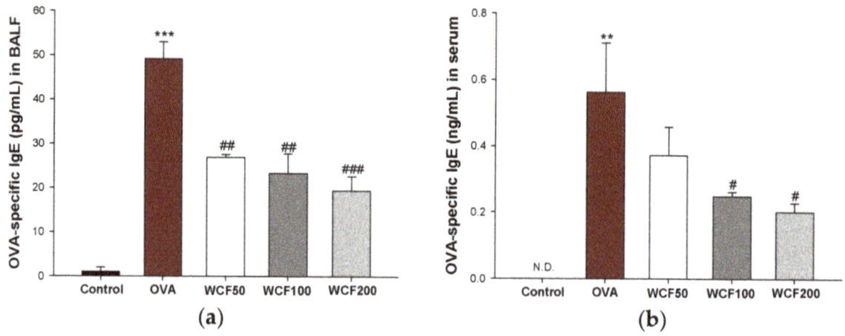

Figure 4. Effect of water extract of *Codium fragile* (WCF) on ovalbumin (OVA)-specific immunoglobulin (Ig)E levels in bronchoalveolar lavage fluid (BALF) (**a**) and serum (**b**) of OVA-induced mice. N.D. means not detected. Data are presented as mean ± SD (n = 5). ** $p < 0.01$ and *** $p < 0.001$: OVA group vs. control group; # $p < 0.05$, ## $p < 0.01$, and ### $p < 0.001$: WCF groups vs. OVA group.

2.6. Effect of WCF on Histopathological Changes in Lung Tissue of OVA-Induced Mice

Histopathological changes were examined to evaluate the effects of WCF on lung inflammation and mucus production in lung tissues. The results of hematoxylin and eosin (H&E) and periodic acid–Schiff (PAS) staining in lung tissues are shown in Figure 5. In asthma models, pathological changes such as inflammatory cell infiltration, increased airway wall thickness, and collagen accumulation are commonly observed. These can affect alveolar size by reducing airway compliance and impeding alveolar airway delivery. Compared with the control group, OVA exposure significantly increased the concentration of inflammatory cells ($p < 0.01$) in the perivascular and peribronchial spaces, as well as the bronchial wall thickness ($p < 0.001$) (Figure 5a,e). Moreover, we confirmed that the alveoli shrunk in the OVA group compared to the control group (Figure 5b,f; $p < 0.001$). Mucus hypersecretion was assessed by detecting PAS-positive cells (Figure 5c,g). As a result, PAS-stained cells were not found in the control group, whereas excessive PAS-positive cells, including goblet cell proliferation, were found in the OVA group ($p < 0.001$). However, WCF intakes restored these histopathological changes such as inflammation scores, bronchial wall thickness, alveolar area, and mucus score compared with the OVA group ($p < 0.01$ or less).

2.7. Effect of WCF on Levels of Antioxidant System in Lung Tissues of OVA-Induced Mice

The levels of malondialdehyde (MDA), reduced glutathione (GSH), and superoxide dismutase (SOD) were examined to evaluate the antioxidant effects of WCF in lung tissues (Figure 6). Excessive inflammatory response leads to the formation of reactive oxygen species (ROS) and a decrease in the antioxidant system. To evaluate OVA-induced oxidative stress, the MDA content was determined (Figure 6a). The MDA content was significantly increased in the OVA group compared with the control group ($p < 0.01$). However, the MDA content was significantly decreased in the WCF100 ($p < 0.05$) and WCF200 ($p < 0.01$) groups compared with the OVA group. We evaluated the effect of OVA exposure on the GSH level and SOD activity, which are antioxidants (Figure 6b,c). The GSH level and SOD activity were significantly reduced in the OVA group compared with the control group ($p < 0.001$). Nevertheless, WCF treatment significantly enhanced the levels of antioxidants compared with the OVA group ($p < 0.01$ or less).

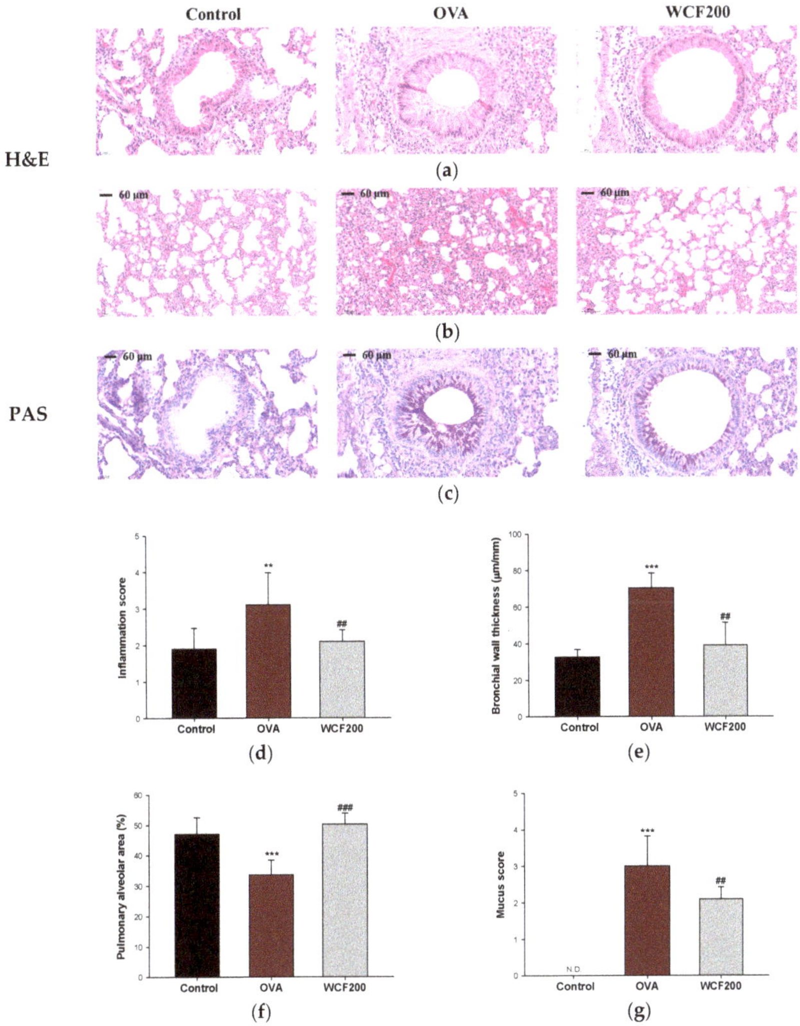

Figure 5. Effect of water extract of *Codium fragile* (WCF) on histopathological changes in lung tissue of ovalbumin (OVA)-induced mice. Representative hematoxylin and eosin (H&E)-stained sections of bronchiole (**a**) and alveoli (**b**), and periodic acid–Schiff (PAS)-stained sections (**c**) of bronchiole in lung tissues. Inflammation score (**d**), bronchial thickness (**e**), pulmonary alveolar area (**f**), and mucus score (**g**). N.D. means not detected. Data are presented as mean ± SD (n = 3). ** $p < 0.01$ and *** $p < 0.001$: control group vs. OVA group; ## $p < 0.01$, and ### $p < 0.001$: OVA group vs. WCF groups.

2.8. Effect of WCF on Activation of Nuclear Factor kB (NF-κB) Pathway in Lung Tissues of OVA-Induced Mice

The expression levels of Toll-like receptor-4 (TLR-4), phospho-NF-κB inhibitor α (p-IκB-α), p-NF-κB, inducible nitric oxide synthase (iNOS), and cyclooxygenase-2 (COX-2) were detected to investigate the effects of WCF on the NF-κB pathway (Figure 7). The NF-κB pathway is activated by TNF-α and IL-1β, which results in the secretion of many inflammatory mediators from cells. OVA exposure significantly increased the levels of TLR-4, p-IκB-α, p-NF-κB, iNOS, and COX-2 compared with the control group ($p < 0.01$ or less). However, the expression levels of TLR-4, p-IκB-α, p-NF-κB, iNOS, and COX-2 in the

WCF200 group were significantly down-regulated compared with the OVA group ($p < 0.05$ or less).

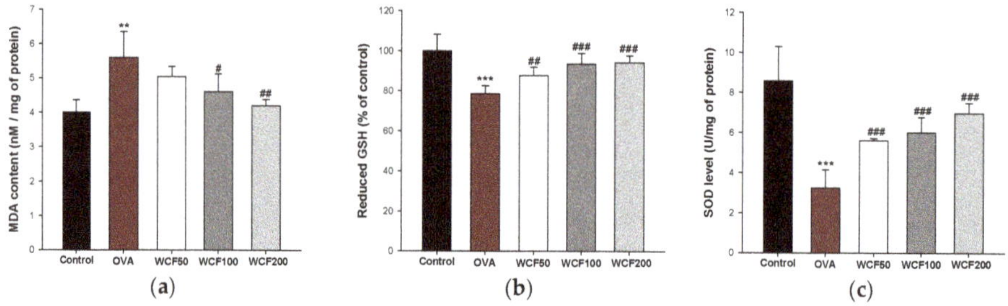

Figure 6. Effect of water extract of *Codium fragile* (WCF) on levels of antioxidant system in lung tissues of ovalbumin (OVA)-induced mice. Malondialdehyde (MDA) content (**a**), reduced glutathione (GSH) (**b**), and superoxide dismutase (SOD) level (**c**). Data are presented as mean ± SD (n = 5). ** $p < 0.01$ and *** $p < 0.001$: OVA group vs. control group; # $p < 0.05$, ## $p < 0.01$, and ### $p < 0.001$: WCF groups vs. OVA group.

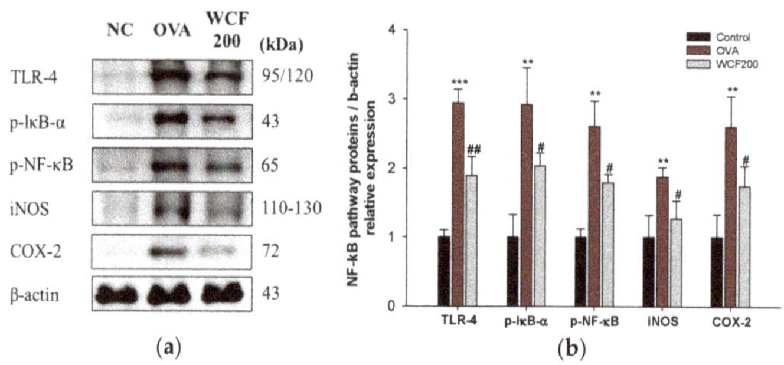

Figure 7. Effect of water extract of *Codium fragile* (WCF) on activation of NF-κB pathway in lung tissues of ovalbumin (OVA)-induced mice. Western blot images (**a**) and relative expression levels of TLR-4, p-IκB-α, p-NF-κB, iNOS, and COX-2 (**b**). Data are presented as mean ± SD (n = 3). ** $p < 0.01$ and *** $p < 0.001$: OVA group vs. control group; # $p < 0.05$ and ## $p < 0.01$: WCF groups vs. OVA group.

2.9. Effect of WCF on Activation of Transforming Growth Factor β (TGF-β)/Smad Pathway in Lung Tissues of OVA-Induced Mice

The expression levels of matrix metalloproteinases (MMP)-2, MMP-9, TGF-β1, p-Smad-2, and p-Smad-3 were examined to confirm the effects of WCF on the TGF-β/Smad pathway (Figure 8). Pulmonary fibrosis progression is closely associated with the TGF-β/Smad pathway, which facilitates fibroblast activation and leads to the accumulation of excessive extracellular matrix. OVA exposure significantly up-regulated the levels of TGF-β1, p-Smad-2, p-Smad-3, MMP-1, MMP-2, and MMP-9 compared with the control group ($p < 0.01$ or less). However, the expression levels of TGF-β1, p-Smad-2, p-Smad-3, MMP-2, and MMP-9 in the WCF200 group were significantly down-regulated compared with the OVA group ($p < 0.05$).

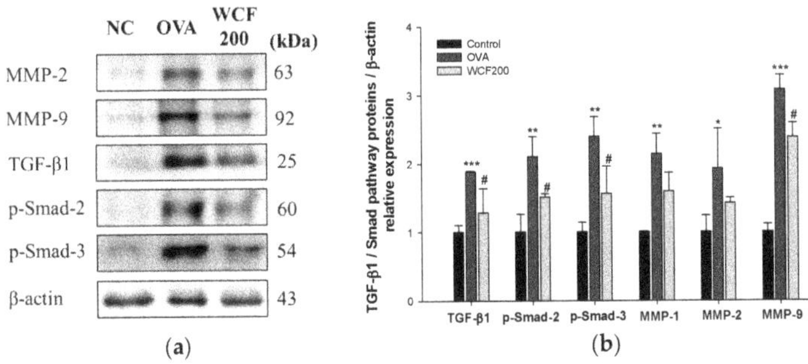

Figure 8. Effect of water extract of *Codium fragile* (WCF) on activation of TGF-β/Smad pathway in lung tissues of ovalbumin (OVA)-induced mice. Western blot images (**a**) and relative expression levels of MMP-2, MMP-9, TGF-β1, p-Smad-2, and p-Smad-3 (**b**). Data are represent mean ± SD (n = 3). * $p < 0.05$, ** $p < 0.01$, and *** $p < 0.001$: OVA group vs. control group; # $p < 0.05$: WCF groups vs. OVA group.

2.10. Effect of WCF on Activation of Apoptosis Pathway in Lung Tissues of OVA-Induced Mice

The expression levels of phospho-Jun N-terminal kinase (p-JNK), B-cell lymphoma 2 (BCL2), BCL-2 associated X (BAX), and caspase (CAS)-3 were measured to investigate the effects of WCF on the apoptosis pathway (Figure 9). Elevated levels of apoptosis-related proteins indicate OVA-induced lung cell damage. OVA exposure significantly increased the levels of p-JNK, BAX, and CAS-3 compared with the control group ($p < 0.01$ or less). In contrast, the expression levels of p-JNK, BAX, and CAS-3 in the WCF200 group significantly decreased compared with the OVA group ($p < 0.05$ or less). There was no significant difference in BCL-2 expression between all groups. However, the BAX/BCL-2 ratio increased in the OVA group compared with the control group ($p < 0.01$). Conversely, the ratio significantly decreased in the WCF200 group compared with the OVA group ($p < 0.05$).

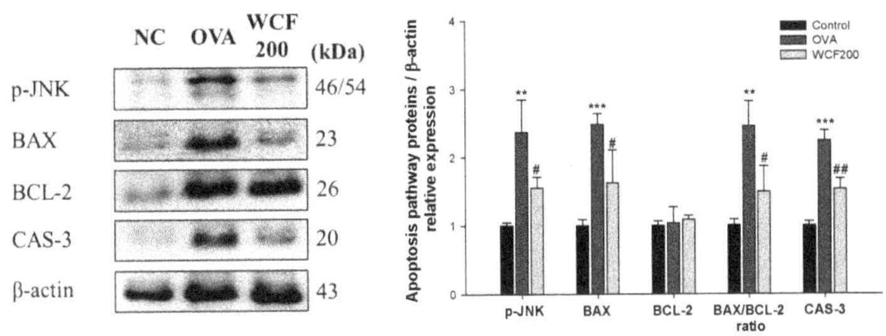

Figure 9. Effect of water extract of *Codium fragile* (WCF) on activation of apoptosis pathway in lung tissues of ovalbumin (OVA)-induced mice. Western blot images (**a**) and relative expression levels of p-JNK, BAX, BCL-2, BAX/BCL-2 ratio, and CAS-3 (**b**). Data are presented as represent mean ± SD (n = 3). ** $p < 0.01$, and *** $p < 0.001$: OVA group vs. control group; # $p < 0.05$ and ## $p < 0.01$: WCF groups vs. OVA group.

3. Discussion

Allergic asthma is a common respiratory disease that, in response to specific allergens, causes airway inflammation and lung damage [3]. When the airway is exposed to an antigen, the antigen is recognized by antigen-presenting cells and T cells are activated. Specifically, the Th2 immune response is activated, promoting eosinophil recruitment and

IgE synthesis by leasing IL-4, IL-5, and IL-13 from bronchial epithelial cells [4]. Subsequently, airway inflammation intensifies, promoting excessive extracellular matrix (ECM) accumulation, leading to airway fibrosis and lung damage [19]. Asthma can be managed through early diagnosis and treatment, but long-term use of current drugs may cause side effects [9]. Accordingly, there is a growing interest in natural products as safer therapeutic alternatives [6]. *C. fragile* has been reported to have immunomodulatory activity as a source of various biologically active compounds, including oleamide [12,16,20]. Therefore, we aimed to evaluate the protective respiratory function effects of WCF in OVA-induced allergic bronchial disorders in mice.

In this study, HPLC-PDA analysis was used to analyze oleamide in WCF. Typically, oleamide, a fatty acid amide derived from the amide form of oleic acid, is analyzed using GC-MS. However, we aimed to develop and validate an HPLC-PDA method for industrial applicability for analyzing oleamide. Consequently, in compliance with AOAC standards, we established an HPLC-PDA method for quantifying oleamide in *C. fragile*. WCF contains significant amounts of oleamide, which has been reported to exhibit anti-allergic, anti-inflammatory, and antioxidant effects [13,15–17]. A previous study has shown that oleamide, a bioactive compound found in the leaves of *Anacardium occidentale*, exhibits bronchodilatory and anti-inflammatory effects [21]. Furthermore, it was reported that oleamide reduced the increased mRNA protein expression of inflammatory mediators COX-2 and iNOS in lipopolysaccharide (LPS)-treated RAW 264.7 cells [17]. Therefore, we expected that WCF containing oleamide would show a positive effect on respiratory function in OVA-induced allergic bronchial disorders in mice.

OVA is the most commonly used irritant to trigger eosinophilic asthma. The OVA-induced mouse model was developed with typical asthma features, including moderate airway hyperresponsiveness, excessive collagen deposition, and inflammation [22]. In this study, OVA exposure increased $CD3^{+}CD4^{+}$ and $CD3^{+}CD8^{+}$ T cells and $CD3^{+}CD4^{+}IL\text{-}4^{+}$ cells in the blood, which was regulated by WCF treatment. The activation of Th2 cells drives the inflammatory response by promoting eosinophil recruitment and IgE production through the release of IL-33, IL-4, IL-5, and IL-13 [22]. Consistent with this mechanism, our results also showed an increase in the number of leukocytes, including eosinophils, as well as OVA-specific IgE levels in the BALF. Th2 cytokines can induce various downstream responses in asthma as well. Specifically, IL-13, in conjunction with IL-4, plays a role in Th2 cell differentiation and contributes to fibrosis by promoting mucin overproduction and thickening of the basement membrane [23]. In this study, severe inflammatory infiltrates around the bronchi, increased bronchial wall thickness, and PAS-positive goblet cells in the lung tissues of OVA-exposed mice were observed. However, WCF intake ameliorated these pathological and histological symptoms of asthma. Therefore, these results suggest that WCF may be used as a preventive agent against OVA-induced respiratory injury by modulating type 2 immune responses.

The molecular mechanisms by which WCF exerts beneficial effects on OVA-induced inflammation and airway remodeling were identified by measuring oxidative stress markers and protein expression in the lung tissues of mice. Recent studies have reported that mast cells regulate allergic airway inflammation through increased TLR4-mediated Th2 cytokine production [24,25]. ROS production increases while antioxidant activity declines under oxidative stress caused by excessive inflammatory responses [26]. ROS accumulation can stimulate NF-κB activation, thereby promoting the production of pro-inflammatory cytokines such as IL-1β and TNF-α [12,25]. Therefore, the TLR-4/NF-κB axis plays an essential role in modulating immune responses and is considered a major contributor to airway inflammation in asthma [27]. In this study, WCF significantly down-regulated the TLR4/NF-κB pathway and oxidative stress stimulated by OVA. Similar findings were observed in an earlier study, where oleamide and *C. fragile* were found to reduce the inflammatory response in LPS-treated RAW264.7 cells by down-regulating NF-κB signaling [17,20]. Furthermore, *C. fragile* reduced inflammatory enzymes such as COX-2 and iNOS against ultraviolet B-induced oxidative stress in HaCaT cells [14]. These results suggest that WCF exhibits an improving effect on respiratory function through the suppression of TLR-4/NF-κB pathway-mediated immune response and oxidative stress.

Airway remodeling refers to the pathological process in which the airway structure is altered and remodeled due to persistent inflammation and damage from chronic asthma or chronic lung disease [19]. In the asthma model, this is associated with thickening of the airway walls due to tissue fibrosis and excessive mucus production. Neutrophils secrete MMP-8 and MMP-9, which activate TGF-β and promote the decomposition of lung tissue and fibrosis around the small airways [28]. TGF-β1 activates Smad-2/3 and forms a complex with Smad-4 to increase the expression of fibrosis-related genes such as α-smooth muscle actin, collagen, and fibronectin [29]. A previous study demonstrated that OVA exposure increases the TGF-β1/Smad pathway, highlighting it as a critical regulator of airway remodeling [19]. Another previous study reported that IL-13 may interact with TGF-β1 to induce pulmonary fibrosis [23]. Additionally, they explained that blocking the signaling of IL-4 or IL-13 could prevent fibrosis while maintaining anti-inflammatory function. Similarly, our study found that the TGF-β1/Smad pathway was up-regulated along with the increase in neutrophils and IL-13 in the OVA group, which was consistent with the histological analysis data. However, WCF intake alleviated MMPs and TGF-β1/Smad pathway expressions. Therefore, these results suggest that the anti-inflammatory effect of WCF is related to the suppression of pulmonary fibrosis.

When ECM degradation is excessive, movement of inflammatory cells is facilitated, which amplifies the inflammatory response and damages the alveolar structure. Consequently, there is a functional loss of lung tissue [30]. Moreover, the increased Th2 immune response caused by OVA can increase oxidative stress and activate the endogenous apoptosis pathway [23]. Increased oxidative stress activates JNK, which increases the pro-apoptotic protein BAX and activates caspases, thereby inducing apoptosis [31]. Indeed, it was reported that BAX and CAS-3 increased, and BCL-2 decreased in idiopathic pulmonary fibrosis patients [32]. This study confirmed that OVA treatment increased apoptosis proteins. These results are thought to be due to complex interactions between inflammation and oxidative stress. However, by down-regulating the apoptosis pathway, WCF treatment ameliorated OVA-induced lung cell damage. Therefore, these results demonstrate that WCF has a potent anti-apoptotic effect based on anti-inflammatory and antioxidant effects that may protect against OVA-induced respiratory damage.

4. Materials and Methods

4.1. Materials and Reagents

High-performance liquid chromatography (HPLC)-grade acetonitrile (ACN), methanol, and water were purchased from Thermo Fisher Scientific (Waltham, MA, USA). Oleamide (08393), OVA (A5503), and aluminum hydroxide (239186) were purchased from Sigma-Aldrich (St. Louis, MO, USA). Antibodies of BV786 anti-mouse CD3e (564379), APC-H7 anti-mouse CD8 (560182), PE anti-mouse IL-4 (562044), and BV421 anti-mouse interferon-gamma (IFN-γ) (563376) and intravenous (IV) catheter (382434; 20 gauge, 1.16 inch) were purchased from BD Biosciences (Franklin Lakes, NJ, USA). PE-Cy7 anti-mouse CD4 (100421) antibody and mouse OVA-specific IgE ELISA kit (439807) were purchased from BioLegend (San Diego, CA, USA).

4.2. Preparation of WCF

C. fragile collected from the coast of Wando-gun (Republic of Korea) was purchased from a local store in July 2024 and washed with tap water until the salinity content was zero. Then, it was dried in a dry oven at 45 °C for 30 h, and its moisture content was kept under 6–9%. The dried *C. fragile* was extracted twice with water (25-fold volume) by reflux at 100 °C for 7 h. Then, the extracts were filtered, concentrated, and then freeze-dried to obtain WCF.

4.3. HPLC with Photodiode Array Detection (HPLC-PDA) Analysis

Oleamide is a bioactive and marker compound of C. fragile. HPLC analysis was conducted to determine oleamide content in WCF and to validate the analytical method. WCF powder was dissolved in 100% methanol to a concentration of 5 mg/mL and extracted by sonication for 30 min. The extract was filtered using a PTFE 0.45 mm syringe filter (Whatman, Maidstone, UK). Oleamide standard sample was also prepared in the same method as concentrations of 5, 10, 20, 50, and 100 μg/mL. The filtrates were analyzed using an HPLC-PDA system (Ultramate 3000 series, Thermo Fisher Scientific) with a YMC-Triart C_{18} column (150 × 4.6 mm, 5 μm particle size, YMC, Seongnam, Republic of Korea) at 40 °C. Mobile phase solvent was prepared with 0.1% formic acid in water (A) and 0.1% formic acid in ACN (B). The solvent condition was set to isocratic elution with 80% B solvent at a flow rate of 1 mL/min for 30 min. The UV spectra were recorded at 203 nm.

4.4. Method Validation

Method validation was used to confirm the accuracy of the analytical method described above. To validate the analytical method for oleamide quantification in WCF, specificity, linearity, sensitivity, accuracy, precision, and recovery were assessed according to the methodology outlined in a prior report [33].

4.5. Animal Experiment Design

4.5.1. Animals

All animal experiments were performed in accordance with the regulations approved by the Institutional Animal Care and Use Committee of Gyeongsang National University (Approval No. GNU-240405-M0076) on 5 April 2024. Female BALB/c mice (4 weeks old) were purchased from Koatech (Pyeongtaek, Republic of Korea). Mice were raised under a stable temperature (22 ± 2 °C) and humidity (55 ± 5%), and a 12 h light/dark cycle condition was used in a semi-specific pathogen-free laboratory.

4.5.2. Immunization and Treatment

After a week of adaptation, mice were randomly assigned into five groups (n = 15/group): (1) normal control, (2) OVA-induced asthma model group (OVA), (3) low dose of WCF treatment (WCF50, 50 mg/kg of body weight (B.W.)), (4) middle dose of WCF treatment (WCF100, 100 mg/kg of B.W.), and (5) high dose of WCF treatment (WCF200, 200 mg/kg of B.W.). As previously described [34], the sensitization and challenge schedule are shown in Figure 10. Briefly, mice were immunized with 20 μg OVA emulsified in 2 mg aluminum hydroxide intraperitoneally in a total volume of 0.2 mL on days 14 and 28, while the control group received the same volume of saline. Mice were challenged with the aerosolized 1% (*w/v*) OVA (0.25 mL/min) by using a nebulizer (Omron, Kyoto, Japan) for 30 min from days 35 to 37. Mice in the WCF treatment group were treated orally with WCF once daily for one week starting on day 31. The control and OVA groups received drinking water instead. Mice were anesthetized with CO_2 on day 38, followed by blood collection via the abdominal aorta.

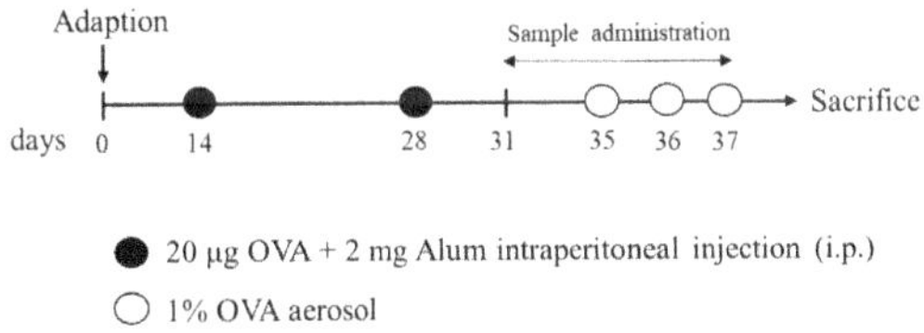

Figure 10. Experimental procedure for ovalbumin (OVA)-induced asthma model and treatment with water extract of *Codium fragile* (WCF).

4.6. Flow Cytometry Fluorescence-Activated Cell Sorting (FACS) Analysis

Sample preparation for flow cytometry analysis was performed as previously described [31]. Briefly, whole blood was stained with the following antibodies to detect T cell populations and intracellular cytokines: BV786 anti-mouse CD3e, PE-Cy7 anti-mouse CD4, APC-H7 anti-mouse CD8, PE anti-mouse IL-4, and BV421 anti-mouse IFN-γ. The stained cells were analyzed by three-color flow cytometry using a BD FACSLyric device (BD Biosciences), and data were processed using BD FACSuite software (BD Biosciences).

4.7. Cell Counting in BALF

BALF was obtained by injecting and aspirating 0.7 mL of sterile phosphate-buffered saline (PBS) through a polyethylene IV catheter inserted into the trachea as described previously with some modifications [35]. This process was repeated twice, and the collected BALF was centrifuged at 300× *g* for 5 min at 4 °C. The cell pellet was used to count leukocytes after resuspending in PBS. Total leukocyte, eosinophils, lymphocytes, neutrophils, and monocytes were analyzed in BALF using an automated cell counter (SYSMEX XN-V, Sysmex Corporation, Kobe, Japan).

4.8. OVA-Specific IgE Level

The blood samples were centrifuged at 10,000× *g* for 10 min at 4 °C, and BALF was centrifuged at 300× *g* for 5 min at 4 °C [31]. The resulting supernatant was used for biochemical analysis. OVA-specific IgE levels in BALF and serum were determined using an ELISA kit according to the manufacturer's recommendations.

4.9. Histopathological Analysis

Lung tissues were fixed in 10% neutral buffered formalin. The fixed lung tissues were sectioned into specimens of appropriate size and approximately 2–3 mm in thickness for histological processing. Then, tissue blocks were made and sectioned into slices approximately 3 μm thick using a Finesse ME Microtome (Thermo Fisher Scientific). Sections were then slide-mounted, dried, deparaffinized, rehydrated, and rinsed with distilled water. The sections were stained with H&E and PAS to assess lung inflammation, bronchial wall thickness, and goblet cell hyperplasia. As described in a previous study [36], inflammation and mucus scores were evaluated on a subjective scale from 0 to 4, and data were collected from five regions per tissue. Briefly, inflammatory cell infiltration was scored on a scale from 0 to 4, where 0 = normal; 1 = few cells; 2 = a one-cell-layer ring; 3 = a 2–4-cell-layer ring; and 4 = a ring more than four cells deep. Goblet cell hyperplasia in the bronchi and bronchioles was assessed as follows using a five-point scale based on the percentage of PAS-positive cells: 0 = <0.5%, 1 = <25%, 2 = 25–50%, 3 = 50–75%, and 4 = >75%. The bronchial wall thickness was calculated by dividing the values measured in four different directions of the bronchiole tube (μm) by the basement membrane length (mm). The alveolar size was assessed by measuring alveolar area (%) using the Image J program (NIH, Bethesda,

MD, USA). The alveolar area and bronchial wall thickness data were collected from three regions per tissue.

4.10. Measurement of SOD, Reduced GSH, and MDA Levels

Antioxidant parameters in lung tissue were measured as previously described [31]. Briefly, lung tissues were homogenized using a bullet blender (New York, NY, USA). The homogenates were centrifuged to collect pellets and supernatants for the determination of SOD, reduced GSH, and MDA levels. SOD activity was determined using a commercially available kit following the protocol provided by the manufacturer (Dojindo Laboratories, Kumamoto, Japan).

4.11. Western Blotting

Sample preparation and experimental procedures followed previously described methods [31]. Briefly, lung tissues were homogenized with lysis buffer containing 1% (*v*/*v*) protease inhibitor using an ultrasonic homogenizer on ice. The obtained homogenates were centrifuged at 13,000× *g* for 10 min at 4 °C. The amount of protein in supernatants was quantified using the Bradford reagent (Bio-Rad, Hercules, CA, USA). Protein samples were subjected to 8–12% SDS polyacrylamide gel and transferred to polyvinylidene fluoride (PVDF) membranes (Millipore, Burlington, MD, USA). To prevent nonspecific binding, membranes were incubated in 5% (*v*/*v*) skim milk for 1 h at room temperature, followed by overnight incubation with primary antibodies at 4 °C. The primary antibodies were removed, and membranes were incubated with secondary antibodies for 2 h at room temperature. Protein signals were detected by ECL and captured using the iBright CL1000 imaging system (Thermo Fisher Scientific). Details of primary and secondary antibodies are shown in Table S1.

4.12. Statistical Analysis

Data were presented as mean ± standard deviation (SD), and 'n' refers to the number of mice in each group. Using the SAS program (Ver. 9.4 SAS Institute, Cary, NC, USA), a one-way ANOVA followed by Tukey's honest significant difference test were conducted to analyze the results. A two-tailed Student's *t*-test was used to test the statistical difference between the two groups. Differences were considered statistically significant at $p < 0.05$. The normality of data distribution was confirmed using the Shapiro–Wilk test (https://www.statskingdom.com).

5. Conclusions

In conclusion, our study demonstrates that WCF improved respiratory dysfunction by inhibiting pulmonary inflammation, oxidative stress, and fibrosis in OVA-induced asthma mice. Its mechanism may be related to regulating the Th2 immune response and the NF-κB and TGF-β1 pathways by oleamide-containing WCF, which suggests that WCF can improve allergic bronchial disorders. These findings suggest that WCF could serve as a potential preventive for allergic respiratory diseases such as asthma. However, as the present study lacks direct comparison with conventional therapies, further research is needed to validate its therapeutic relevance and to identify the major active compounds responsible for its effects.

Supplementary Materials: The following supporting information can be downloaded at https://www.mdpi.com/article/10.3390/md23050221/s1, Table S1. Information on primary and secondary antibodies used in Western blotting.

Author Contributions: Conceptualization, H.J.H. and H.L.L.; methodology, H.L.L.; software, I.Y.K. and H.J.C.; validation, H.L.L. and Y.H.J.; formal analysis, I.Y.K. and H.L.L.; investigation, Y.H.J., Y.M.H. and H.R.N.; data curation, H.J.C., Y.H.J. and H.L.L.; writing—original draft preparation, H.L.L.; writing—review and editing, H.J.H.; supervision, H.J.H.; project administration, H.J.H.; funding acquisition, H.J.H. All authors have read and agreed to the published version of the manuscript.

Funding: This study was supported by the 'Leaders in INdustry-university Cooperation (LINC) 3.0' (2019) apostrophe project, which is funded by the Ministry of Education and the National Research Foundation of Korea, and Korea Institute of Marine Science & Technology Promotion (KIMST), funded by the Ministry of Oceans and Fisheries (2017029713), Republic of Korea.

Institutional Review Board Statement: All animal experimental protocols were approved by the Institutional Animal Care and Use Committee of Gyeongsang National University (approval number: GNU-180927-M0050, 27 September 2018).

Data Availability Statement: The data presented in this study are available upon request from the corresponding author.

Acknowledgments: This study was supported by the 'Leaders in INdustry-university Cooperation (LINC) 3.0' (2019) apostrophe project, which is funded by the Ministry of Education and the National Research Foundation of Korea, and Korea Institute of Marine Science & Technology Promotion (KIMST), funded by the Ministry of Oceans and Fisheries (2017029713), Republic of Korea.

Conflicts of Interest: The authors declare no conflicts of interest.

References

1. Labaki, W.W.; Han, M.K. Chronic respiratory diseases: A global view. *Lancet Respir. Med.* **2020**, *8*, 531–533. [CrossRef]
2. Dey, S.; Eapen, M.S.; Chia, C.; Gaikwad, A.V.; Wark, P.A.; Sohal, S.S. Pathogenesis, clinical features of asthma COPD overlap, and therapeutic modalities. *Am. J. Physiol.-Lung Cell. Mol. Physiol.* **2022**, *322*, L64–L83. [CrossRef]
3. Witt, A.; Douglass, J.A.; Harun, N.S. Overview of recent advancements in asthma management. *Intern. Med. J.* **2022**, *52*, 1478–1487. [CrossRef]
4. Hammad, H.; Lambrecht, B.N. The basic immunology of asthma. *Cell* **2021**, *184*, 1469–1485. [CrossRef]
5. Wang, M.-C.; Huang, W.-C.; Chen, L.-C.; Yeh, K.-W.; Lin, C.-F.; Liou, C.-J. Sophoraflavanone G from *Sophora flavescens* ameliorates allergic airway inflammation by suppressing Th2 response and oxidative stress in a murine asthma model. *Int. J. Mol. Sci.* **2022**, *23*, 6104. [CrossRef]
6. Timalsina, D.; Pokhrel, K.P.; Bhusal, D. Pharmacologic activities of plant-derived natural products on respiratory diseases and inflammations. *BioMed Res. Int.* **2021**, *2021*, 1636816. [CrossRef]
7. Jasemi, S.V.; Khazaei, H.; Morovati, M.R.; Joshi, T.; Aneva, I.Y.; Farzaei, M.H.; Echeverría, J. Phytochemicals as treatment for allergic asthma: Therapeutic effects and mechanisms of action. *Phytomedicine* **2024**, *122*, 155149. [CrossRef]
8. Agache, I.; Rocha, C.; Beltran, J.; Song, Y.; Posso, M.; Solà, I.; Jutel, M. Efficacy and safety of treatment with biologicals (benralizumab, dupilumab and omalizumab) for severe allergic asthma: A systematic review for the EAACI Guidelines-recommendations on the use of biologicals in severe asthma. *Allergy* **2020**, *75*, 1043–1057. [CrossRef]
9. Ramírez-Jiménez, F.; Pavón-Romero, G.F.; Velásquez-Rodríguez, J.M.; López-Garza, M.I.; Lazarini-Ruiz, J.F.; Gutiérrez-Quiroz, K.V.; Teran, L.M. Biologic therapies for asthma and allergic disease: Past, present, and future. *Pharmaceuticals* **2023**, *16*, 270. [CrossRef]
10. Amaral-Machado, L.; Oliveira, W.N.; Moreira-Oliveira, S.S.; Pereira, D.T.; Alencar, E.N.; Tsapis, N.; Egito, E.S.T. Use of natural products in asthma treatment. *Evid.-Based Complement. Altern. Med.* **2020**, *2020*, 1021258. [CrossRef]
11. Karthikeyan, A.; Joseph, A.; Nair, B.G. Promising bioactive compounds from the marine environment and their potential effects on various diseases. *J. Genet. Eng. Biotechnol.* **2022**, *20*, 14. [CrossRef]
12. Kim, T.Y.; Kim, J.M.; Lee, H.L.; Go, M.J.; Joo, S.G.; Kim, J.H.; Lee, H.S.; Jeong, W.M.; Lee, D.Y.; Kim, H.-J. *Codium fragile* suppressed chronic $pm_{2.5}$-exposed pulmonary dysfunction via TLR/TGF-β pathway in BALB/c mice. *Antioxidants* **2023**, *12*, 1743. [CrossRef]
13. Jang, A.-y.; Choi, J.; Rod-In, W.; Choi, K.Y.; Lee, D.-H.; Park, W.J. In vitro anti-inflammatory and skin protective effects of *Codium fragile* extract on macrophages and human keratinocytes in atopic dermatitis. *J. Microbiol. Biotechnol.* **2024**, *34*, 940. [CrossRef]
14. Lee, C.; Park, G.H.; Ahn, E.M.; Kim, B.-A.; Park, C.-I.; Jang, J.-H. Protective effect of *Codium fragile* against UVB-induced pro-inflammatory and oxidative damages in HaCaT cells and BALB/c mice. *Fitoterapia* **2013**, *86*, 54–63. [CrossRef]
15. Akarsha, B.; Krishnakumar, G.; Khandige, P.S. Hepatoprotective potency of *Lagenandra toxicaria* and *Ariopsis peltata* against CCl_4 induced liver fibrosis in Wistar rats. *Plant Sci. Today* **2022**, *9*, 855–866. [CrossRef]

16. Meinita, M.D.N.; Harwanto, D.; Choi, J.-S. A concise review of the bioactivity and pharmacological properties of the genus *Codium* (Bryopsidales, Chlorophyta). *J. Appl. Phycol.* **2022**, *34*, 2827–2845. [CrossRef]
17. Moon, S.-M.; Lee, S.A.; Hong, J.H.; Kim, J.-S.; Kim, D.K.; Kim, C.S. Oleamide suppresses inflammatory responses in LPS-induced RAW264.7 murine macrophages and alleviates paw edema in a carrageenan-induced inflammatory rat model. *Int. Immunopharmacol.* **2018**, *56*, 179–185. [CrossRef]
18. AOAC INTERNATIONAL. *AOAC Official Methods of Analysis*; Appendix F: Guidelines for Standard Method Performance Requirements; AOAC INTERNATIONAL: Rockville, MD, USA, 2016; pp. 1–17.
19. Shen, Q.-Y.; Wu, L.; Wei, C.-S.; Zhou, Y.-N.; Wu, H.-M. Sevoflurane prevents airway remodeling via downregulation of VEGF and TGF-β1 in mice with OVA-induced chronic airway inflammation. *Inflammation* **2019**, *42*, 1015–1022. [CrossRef]
20. Lee, S.A.; Moon, S.-M.; Choi, Y.H.; Han, S.H.; Park, B.-R.; Choi, M.S.; Kim, J.-S.; Kim, Y.H.; Kim, D.K.; Kim, C.S. Aqueous extract of *Codium fragile* suppressed inflammatory responses in lipopolysaccharide-stimulated RAW264.7 cells and carrageenan-induced rats. *Biomed. Pharmacother.* **2017**, *93*, 1055–1064. [CrossRef]
21. Awakan, O.J.; Malomo, S.O.; Adejare, A.A.; Igunnu, A.; Atolani, O.; Adebayo, A.H.; Owoyele, B.V. Anti-inflammatory and bronchodilatory constituents of leaf extracts of *Anacardium occidentale* L. in animal models. *J. Integr. Med.* **2018**, *16*, 62–70. [CrossRef]
22. Yi, L.; Zhou, Y.; Song, J.; Tang, W.; Yu, H.; Huang, X.; Shi, H.; Chen, M.; Sun, J.; Wei, Y. A novel iridoid glycoside leonuride (ajugol) attenuates airway inflammation and remodeling through inhibiting type-2 high cytokine/chemokine activity in OVA-induced asthmatic mice. *Phytomedicine* **2022**, *105*, 154345. [CrossRef] [PubMed]
23. Gieseck III, R.L.; Wilson, M.S.; Wynn, T.A. Type 2 immunity in tissue repair and fibrosis. *Nat. Rev. Immunol.* **2018**, *18*, 62–76. [CrossRef]
24. Dominguez-Flores, A.; López, G.M.R.; Soria-Castro, R.; López-Santiago, R.; Rodríguez-Cortés, O.; Pérez-Tapia, S.M.; Chávez-Blanco, A.D.; Estrada-Parra, S.; Flores-Mejía, R.; Chacón-Salinas, R. *Brucella abortus* induces mast cell activation through TLR-2 and TLR-4. *Microb. Pathog.* **2023**, *176*, 106005. [CrossRef] [PubMed]
25. Helal, M.G.; Megahed, N.A.; Abd Elhameed, A.G. Saxagliptin mitigates airway inflammation in a mouse model of acute asthma via modulation of NF-κB and TLR4. *Life Sci.* **2019**, *239*, 117017. [CrossRef] [PubMed]
26. Fatani, S.H. Biomarkers of oxidative stress in acute and chronic bronchial asthma. *J. Asthma* **2014**, *51*, 578–584. [CrossRef]
27. Zou, S.; Hong, J.; Liu, D.; Lai, G.; Ye, J.; Song, Y. Enhanced effect of catalpol on specific immune therapy in treatment of asthmatic mice. *Am. J. Transl. Res.* **2019**, *11*, 2463.
28. Mahalanobish, S.; Saha, S.; Dutta, S.; Sil, P.C. Matrix metalloproteinase: An upcoming therapeutic approach for idiopathic pulmonary fibrosis. *Pharmacol. Res.* **2020**, *152*, 104591. [CrossRef]
29. Chen, H.; Chen, Q.; Jiang, C.-m.; Shi, G.-Y.; Sui, B.-w.; Zhang, W.; Yang, L.-z.; Li, Z.-y.; Liu, L.; Su, Y.-m. Triptolide suppresses paraquat induced idiopathic pulmonary fibrosis by inhibiting TGFB1-dependent epithelial mesenchymal transition. *Toxicol. Lett.* **2018**, *284*, 1–9. [CrossRef]
30. Sutherland, T.E.; Dyer, D.P.; Allen, J.E. The extracellular matrix and the immune system: A mutually dependent relationship. *Science* **2023**, *379*, eabp8964. [CrossRef]
31. Lee, H.L.; Kim, J.M.; Go, M.J.; Kim, T.Y.; Joo, S.G.; Kim, J.H.; Lee, H.S.; Kim, H.-J.; Heo, H.J. Protective effect of *Lonicera japonica* on $PM_{2.5}$-induced pulmonary damage in BALB/c mice via the TGF-β and NF-κB pathway. *Antioxidants* **2023**, *12*, 968. [CrossRef]
32. Shang, Q.; Zhu, L.; Shang, W.; Zeng, J.; Qi, Y. Dioscin exhibits protective effects on in vivo and in vitro asthma models via suppressing TGF-β1/Smad2/3 and AKT pathways. *J. Biochem. Mol. Toxicol.* **2022**, *36*, e23084. [CrossRef] [PubMed]
33. Drakopanagiotakis, F.; Xifteri, A.; Polychronopoulos, V.; Bouros, D. Apoptosis in lung injury and fibrosis. *Eur. Respir. J.* **2008**, *32*, 1631–1638. [CrossRef] [PubMed]
34. Seo, J.-H.; Kim, J.-E.; Shim, J.-H.; Yoon, G.; Bang, M.-A.; Bae, C.-S.; Lee, K.-J.; Park, D.-H.; Cho, S.-S. HPLC analysis, optimization of extraction conditions and biological evaluation of *Corylopsis coreana* Uyeki Flos. *Molecules* **2016**, *21*, 94. [CrossRef]
35. Lee, J.-A.; Lee, M.-Y.; Seo, C.-S.; Jung, D.Y.; Lee, N.-H.; Kim, J.-H.; Ha, H.; Shin, H.K. Anti-asthmatic effects of an *Amomum compactum* extract on an ovalbumin (OVA)-induced murine asthma model. *Biosci. Biotechnol. Biochem.* **2010**, *74*, 1814–1818. [CrossRef]
36. Kim, D.I.; Song, M.-K.; Lee, K. Comparison of asthma phenotypes in OVA-induced mice challenged via inhaled and intranasal routes. *BMC Pulm. Med.* **2019**, *19*, 241. [CrossRef]

marine drugs

MDPI

Article

Chondroitin Sulfate Nanovectorized by LC-PUFAs Nanocarriers Extracted from Salmon (*Salmo salar*) by Green Process with Decreased Inflammatory Marker Expression in Interleukin-1β-Stimulated Primary Human Chondrocytes In Vitro Culture

Louis Pruvost [1], Maureen Gerlei [1], Cédric Paris [1], Émilie Velot [2], Cyril J.-F. Kahn [1], Arnaud Bianchi [2] and Michel Linder [1,*]

[1] LIBio, Université de Lorraine, F-54000 Nancy, France; louis.pruvost@univ-lorraine.fr (L.P.); maureen.gerlei@univ-lorraine.fr (M.G.); cedric.paris@univ-lorraine.fr (C.P.); cyril.kahn@univ-lorraine.fr (C.J.-F.K.)

[2] CNRS, IMoPA, Université de Lorraine, F-54000 Nancy, France; emilie.velot@univ-lorraine.fr (É.V.); arnaud.bianchi@univ-lorraine.fr (A.B.)

* Correspondence: michel.linder@univ-lorraine.fr; Tel.: +33-3-72-74-41-03

Abstract: Chondroitin sulfate (CS), a glycosaminoglycan, supports health through various physiological functions, including tissue protection, bone growth, and skin aging prevention. It also contributes to anticoagulant or anti-inflammatory processes, with its primary clinical use being osteoarthritis treatment. This study presents the results of the valorization of lipids and CS, both extracted from salmon co-products through enzymatic processes. The polar lipids, naturally rich in long-chain fatty acids (docosahexaenoic acid DHA C22:6 n-3 and eicosapentaenoic acid EPA C20:5 n-3), and the CS, primarily located in the nasal cartilage, were separated and concentrated before being characterized using various techniques to determine functional and lipid composition. These compounds were then used to formulate liposomes of 63 to 95 nm in size composed of 19.38% of DHA and 7.44% of EPA and encapsulating CS extract with a Δdi-4S/Δdi-6S ratio of 0.53 at 2 weight masses (10–30 kDa and >30 kDa) or CS standard all at two different concentrations. Liposomes were tested on human chondrocytes in inflamed conditions. Thus, compatibility tests, the expression of various inflammation markers at transcriptional and molecular levels, nitrites, and the amount of collagenase produced were analyzed. The results showed that CS, in synergy with the liposomes, played a positive role in combating chondrocyte inflammation even at a low concentration.

Keywords: liposome; chondroitin sulfate; phospholipid; *Salmo salar*; enzymatic hydrolysis; anti-inflammatory; encapsulation

1. Introduction

According to the Food and Agriculture Organization of the United Nations (FAO) report "The State of World Fisheries and Aquaculture" (2024) [1], the fisheries and aquaculture sector (mainly the production of fish, mollusks, and crustaceans) accounted for 185 million tons globally in 2022. This production generated 20 million tons of by-products (heads, viscera, skeletons) [2], which represent a very interesting and widely available source for biomolecule extraction. This is particularly true for salmon, which is highly consumed worldwide [1]. The heads generated by the aquaculture sector (*Salmo salar*) are a source of long-chain polyunsaturated fatty acids (LC-PUFAs), mainly eicosapentaenoic acid (EPA; C20:5 n-3) and docosahexaenoic acid (DHA; C22:6 n-3), as well as cartilage rich in chondroitin sulfate (CS). These LC-PUFAs, present in the form of triacylglycerols but also polar lipids (phospholipids), have numerous preventive and therapeutic effects on brain function, cardiovascular diseases, and inflammation. Current recommendations for

EPA and DHA intake for general health are typically 400 to 500 mg/day as a combination of both fatty acids (French Agency of Food Administration, AFSSA) [3].

Moreover, salmon heads are rich in polar lipids, particularly phospholipids, which are highly valued for their ability to form liposomes due to their amphipathic properties [4]. In most cases, the core of the vesicle and its surface are hydrophilic, thanks to lipids that self-assemble to form a lipid bilayer, while the space between the two layers of phospholipids is hydrophobic. However, some liposomes can be unilamellar [5]. This particular structure allows for the encapsulation of hydrophilic molecules in the aqueous core or hydrophobic molecules in the membrane. These molecules can contain therapeutic or nutritional active ingredients for applications in cosmetics, pharmacology, or even for the food industry [6].

Glycosaminoglycans from salmon cartilage are increasingly being studied for their interesting properties in attenuating inflammatory responses, limiting angiogenesis, and aging phenomena [7]. Found in the cartilage of the salmon's nasal area, glycosaminoglycans are negatively charged polysaccharides, classified based on the sugars that make up their structure [8].

Among these compounds, CS has a wide range of physiological functions and clinical applications [9]. CS exhibits anticoagulant [10], antioxidant [11], antibacterial [12], and anti-inflammatory activities [13]. The most common clinical application of CS is in the treatment of osteoarthritis [14]. Osteoarthritis is the most common musculoskeletal disease, associated with cartilage degeneration. More than 300 million patients worldwide are affected [15]. CS is part of the SYSADOA (Symptomatic Slow-Acting Drugs for Osteoarthritis) treatments [16]. Indeed, even though the osteoarthritis mechanisms are not fully understood, it was reported in the literature that low-grade joint inflammation participates in this progressive disease [17,18]. Pro-inflammatory cytokines, such as interleukin (IL)-1β, promote the degeneration of the hyaline extracellular matrix by increasing its degradation and preventing its synthesis. Thus, this catabolic process induces an articular chondrocyte altered phenotype and prevents cells from restoring the extracellular matrix equilibrium [10]. Cyclooxygenase (COX)-2, microsomal prostaglandin E2 synthase (mPGES-1), and inducible nitric oxide synthase (iNOS) are among the mediators of inflammation induced by IL-1β [19,20]; monitoring their level of expression reflects the level of inflammation induced by IL-1β. Moreover, COX-2 and mPGES-1 are both responsible for prostaglandin E2 (PGE2) synthesis, while iNOS produces nitric oxide (NO), which both take part in extracellular matrix catabolism, leading to cartilage degradation [21,22]. In addition, matrix metalloproteinases (MMPs), which are responsible for the degenerative part in osteoarthritis pathology, are also good markers of degeneration activity after inflammatory stimulation.

CS is composed of repeating disaccharide units $[\rightarrow 4)$-β-D-GlcA-$(1\rightarrow 3)$-β-D-GalNAc-$(1\rightarrow]_n$, where GlcA corresponds to glucuronic acid and GalNAc to N-acetylgalactosamine (Table 1). The disaccharide units can be classified into the following five groups based on the arrangement of sulfate groups within the disaccharide (number and position of sulfate groups): GlcA-GalNAc (CS-0 unit), GlcA-GalNAc(4S) (CS-A unit), GlcA-GalNAc(6S) (CS-C unit), GlcA(2S)-GalNAc(6S) (CS-D unit), and GlcA-GalNAc(4S,6S) (CS-E unit) [7].

The degree of sulfation and the molecular weight of CS chains can vary depending on the tissue of origin, the age, and the species of the animal. Generally, tissues from terrestrial animals are richer in CS-0 and CS-A units (>60%) and have lighter CS chains (14 to 26 kDa). For marine species, CS chains are heavier (up to 70 kDa), with more complex disaccharides like CS-C, CS-D, and CS-E (proportions vary depending on the species) [23].

Table 1. Specific information regarding CS bioactivities.

Molecule	Formula	Sources	Potential Application	References
CS-O	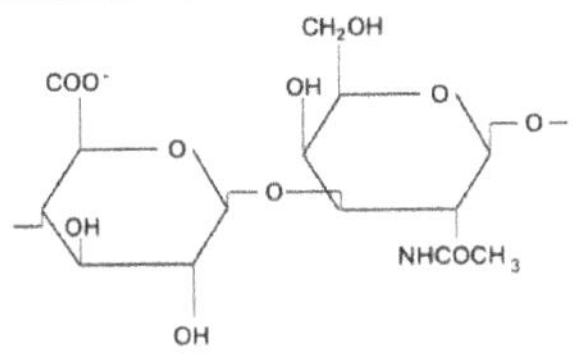	Shark fins, human, synthetic	Anti-inflammatory, osteoarthritis, biotechnology precursor	[24–26]
CS-A	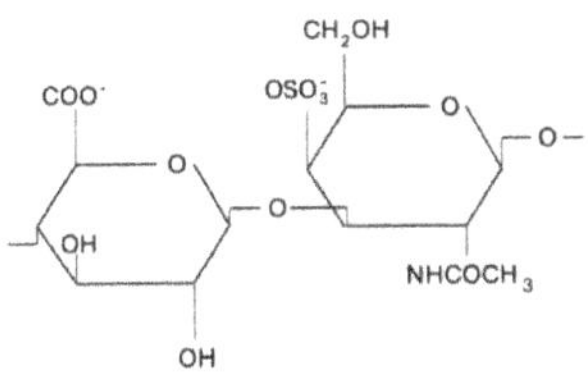	Shark fins, bovine trachea, sturgeon notochord	Anti-inflammatory, repair the central nervous system, malarial vaccine	[27–29]
CS-C	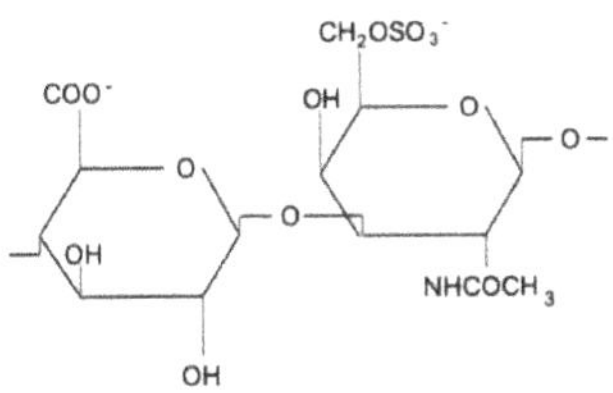	Unknown	Anti-tumor	[30]
CS-E	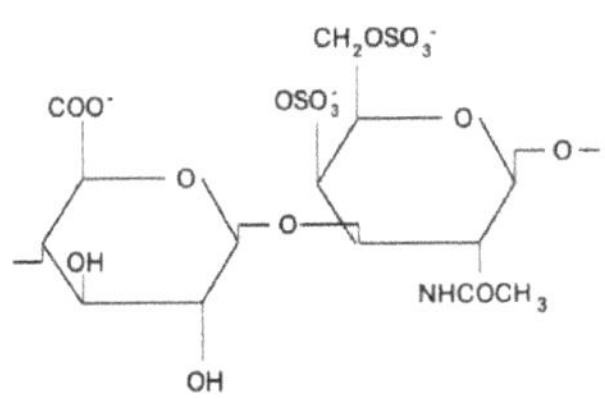	Unknown	Anti-thrombus, anti-viral, anti-inflammatory	[31–33]

Since liposomes have increased the bioavailability of molecules (transforming growth factor beta 1 (TGF-β1), antioxidants), chondrocyte in particular [34–36], the choice was made to vectorize CS to decrease the inflammatory effect of IL-1β. In addition, the properties of nanoliposomes were enhanced by the choice of phospholipid origin. Indeed, marine phospholipids are naturally rich in LC-PUFAs such as DHA, also known to have a reduced inflammation effect [37–39].

The objective of the present study is to perform an enzymatic extraction of chondroitin sulfate (CS) and polar lipids from salmon heads, characterize them, and then formulate liposomes naturally rich in LC-PUFAs. Fractions of CS obtained through ultrafiltration will be encapsulated within these liposomes. These liposome formulations are then applied to chondrocytes cultured under inflammatory conditions to study their ability to decrease the expression of inflammatory markers.

2. Results

2.1. FT-IR Spectroscopy of CS and Lipids Analyses

According to Kai-Ruei Yang et al. [40], the Fourier Transform Infrared (FTIR) technique is regularly used to characterize the functional groups of CS. The FTIR spectra of the marine CS standard (Sigma-Aldrich, International standard, Saint-Quentin-Fallavier, France), as well as CS extracted from salmon, were measured from 4000 cm^{-1} to 400 cm^{-1} at a resolution of 6 cm^{-1} (Figure 1b, Table 2). The CS extracted from salmon heads (*Salmo salar*) exhibit a similar spectrum to that of the standard. The peak observed at 3412 cm^{-1} originated from the stretching vibrations of hydroxyl and carboxyl groups, while bands observed at 2920 cm^{-1} and 2850 cm^{-1} were assigned to the stretching and bending vibrations of C-H bonds [41]. The peaks detected at 1410 cm^{-1} and 1625 cm^{-1} were indicative of stretching vibrations associated with C-O bonds, [41]. The bands at, respectively, 1550, 1373, and 1220 cm^{-1} correspond to N-H bending vibration, C-O symmetric vibration, and S-O stretching vibration [42]. According to Garnjanagoonchorn et al. [43], analysis of the spectra of chondroitin-4-sulfate and chondroitin-6-sulfate standards indicated the existence of peaks observed at 857 and 826 cm^{-1}. It probably corresponds to the peaks observed at 858 and 820 cm^{-1}.

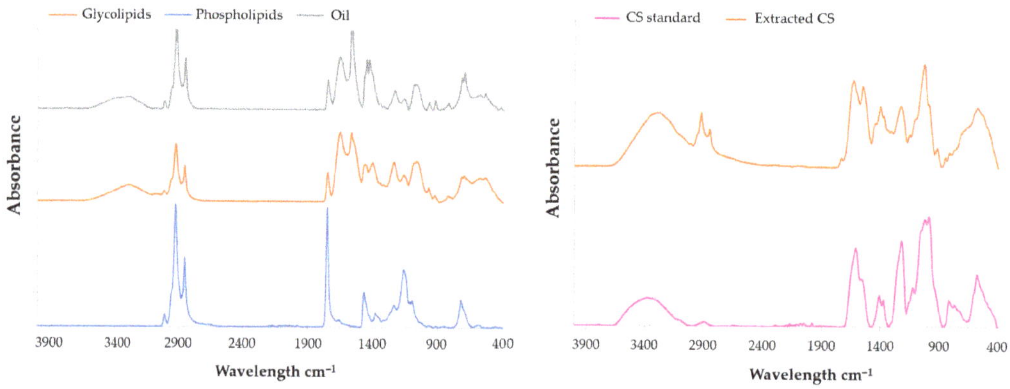

(a) (b)

Figure 1. FT-IR spectra of (**a**) CS and (**b**) lipids all extracted from *Salmo salar* heads by enzymatic hydrolysis.

Table 2. Wavenumber (cm^{-1}) of FT-IR spectra of CS and lipids extracted from *Salmo salar* heads by enzymatic hydrolysis.

Chondroitin Sulfate		Lipids	
Bond	Wavenumber (cm^{-1})	Bond	Wavenumber (cm^{-1})
-OH, H_2O	3400	-H-OO	3250
-CH	2920	-CH	3005
-CH	2850	$-CH_3$	2958
-C-O	1625	$-CH_2$	2920
-NH	1550	$-CH_3$	2850
-CO	1373	$-CH_2$, $-CH_3$	1450
-CO	1410	Ester -CO	1080
-SO	1220	($-CH_2-$, -HC=CH-(*cis*))	720

The lipid analyses of salmon by FTIR were conducted using the same parameters as the CS analysis. Lipids spectra are presented in Figure 1a and Table 2. The infrared spectra of the samples exhibited a large absorption band at 3250 cm^{-1} (indicative of hydroperoxides), 3017 cm^{-1} (corresponding to =C−H (*cis*) stretching), 2920 cm^{-1} (attributed to $-CH_2$ stretching asymmetry), and 2850 cm^{-1} (associated with methyl $-CH_3$ stretching symmetry) according to Wan et al. [44]. Peaks at wavenumber of 1450, 1080, and 720 cm^{-1} correspond, respectively, to CH_2, CH_3, esters of the C-O group, and *cis*-disubstituted olefins [44].

2.2. HPLC-MS Characterization of CS Disaccharides

A liquid chromatography analysis coupled to UV-Vis absorbance and tandem mass spectrometry (MS/MS) was initially performed on a reference mixture of hydrolyzed CS to unambiguously identify the retention times (RTs) of the two compounds of interest, i.e., Δdi-4S ($RTUV_{240}$ = 2.6 min) and Δdi-6S ($RTUV_{240}$ = 3.6 min) [45]. Then, a robust semi-quantitative UV_{240} study of Δdi-4S and Δdi-6S was performed on our sample assuming a strictly similar response of the two compounds under these conditions and checking beforehand that the peak areas were indeed located in a linear portion of the calibration range (Figure 2b, Appendix A).

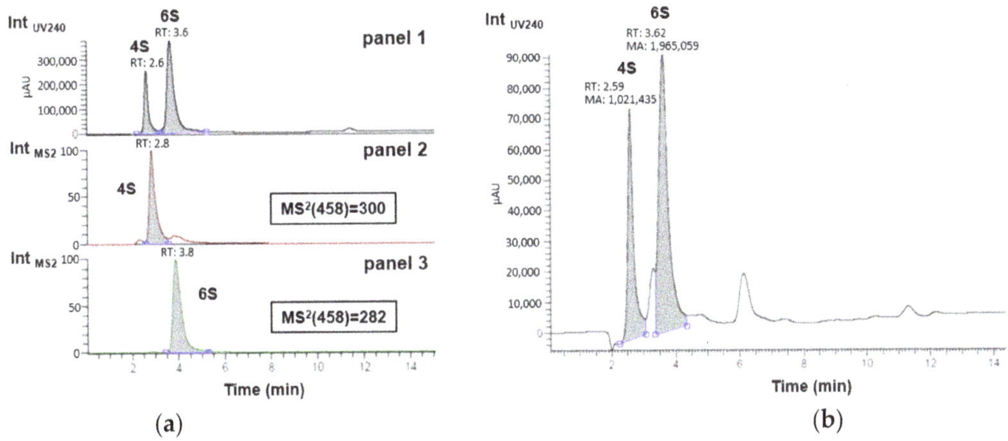

Figure 2. Monitoring Δdi-4S and Δdi-6S disaccharides in (**a**) reference mixture of hydrolyzed commercial marine CS by UV_{240} in panel 1 and by MS^2 in panels 2 (specific screening of delta Δdi-4S with daughter ion m/z = 300) and 3 (specific screening of delta Δdi-6S with daughter ion m/z = 282); and in (**b**) sample of interest by UV_{240} for semi-quantitative evaluation.

As shown in Figure 2b, taking into account only the Δdi-4S and Δdi-6S peaks, their relative percentages are 35% and 65%, respectively. By approximation, taking care of the entire area (with both non-identified peak areas, 222,289 for the peaks between Δdi-4S and Δdi-6S peaks and 345,913 for the peak after Δdi-6S peak) of the sample and not only Δdi-4S and Δdi-6S peaks, it is possible to say that by semi-quantification the extracted sample contains 29% of Δdi-4S and 54% of Δdi-6S approximately. When comparing these results with those presented by Uchisawa et al. [46], the findings are close (30% for Δdi-4S and 60% for Δdi-6S). The composition of disaccharides could likely vary with diet, the origin of the salmon, or the extraction process. It is increasingly recognized that an increase in the proportion of the 6S isomer is linked to enhanced therapeutic efficacy against osteoarthritis. This action is partly based on its anti-inflammatory capacity [33]. Since marine CS samples are rich in the 6S isomer, this explains why they are predominantly used for this application [47]. In the sample, this higher level of Δdi-6S compared to Δdi-4S, typical of marine sources, is observed. The concentration ratio of Δdi-4S/Δdi-6S is 0.53 in the CS extracted from salmon. In the work of Uchisawa et al. [46], the ratio between Δdi-4S and Δdi-6Sis is about 0.51, which is pretty close to the experimental results. These two most common disaccharide categories are increasingly used to link CS activity to their composition [33]. This Δdi-4S/Δdi-6S ratio can therefore be connected to anti-inflammatory activity, as shown by the results in Figures 4 and 5.

2.3. *Lipid TLC-FID (Iatroscan®) Analysis*

Phospholipids from *Salmo salar* heads were determined using Iatroscan® in the polar lipid fraction. The results reveal that the fraction contains 14.52 ± 1.41% phosphatidylethano
lamine, 1.13 ± 0.11% sterols, 64.66 ± 0.04% phosphatidylcholine, 1.32 ± 0.08% sphin-

gomyelin, 4.77 ± 0.75% lysophosphatidylcholine, and 13.59 ± 2.30% of other polar lipids and non-lipidic compounds.

2.4. GC-FID Analysis of Lipids

The fatty acid composition of the three lipid fractions (Triacylglycerol (TAG), glycolipids, and phospholipids) from salmon heads (*Salmo salar*) was determined by gas chromatography coupled with a flame ionization detector (GC-FID) (Table 3) after separation on a silica column. The three fractions exhibit significant differences in their fatty acid composition. The oil fraction contains a high amount of monounsaturated fatty acids (44.10%), particularly oleic acid (28.88%). It also has the highest levels of dienes (8.27%) and trienes (12.01%). However, this fraction is low in long-chain fatty acids such as tetraenes (1.55%) and pentaenes (7.15%). The highest content of saturated fatty acids, mainly composed of palmitic acid in all three fractions, is found in the glycolipids (30.02%). The compositions of phospholipids and glycolipids are very similar and show interesting levels of long-chain fatty acids. The phospholipid fraction has the highest pentaene content (10.59%), primarily composed of EPA (7.44%). It is also the fraction with a significantly higher DHA content compared to the other fractions, with 19.38%. This high level of long-chain fatty acids enhances membrane fluidity in liposomes, facilitating membrane fusion with cells [48].

Table 3. Fatty acids composition of different lipid fractions extracted (% of total fatty acids) from *Salmo salar* heads by enzymatic hydrolysis.

Fatty Acids	TAG	Glycolipids	Phospholipids
C14:0	3.68 ± 0.03	1.68 ± 0.10	2.71 ± 0.14
C15:0	0.12 ± 0.01	0.27 ± 0.01	0.25 ± 0.25
Iso C16:0	0.22 ± 0.01	0.49 ± 0.01	0.40 ± 0.01
C16:0	10.80 ± 0.01	18.97 ± 0.05	17.15 ± 0.30
C18:0	2.27 ± 0.04	5.53 ± 0.01	4.90 ± 0.08
C20:0	0.57 ± 0.02	1.88 ± 0.02	2.20 ± 0.01
Σ Saturates	**17.66**	**30.02**	**27.61**
C16:1 n-9	4.99 ± 0.01	2.96 ± 0.06	2.52 ± 0.07
C18:1 n-9	28.88 ± 0.12	21.02 ± 0.01	18.10 ± 0.19
C18:1 n-7	0.23 ± 0.01	0.33 ± 0.01	0.31 ± 0.01
C20:1 n-11	7.99 ± 0.13	4.19 ± 0.09	3.57 ± 0.15
C20:1 n-9	1.46 ± 0.07	0.57 ± 0.08	0.63 ± 0.11
C20:1 n-7	0.17 ± 0.01	0.19 ± 0.03	0.25 ± 0.05
C22:1 n-9	0.38 ± 0.02	0.40 ± 0.02	0.55 ± 0.04
Σ Monoenes	**44.10**	**29.66**	**25.93**
C16:2 n-6	0.19 ± 0.01	0.34 ± 0.05	0.32 ± 0.01
C16:2 n-4	0.36 ± 0.01	0.72 ± 0.01	0.54 ± 0.01
C18:2 n-7	0.30 ± 0.02	0.16 ± 0.01	0.14 ± 0.01
C18:2 n-6	7.24 ± 0.01	3.96 ± 0.01	3.66 ± 0.04
C18:2 n-4	0.18 ± 0.01	0.26 ± 0.02	0.20 ± 0.01
Σ Dienenes	**8.27**	**5.44**	**4.86**
C16:3 n-4	0.55 ± 0.02	0.53 ± 0.01	0.47 ± 0.02
C18:3 n-6	0.20 ± 0.02	0.12 ± 0.01	0.13 ± 0.01
C18:3 n-4	2.70 ± 0.10	1.63 ± 0.01	1.59 ± 0.02
C18:3 n-3	8.33 ± 0.04	4.63 ± 0.01	3.90 ± 0.05
C18:3 n-1	0.23 ± 0.01	0.25 ± 0.01	0.23 ± 0.01
Σ Trienenes	**12.01**	**7.16**	**6.32**
C16:4 n-1	0.27 ± 0.05	0.36 ± 0.02	0.31 ± 0.09
C18:4 n-3	0.59 ± 0.02	0.61 ± 0.01	0.59 ± 0.02
C22:4 n-6	0.69 ± 0.01	2.93 ± 0.01	2.56 ± 0.12
Σ Tetraenes	**1.55**	**3.90**	**3.46**
C20:5 n-3	4.89 ± 0.03	5.79 ± 0.02	7.44 ± 0.03
C21:5 n-3	0.44 ± 0.01	0.63 ± 0.01	0.84 ± 0.07
C22:5 n-3	1.82 ± 0.04	1.94 ± 0.05	2.31 ± 0.04

Table 3. *Cont.*

Fatty Acids	TAG	Glycolipids	Phospholipids
Σ Pentaenes	**7.15**	**8.36**	**10.59**
C22:6n-3	7.12 ± 0.03	13.64 ± 0.02	19.38 ± 0.40
Σ n-6	8.32	7.35	9.06
Σ n-3	23.19	27.24	34.46
n-6/n-3	0.36	0.27	0.26
EPA/DHA	0.69	0.42	0.38

In comparison, the flesh of Norwegian salmon does not exhibit the same proportions of LC-PUFAs. The DHA and EPA levels are very low (3.94% and 2.19%, respectively). The major fatty acid is oleic acid, at 44%, which is very high. This highlights the advantage of using salmon heads for lipid extraction, as this part of the fish is richer in LC-PUFAs n-3 than the muscle [49]. The high oleic acid content found in the fatty acid composition of salmon (28.88% in oil, 21.02% in glycolipids, and 18.1% in phospholipids) corresponds to the increased intake of vegetable fatty acids in farmed salmon diets. This phenomenon also reduces the amount of omega-3 PUFAs, such as EPA and DHA [49]. In an earlier study from 2006, DHA and EPA levels were higher, at 18.2% and 8.2%, respectively. Additionally, the oleic acid content was lower at 15.6% [50]. This comparison thus shows that the evolution of farmed salmon diets impacts the levels of beneficial omega-3 PUFAs.

2.5. DLS Analysis of Liposome-Chondroitin Sulfate

The results of the characterization of L-CS are presented in Table 4. Surprisingly, it is the fraction with the least pure and heaviest CS (L-CSh1) that produces the smallest liposomes (65 nm). It would have been more logical to observe that the smallest would be the empty liposomes, but this is not the case (87 nm). Moreover, it is the smallest fraction with the lowest concentration of CS (L-CSl2) that shows the largest liposomes (94 nm). It is possible that the encapsulation or organization of compounds around the liposome compressed the liposome, making it smaller, just like in the work of Hanachi et al. where the encapsulation of peptides reduced the size of the liposome [51]. This could explain why the largest particles result in smaller liposomes. As for the ζ potential, the values are negative and centered around −20 mV. This negativity is favorable for particle stability due to the repulsion of negative charges. Zhang et al.'s work [52] shows L-CS with a size around 140 nm, which is larger than the values obtained here. This difference can be explained by the sonicator treatment, which creates smaller liposomes.

Table 4. Size, ζ potential, and Polydispersity Index (PdI) of different liposome formulations with or without CS.

	Day 0			Day 7		
Samples	**Size (nm)**	**ζ Potential (mV)**	**PdI**	**Size (nm)**	**ζ Potential (mV)**	**PdI**
L-E	87.91 ± 3.19	−20.60 ± 0.79	0.26 ± 0.01	95.12 ± 9.44	−28.60 ± 0.66	0.268 ± 0.07
L-CSl1	82.07 ± 0.98	−20.30 ± 0.76	0.21 ± 0.01	123.56 ± 2.54	−39.00 ± 0.46	0.282 ± 0.01
L-CSl2	94.01 ± 0.99	−21.20 ± 1.20	0.21 ± 0.01	148.33 ± 2.80	−42.60 ± 0.58	0.247 ± 0.03
L-CSh1	65.76 ± 1.95	−16.20 ± 0.32	0.25 ± 0.01	74.41 ± 4.83	−36.10 ± 0.43	0.310 ± 0.06
L-CSh2	84.59 ± 1.12	−19.90 ± 0.75	0.22 ± 0.01	173.33 ± 2.41	−37.30 ± 0.28	0.364 ± 0.01
L-CSs1	74.76 ± 0.34	−19.30 ± 0.10	0.24 ± 0.01	144.13 ± 3.65	−47.70 ± 0.80	0.254 ± 0.01
L-CSs2	84.03 ± 0.88	−15.50 ± 0.43	0.22 ± 0.01	132.96 ± 2.55	−38.60 ± 0.55	0.389 ± 0.01

L-E: empty liposomes; L-CSh1: liposomes with more than 30 kDa CS at 1%; L-CSh2: liposomes with more than 30 kDa CS at 0.2%; L-CSl1: liposomes with CS between 10 and 30 kDa CS at 1%; L-CSl2: liposomes with CS between 10 and 30 kDa CS at 0.2%; L-CSs1: liposomes with standard CS at 1%; L-CSs2: liposomes with standard CS at 0.2%.

However, this smaller size is advantageous for the stability of the liposome and the release of its content at the level of cell membranes [53]. The same measurements were taken 7 days after formulation to study the evolution of size and ζ potential.

The sizes significantly increased. Only the value for the empty liposome showed little increase; this indicates that CS reduces the stability of the liposomes. The ζ potential also decreased significantly and nearly doubled for all the samples. This strong increase in negativity can be explained by the release of CS, which are negatively charged. The Polydispersity Index (PdI) also increased substantially due to the creation of new liposome sizes (following system destabilization) and the release of CS tending toward a multimodal size liposome distribution. Nonetheless, these values after 7 days are close to those found in the literature, around 140 nm [52].

2.6. Anti-Inflammatory Study of Chondroitin Sulfate-Liposomes on Human Chondrocytes

The results presented in Figure 3 show the study of the biocompatibility of L-CS with chondrocytes. Cytotoxicity (A) was analyzed by Lactate Deshydrogenase (LDH) assay. The results indicate that an excessively high concentration of L-CS (1%) causes cell damage compared to the control. This effect is observed for all three categories of CS. At a concentration of 0.2%, no significantly higher toxicity levels compared to the control are noted. Cellular respiration was studied by evaluating metabolic activity with MTT (3-(4,5-dimethylthiazol-2-yl)-2,5-diphenyltetrazolium bromide) assay (B). Again, L-CS at 1% shows significantly lower mitochondrial respiration activity than the control. In contrast, L-CS at 0.2% results in a slight increase in mitochondrial activity compared to L-CS at 1%. Finally, the DNA quantity was analyzed to assess cell growth (C). L-CS at 1% leads to a significant decrease in DNA quantity, whereas L-CS at 0.2% shows a slight increase in DNA quantity compared to the control. These results demonstrate that using L-CS at 1% has a negative effect on cell growth and survival, while a lower concentration of 0.2% does not show this negative effect compared to the control and even shows a positive effect in some cases. Therefore, subsequent studies will be conducted using the 0.2% fraction of L-CS.

The results of the effects of L-CS treatment on chondrocytes cultured under inflammatory conditions induced by IL-1β for different inflammatory pathways are presented in Figure 4. The expression of the COX-2 enzyme gene is shown in Figure 4A. The results indicate that each L-CS fraction significantly reduces inflammation compared to the control, with the reduction being most pronounced for the 10–30 kDa CS fraction. The expression of the mPGES-1 enzyme gene is analyzed in Figure 4B, showing results similar to those in Figure 4A. All L-CS fractions significantly reduce inflammation compared to the control, with an increased effect for the 10–30 kDa CS fraction. In Figure 4C, PGE2 concentration is measured, confirming the results of Figure 4A,B, with the 10–30 kDa CS fraction again showing the most substantial results. Figure 4D analyzes the expression of the iNOS gene, confirming the previous observations, as all L-CS fractions have a significant positive effect on IL-1β-induced inflammation. These results further emphasize that the 10–30 kDa CS fraction strongly reduces inflammation compared to other fractions.

Following the study of iNOS gene expression, nitrates produced by this enzyme during inflammation are measured in Figure 4E. These results are consistent with iNOS gene expression, as expected. Finally, Figure 4F tracks the expression of the aggrecan gene. In this case, inflammation reduces gene expression, and only the >30 kDa CS fraction at 0.2% shows a significant effect on increasing aggrecan expression compared to the controls. Interestingly, throughout the results, nanoliposomes without CS exhibit a significant intrinsic decrease in inflammatory markers, which is further enhanced in the presence of 0.2% CS, particularly for the 10–30 kDa fraction. This suggests a possible synergistic effect between the polar lipids in the liposomes and the CS in reducing inflammation.

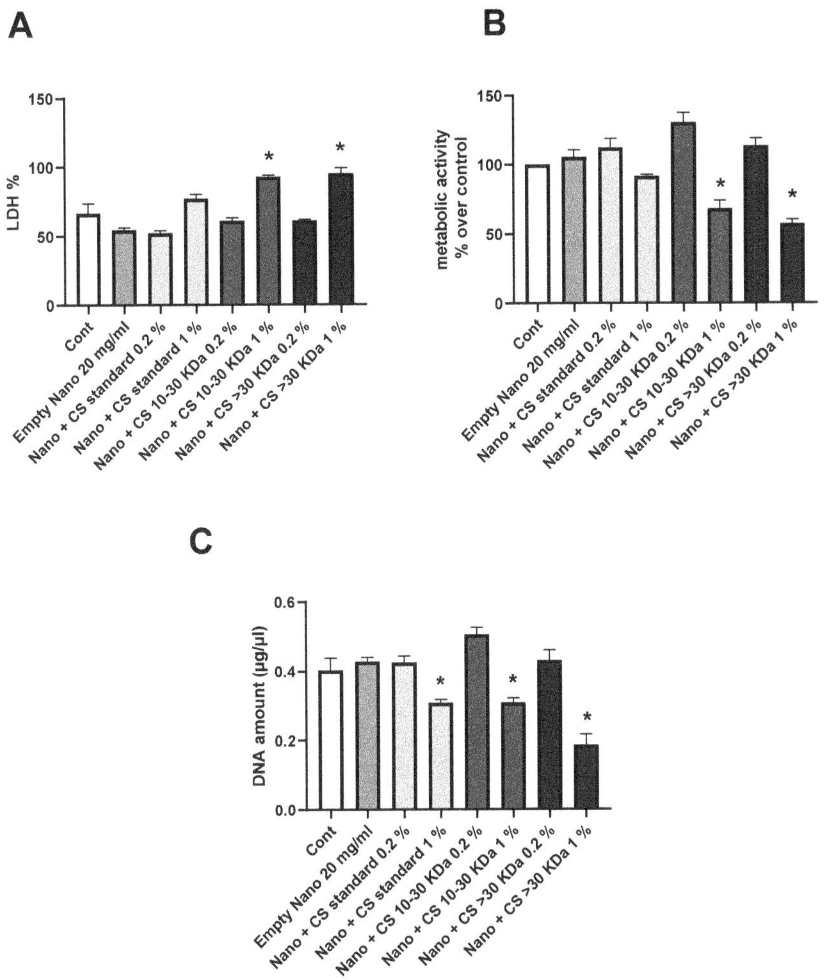

Figure 3. Biocompatibility of liposomes with CS with human chondrocytes. Human chondrocytes exposed to nanoliposomes (250 µg/mL) or nanoliposomes and CS extracts (250 µg/mL + 125 or 25 µg/mL) for 1 days. (**A**) Lactate Deshydrogenase (LDH) release determined as described under Section 3. Metabolic activity assessed using MTT assay. (**B**) Cell metabolic activity results on different membranes presented in % vs. control results (as 100%). (**C**) DNA concentrations measured to estimate proliferation of cells. Results shown are mean ± SD of at least four individual experiments. *: $p < 0.01$, compared to control.

These findings support those published by Chang et al. and Nguyen et al., demonstrating the anti-inflammatory effects of CS [54]. Here, we show that CS amplifies the intrinsic effects of empty nanoliposomes. Further studies are needed to confirm that these nanoliposomes extend the lifespan of CS and prevent their degradation in vivo in the joint site [55].

We also show that CS > 30 kDa have the strongest anti-inflammatory properties, which supports a recent study suggesting that low kDa CS (A and B) are present at non-inflamed sites, while CS < 30 kDa (C, D, and E) are more prevalent at highly inflamed sites [56].

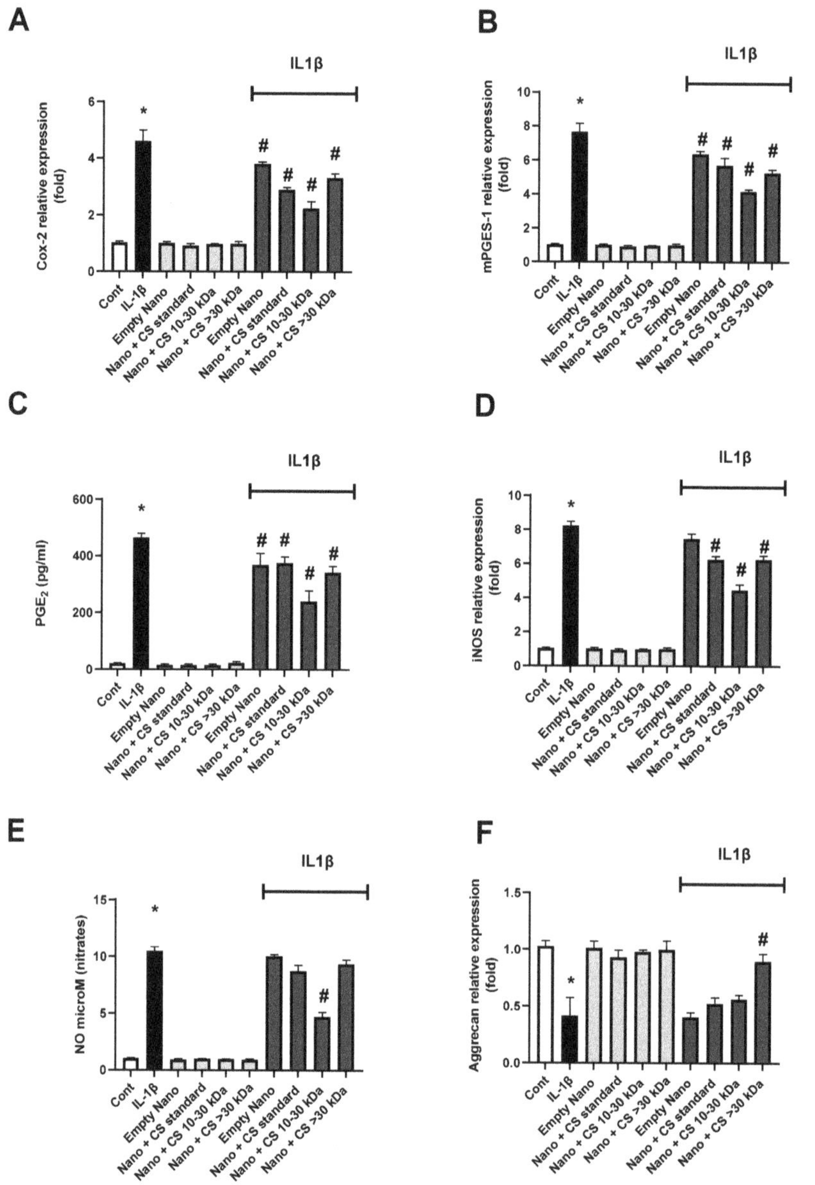

Figure 4. Effect of nanoliposomes/CS exposure on IL-1β-stimulated Cox/mPGES pathways. Human chondrocytes stimulated or not with 1 ng/mL IL-1β and exposed to nanoliposomes (250 µg/mL) or nanoliposomes and CS extracts (250 µg/mL + 25 µg/mL). For (**A**,**B**,**D**,**F**), culture conditions performed for 6 h for early inflammation markers (COX-2 and iNOS mRNA) and 24 h (Aggrecan and mPGES-1 mRNA). Total RNA extracted, then reverse transcribed into cDNA and analyzed by Real-Time Polymerase Chain Reaction (RT-PCR). Relative abundance of Cox-2, mPGES, iNOS, and Aggrecan mRNAs normalized to Retinitis Pigmentosa 29 (RP29) mRNA. Comparison made by using ΔCt method with fold value of reference = 1. Results shown are mean ± SD of at least four individual experiments (*: $p < 0.01$ vs. control; #: $p < 0.01$ versus IL-1β). For (**C**,**E**), culture conditions performed for 48 h for PGE2 and of nitrites (*: $p < 0.01$ vs. control; #: $p < 0.01$ vs. IL-1β).

To assess the anti-catabolic effect induced by IL-1β, the expression and quantity of metalloproteinases (MMPs) 1, 3, and 13—responsible for the turnover and/or degradation of the cartilage extracellular matrix—were evaluated. The expression and quantity of MMP1 are shown in Figure 5A,C, where both extracted L-CS fractions exhibit significant effects. Unlike previous studies on inflammatory pathways, it is the CS > 30 kDa 0.2% fraction that shows the best effect, although expression and production levels remain distant from those of the non-inflamed control. Another MMP, MMP3 was studied similarly in Figure 5B,D. Again, it is worth noting that the fraction containing the longest CS chains is much more effective on enzymatic activity than the 10–30 kDa fraction. This level is comparable to that of the control, indicating that this fraction is very effective on MMP3. Finally, the results of the same experiment on MMP13 are shown in Figure 5E,F. Similarly to the previous results, L-CS reduces both gene expression and MMP13 concentration. This efficacy is further enhanced with the CS > 30 kDa 0.2% fraction. Notably, in this case, the nanoliposomes without CS had no effect on these inflammation parameters, suggesting that polar lipids have little to no impact on MMP production in the cell renewal process.

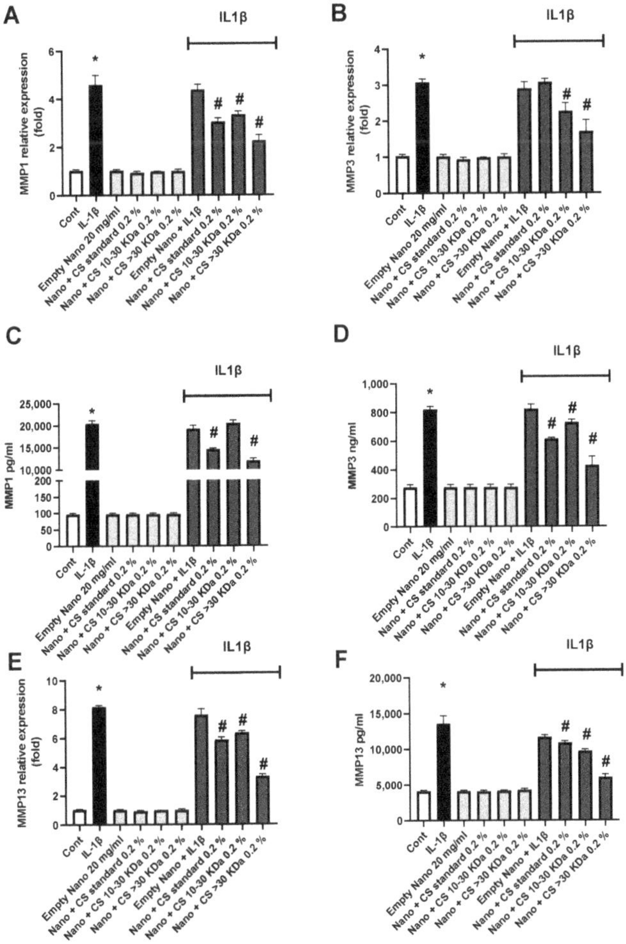

Figure 5. The effect of nanoliposomes/CS exposure on IL-1β-stimulated MMPs. Human chondrocytes were stimulated or not with 1 ng/mL IL-1β and exposed to nanoliposomes (250 μg/mL)

or nanoliposomes and CS extracts (250 µg/mL+ 25 µg/mL). For (**A**,**B**,**E**), total RNA was extracted after 24 h stimulation then reverse transcribed into cDNA and analyzed by RT-PCR. The relative abundance of MMP1, MMP3, and MMP13 mRNAs was normalized to RP29 mRNA. Comparison was performed using the ΔCt method with the fold value of reference = 1. The results shown are the mean ± SD of at least four individual experiments (*: $p < 0.01$ vs. control; #: $p < 0.01$ vs. IL-1β). For (**C**,**D**,**F**) levels of MMP1, 3, and 13 after 48 h of stimulation (*: $p < 0.01$ vs. control; #: $p < 0.01$ vs. IL-1β).

The data presented in Figure 5 confirm the strong efficacy of the CS > 30 kDa 0.2% fraction in reducing MMP expression and concentration. Interestingly, the anti-catabolic effects of CS < 30 kDa appear to be stronger, contrary to what was observed for the anti-inflammatory side. This aspect will be explored in greater depth in future research. However, our results align with those obtained by Li et al.'s team [57].

3. Materials and Methods

3.1. Reagent

Fresh salmon (*Salmo salar*) heads were sourced from a local processing plant and stored at −20 °C. Before use, the heads were thawed overnight at 4 °C. Alcalase® 2.4 L (EC.3.4.21.14a; Novozymes A/S, Bagsvaerd, Denmark), along with sodium hydroxide (NaOH) and hydrochloric acid (HCl), Neutrase® 0.8 L (neutral protease, EC.3.4.24.4f, Novo Nordisk, Bagsvaerd, Denmark, food-grade enzyme), ethanol (C_2H_6O), chloroform ($CHCl_3$), methanol, (CH_3OH), hexane (C_6H_{14}), boron trifluoride (BF_3), Tris base, CS marine standard, chondroitinase ABC, ammonium acetate, and acetonitrile were purchased from Sigma-Aldrich® (Merck KGaA, Darmstadt, Germany) unless specified otherwise.

3.2. Extraction of Chondroitin Sulfate and Lipids from Salmon Heads (Salmo salar)

3.2.1. Enzymatic Extraction

Total lipids and CS were extracted by green solvent-free processes from 12 kg heads of Atlantic salmon (*Salmo salar*), according to Linder et al. [58] with modifications. To extract the compounds of interest, the salmon heads will be subjected to a double enzymatic hydrolysis in order to extract the lipid fraction on one hand and the cartilaginous fraction containing chondroitin sulfate present in the salmon head on the other hand.

The substrate was thawed before being placed in a thermostatic reactor under agitation with water 1:1 (*v*/*v*). After addition of the enzyme Neutrase® 0.8 L (neutral protease, EC.3.4.24.4f, Novo Nordisk, Bagsvaerd, Denmark, food-grade enzyme) to the reaction medium (50 °C, pH 7.5), the reaction is controlled by the "pH-stat" method for 15 min. At the end of hydrolysis, the enzyme is inactivated (90 °C, 10 min). This first step allows the cartilaginous fraction of the head to be recovered after filtration, free from the lipid and protein fractions.

The CS-rich cartilaginous parts of the salmon nasal fraction are then subjected to a second hydrolysis to release the CS in the presence of Alcalase® 2.4 L protease (Novo Nordisk, Bagsvaerd, Denmark) for 40 min at 55 °C and pH 8. The reaction is controlled by the pH-stat method, as with the first hydrolysis, by the addition of a sodium hydroxide solution (2N). The enzyme is then inactivated by heat treatment at 90 °C for 10 min.

Both reaction mixtures are filtered with an inox filter of 300 mesh to remove the solid structures and centrifuged using a Beckman Coulter® Rotor J-10 (Beckman Coulter®, Brea, CA, USA) at 20 °C, 14,334× *g* for 20 min to obtain four different phases: oil, emulsified lipids, proteolysis, and a heavy fraction rich in peptides. The peptide phase is freeze-dried with a Christ® Beta 1–8 Lyophilisator (Grosseron, France) and stored at −20 °C under vacuum in plastic bags.

3.2.2. Purification of CS Fraction

Proteolytics CS are precipitated to ethanol using the method presented in the review of José Antonio Vasquez et al. [2]. A solution of 50% ethanol diluted in water with 0.2 M NaOH is added to the freeze-dried peptidic fraction in proportions of 1:1.

The mixture is stirred for 1 h at 20 °C, before being centrifuged at 6371× *g* with J-10 rotor for 20 min. The unit containing the precipitated CS is recovered and re-suspended in distilled water. The precipitation step is repeated 3 times before the samples are freeze-dried. An AMICON® (Amicon® stirred cell, Merck KGaA, Darmstadt, Germany) with 200 mL membrane filtration stage with Ultracel® cellulose membranes (Ultrafiltration disks, Merck, Jaffrey, NH, USA) of 10 and 30 kDa yields were used. Then, the 10 to 30 kDa and greater than 30 are freeze-dried. These fractions are diluted in distilled water at a concentration of 30 g/L to prevent clogging of the membrane. The separate phases are recovered and re-suspended in water before being freeze-dried and stored at 4 °C before analysis.

3.2.3. Separation of Lipid Classes and Purification of Phospholipids

The different lipid fractions, neutral and polar, were separated by centrifugation (20 °C, 20 min, 14,334× *g*) and purified using the appropriate solvents. Regarding polar lipids, a freeze-drying step is performed to remove water given the amphipathic character of the polar lipids.

The recovery of the residues contained in the peptide fraction obtained as a result of hydrolysis is carried out according to Folch et al. [59]. The powder resulting from the hydrolysis of the heads is solubilized in a mixture of chloroform/methanol (99.9%) in proportions 2:1 (v/v), respectively. The solution is then filtered through a sintered glass (Robu-Glas® borosilicat por. 4, Hattert, Germany) under vacuum. The lipid solution is then evaporated at 40 °C in the dark and under nitrogen by Rotavapor R-205, with a vacuum connector V-800, and a pumpV-500 BUCHI (BUCHI Sarl, Villebon-sur-Yvette, France). The recovered lipid fractions are subjected to glacial acetone precipitation at −20 °C to separate the neutral and polar lipid fractions according to Zhu et al. [60].

3.3. *FT-IR Spectroscopy Analysis of CS and Lipids*

The analyses are performed in Infrared to Fourier Transform Attenuated Total Reflection (FTIR-ATR) mode at 22 °C in a Tensor 27 mid-FTIR Bruker spectrometer (Brüker, Karlsruhe, Germany), equipped with a DTGS detector (Mercury-Cadmium-Tellure, Brüker, Karlsruhe, Germany) and an ATR A537-L11 optical cell. The diaphragm was set to 6 mm, with a scanning speed of 10 KHz. There were 128 scans performed by analysis, from 400 to 4000 cm^{-1} with a spectral resolution of 6 cm^{-1} according to Chihaoui et al. [61] with modifications.

3.4. *Digestion of CS and Semi-Quantitative Analysis of Δdi-4S and Δdi-6S by HPLC-MS*

CS disaccharides were obtained by chondroitinase ABC digestion according to Takeda et al. [62]. Then, 1 mg of the extracted CS samples was diluted in 1 mL of Tris-HCl buffer at pH 8. After the addition of chondroitinase ABC, the mixture is placed at 37 °C for 24 h. The sample is centrifugated, and supernatant is collected for analysis. The same procedure is realized with a marine CS commercial standard, which is becoming a disaccharide reference mixture for the calibration curve.

The qualitative and semi-quantitative analysis of Δdi-4S and Δdi-6S were conducted on an HPLC-MS system (Thermo Scientific, San Jose, CA, USA) consisting of a quaternary solvent delivery pump connected to a photodiode array detector (PDA) and a LTQXL mass spectrometer equipped with an atmospheric pressure ionization interface operating in electrospray negative ion mode (ESI–).

Ten microliters of chondroitin hydrolysis sample were injected on a Hypercarb column (100 × 2.1 mm, 5 μm, Thermo Fisher Scientific) maintained at 40 °C during the run. Mobile phase A was ammonium acetate in water at pH 11 and mobile phase B was pure acetonitrile.

The flow rate was set at 0.2 mL/min. Sulfate disaccharides were eluted by an isocratic step at 6% B for 1.5 min, followed by a linear gradient from 6 to 11% B over 9 min.

Mass spectrometry (MS) conditions were as follows: spray voltage was set at −4.5 kV; source gasses were set (in arbitrary units. min^{-1}) for sheath gas, auxiliary gas and sweep gas at 29, 0.5, and 1, respectively; capillary temperature was set at 280 °C; capillary voltage was set at −45 V; and tube lens, split lens, and front lens voltages were set at −77 V, 60 V, and 9 V, respectively. Ion optics parameters were optimized by automatic tuning using ΔCS-4S and ΔCS-6S present in chondroitin hydrolysis solution (0.5 g/L) infused in mobile phase at a flow rate of 5 μL/min. Full scan MS (100 to 1000 *m*/*z*) and MS/MS spectra were performed on an LTQ analyzer (Linear Trap Quadrupole). Raw data were processed using the XCALIBUR software program (version 2.1, http://www.thermoscientific.com (accessed on 15 October 2024).

3.5. TLC-FID (Iatroscan®) Analysis of Lipids

The lipid fraction analysis was performed by Iatroscan® MK-5 thin-layer chromatogra phy–flame ionization detection (TLC-FID) (Iatron Laboratories Inc., Tokyo, Japan). The samples are diluted in a mixture of chloroform/methanol (99.9%; 2:1 *v*/*v*) to obtain a concentration of 5 mg/mL. A sample (1 μL) was deposited in tripliquat on chromarods S-III (Iatroscan laboratory Inc, Tokyo, Japan). The migration was conducted for 20 min in a solution of hexane/diethyl ether/formic acid (80:20:0.2 *v*/*v*/*v*), then oven-dried for 1 min at 100 °C, and finally scanned by the Iatroscan® analyzer. A second migration in a chloroform/methanol/ammonia mixture (65/35/5 *v*/*v*/*v*) allows for the detection of the different phospholipids. Hydrogen and air flows are maintained at 160 and 2 mL per minute at 20 °C, respectively. Peak recording and integration were performed with ChromStar® software 4.14 (SCPA, Weyhe-Leeste, Germany). Triglyceride, diglyceride, and monoglyceride standards were used to perform the calibration range (Sigmal-Aldrich, St. Louis, MO, USA).

3.6. Fatty Acid Composition Analysis by GC-FID

The fatty acid composition of the different lipid classes is achieved by gas chromatography coupled with a flame ionization detector (GC-FID) according to the method of Li et al. [33] with modifications. The samples are methylated according to the technique of Morrisson and Smith [63]. Esterification is performed by diluting 0.1 g of lipids in 1.5 mL of hexane and 1.5 mL in a mixture of boron/methanol trifluore (8% of BF_3). The samples were analyzed by CPG-FID SHIMADZU 2010 (Kyoto, Japan), coupled with a flame ionization detector and equipped with a silica capillary column (60 m, 0.2 mm i.d. 0.25 μm film thicknesses, SPTM2380 Supelco, Bellfonte, PA, USA). The injector and detector temperature are set at 250 °C. During the first 3 min, the column temperature reaches 120 °C. It is then increased to 180 °C at a speed of 40 °C per minute for 2 min, then maintained at 220 °C for 25 min. The data were performed with Shimadzu "GC solution" software 2.41.00 (Kyoto, Japan). The identification of fatty acids is carried out using standard mixtures from marine PUFA1 and animal PUFA2 sources, respectively (Supelco, Sigma–Aldrich, Bellefonte, PA, USA).

3.7. Formulation of L-CS

Liposomes are formulated according to the thin lipid film hydration method according to Bingham in 1961. For the lecithin concentration of liposomal dispersion to be 2%, 160 mg of lecithin is accurately weighed and diluted in chloroform/methanol (2:1 *v*/*v*) in a flask according to Hanachi et al. [51]. The thin film is formed by evaporation with Rotavapor R-205, with a vacuum connector V-800, and a pumpV-500 BUCHI (BUCHI Sarl, Villebon-sur-Yvette, France). The film is then rehydrated overnight at 4 °C under agitation with a solution containing CS diluted in 8 mL of ultrapure water. The samples are then sonicated with a sonicator (sonicator probe, Sonics & Materials Inc., CT, USA) for 8 min (1 s «on»/1 s «off») at 40 °C, 40% amplitude, and at a frequency of 20 kHz.

Different types of liposomes are formed for characterization and cell study: empty liposomes (L-E); liposomes containing the marine CS standard with two concentrations: 1.0% (L-CSs1) and 0.2% (L-CSs2); and liposomes containing CS extracted from salmon heads greater than 30 kDa at 1% (L-CSh1) and 0.2% (L-CSh2) and between 10 and 30 kDa at 1.0% (L-CSl1) and 0.2% (L-CSl2).

3.8. *DLS Analysis of L-CS*

To analyze the size, Polydispersity Index (PdI), and liposome charge (potential ζ), the sample was analyzed by DLS (Zetasizer Nano ZS, Malvern, UK). For this, the liposome sample is diluted twice in ultra-pure water. The dilution is transferred to a micro vessel (UV-Cuvette micro, BRAND GMBH + CO. KG, Wertheim, German) for size measurement using Zetasizer software V2.41 (ZetaSizer; Malvern Instrument Ltd., Malvern, UK). For load measurement, the sample is analyzed in a capillary vessel DTS1070 (Malvern Instrument Ltd.) using the Zetasizer software. Size, potential ζ, and PdI were measured at 25 °C, with an absorbance of 0.01 at a fixed diffusion angle of 173° and a refractive index of 1.471.

3.9. *Anti-Inflammatory Study of CS-Liposomes on Human Chondrocytes*

3.9.1. Collection and Culture of Chondrocytes

All specimen collection and all procedures conducted were approved by the Ethics Committee of the Nancy University Hospital (CHU) (agreement #UF 9607-CPRC 2005) and conducted in conformity with the declaration of Helsinki. Femoral condyles and tibial plateaus were obtained from 6 osteoarthritis patients (aged 70 ± 9 years, mean ± SD; M/F: 3/11). For in vitro studies, chondrocytes were released from cartilage pieces by sequential enzymatic digestions with collagenase (1.5 mg/mL) and pronase® (2 mg/mL). They were cultured in DMEM (Dulbecco's Modified Eagle Medium, Gibco™, Life Technologies GmbH, Darmstadt, Germany) containing 4.5 g/L glucose and 10% fetal calf serum (Gibco, Villebon-sur-Yvette, France) for the first 24 h, and then in DMEM containing 1 g/L glucose and 10% fetal calf serum until 70% confluence and then stimulated. The cells were collected after 6 and 24 h for RNA extraction, and supernatants after 48 h for ELISAs.

3.9.2. Study Design

Human chondrocytes were stimulated with 1 ng/mL of IL-1β for 6, 24, or 48 h with or without 250 μg/mL of liposomes empty or with CS encapsulated at 125 μg/mL (1%) or 25 μg/mL (0.2%) in the culture medium. Supernatants were frozen immediately and kept at −80 °C until use and were assayed individually for the nitrites assay and specific ELISAs. As the transcription of the inflammation markers COX-2 and iNOS was early [55], we first measured their expression after 6 h of cell culture. Then, we measured the expression of mPGES-1 [64] after 24 h. Finally, as PGE2 is an end product of the COX-2 and mPGES-1 pathways, and NO for iNOS [65,66], they were quantified after 48 h of cell culture.

3.9.3. Biocompatibility Assays

To evaluate the impact of nanoliposomes on cell behavior, different parameters were estimated: cytotoxicity, cell metabolic activity, and cell proliferation.

The cytotoxicity test was performed using the Cytotoxicity Detection KitPLUS (LDH) (#04744926001; Roche, Boulogne-Billancourt, France) according to the manufacturer's instructions. This assay is based on the measurement of LDH activity released from the cytosol of damaged cells. Three controls are included: background control (assay medium), low control (untreated cells), and high control (maximum LDH release). The absorbance was read on a spectrophotometer at 490 nm (Varioskan® Flash, Thermo Scientific, Illkirch, France). To determine the experimental absorbance values, the average absorbance values of the triplicate samples and controls were calculated and subtracted from the absorbance values of the background control. The percentage of cytotoxicity was determined over the value of the high control (fixed to 100).

Cell proliferation was assessed after 3, 5, or 7 days of chondrocyte culture using Hoechst assay, which allows for cell DNA quantification. Briefly, chondrocytes were harvested from 12-well plates and suspended in 100 μL of Hoechst buffer (10 mM TRIS, 1 mM EthyleneDiamineTetraacetate Acid (EDTA), and 0.1 M of NaCl, pH 7.4) before 5 series of freezing (liquid nitrogen)/thawing (60 °C, 5 min) cycles for lysing cells and releasing their DNA into solution. Black fat-bottom plates with a low fluorescent background were used to perform the assay and a calf thymus DNA standard curve was used for quantification. The samples were mixed with 2 μL of the Hoechst solution (0.1 μg/mL in final concentration) and the measurements of the DNA samples and standards were performed by fluorescence spectrophotometry (360 nm excitation/460 nm emissions, Varioskan® Flash, Thermo, Illkirch, France). The DNA concentration (μg/mL) of each sample was based on its fluorescence measurement relative to the standard curve.

Cell metabolic activity was measured using MTT (3-(4,5-dimethylthiazol-2-yl)-2,5-diphenyltetrazolium bromide) assay as described elsewhere. Then, 50 μL of the MTT solution was added to 200 μL of the cell culture medium. Briefly, chondrocytes were incubated for 4 h (5% CO_2, 95% humidity at 37 °C) to allow the yellow dye to be transformed into blue formazan crystals by the mitochondrial dehydrogenases. The supernatant was removed, and this insoluble product was protected from light and dissolved by the addition of 200 μL Dimethylsulfoxid (DMSO) and gently mixed at 37 °C for 5 min. The supernatants were removed, protected from light, centrifuged, and their absorbance was read within 30 min using a Varioskan® Flash (Thermo Fisher Scientific, Illkirch, France) at 540 nm. The control condition for chondrocyte metabolic activity was used as the reference value.

3.9.4. Nitrites Assay

NO production was estimated spectrophotometrically by measuring the accumulation of nitrites in culture supernatants by the Griess reaction. Briefly, 100 μL of culture supernatant were mixed with 100 μL of the Griess reagent (1% of sulfanilamide in 2.5% H_3PO_4 and 0.1% of N-Naphtylethylenediamine dihydrochloride in H_2O, *v*/*v*) for 5 min at room temperature in microtiter plates. The absorbance was measured at 550 nm with a microplate reader (Multiskan, Labsystems, Cergy Pontoise, France), and nitrite concentrations were calculated with a standard curve of sodium nitrite ranging from 0 to 50 μM. The limit of quantification of this method was determined to be 1 μM of nitrites.

3.9.5. Immuno-Enzymatic Assays (ELISAs)

As mentioned above, the effect of IL-1β and/or nanoliposomes on the level of several proteins secreted by chondrocytes was controlled by enzyme-linked immunosorbent assays (ELISAs). After stimulations, supernatants were collected and centrifuged 5 min at 600 g and analyses were performed according to the kit manufacturer's instructions for MMP1, MMP3, and MMP13 levels (DuoSet® ELISA, R&D systems, Abingdon, UK—Human Total MMP1, Human Total MMP3, and Human Pro-MMP13) and PGE2 levels (Prostaglandin E2 Parameter Assay Kit, Bio-Techne, Abingdon, UK).

3.9.6. RNA Extraction and Reverse Transcription-Polymerase Chain Reaction Analysis

Total RNA was isolated using RNeasy plus mini kit® (Qiagen, Hilden, Germany), which allows for the total removal of genomic DNA with an on-column DNase. Then, 500 ng of the total RNA were reverse-transcribed for 90 min, at 37 °C in a 20 μL reaction mixture containing 5 mM dNTP, 0.2 μg/μL random hexamer primers, 250 mM Tris-HCl-pH 8.3, KCl 375 mM, $MgCl_2$ 15 mM, and 200 units of Moloney Murine Leukemia Virus reverse transcriptase (Invitrogen, Austin, TX, USA).

3.9.7. Real-Time Quantitative Polymerase Chain Reaction

Real-time PCR was performed by the Step One Plus (Applied Biosystems, France) technology using specific primers (Table 5) and iTAQ SYBRgreen master mix system (Biorad, Steenvoorde, Combes-La-Ville, France). All reagents used for RT-PCR were added at the concentrations recommended by the manufacturer. Melting curve was performed to determine the melting temperature of the specific PCR products and, after amplification, the product size was checked on a 1% agarose gel stained with Gel Red (Biotium, Interchim, Montluçon, France). The mRNA levels of the gene of interest and of the ribosomal protein 29 (RPS29), chosen as a housekeeping gene in order to normalize gene expression, were determined in parallel for each sample. Quantification was determined using the $\Delta\Delta$Ct method and the results were expressed as fold expression over the control.

Table 5. Sequences of specific primers for RT-PCR analyses.

Genes	Sequences 5′-3′
Agg	Fwd: CTC-TAA-CCG-CCA-CGG-TCT-GA Rev: ACT-AGC-ATG-ATT-GGT-ATC-AC
COX-2	Fwd: GCT-GGA-ACA-TGG-AAT-TAC-CCA Rev: CTT-TCT-GTA-CTG-CGG-GTG-GAA
mPGES-1	Fwd: TGG-TCA-TCA-AGA-TGT-ACG-TGG-T Rev: GGG-TCG-CTC-CTG-CAA-TAC-T
iNOS	Fwd: TGC-AAT-GAA-TGG-GGA-AAA-AG Rev: ATT-CTG-CTG-CTT-GCT-GAG-GT
MMP1	Fwd: AGG-TCT-CTG-AGG-GTC-AAG-CA Rev: CTG-GTT-GAA-AAG-CAT-GAG-CA
MMP3	Fwd: GCA-GTT-TGC-TCA-GCC-TAT-CC Rev: GAG-TGT-CGG-AGT-CCA-GCT-TC
MMP13	Fwd: TGG-TGG-TGA-TGA-AGA-TGA-TTT Rev: TCT-AAG-CCG-AAG-AAA-GAC-TGC
RP29	Fwd: GGG-TCA-CCA-GCA-GCT-GTA-CT Rev: CCG-ATA-TCC-TTC-GCG-TAC-TG

Agg—aggrecan; COX-2—cyclooxygenase-2; mPGES-1—microsomal prostaglandin E2 synthase-1; iNOS—inducible nitric oxide synthase; Fwd—forward primer; RT-PCR—real-time polymerase chain reaction; Rev—reverse primer; RP—ribosomal protein; MMP1, 3, and 13—metalloproteinase 1, 3, and 13.

3.9.8. Statistical Analysis

All experiments were performed and analyzed in triplicates. The results are expressed as the mean ± SEM. Statistical analyses were performed with GraphPad Prism 6 (GraphPad Software Inc., San Diego, CA, USA) using either one-way ANOVA followed by Bonferroni's post hoc test or unpaired T-test, with Welch's correction when variances were significantly different. p values lower than 0.05 were considered significant for physicochemical analyses and 0.01 for biomolecular analyses.

Figure 6 summarizes the valorization of by-products from the fishing industry, particularly the use of salmon heads (*Salmo salar*) as a source of phospholipids naturally rich in LC-PUFAs and chondroitin sulfate present in the nasal region of cartilage tissue. The results showed that CS, in synergy with the LC-PUFAs present in the phospholipids of the liposomes, played a positive role in combating human chondrocyte inflammation even at low concentrations.

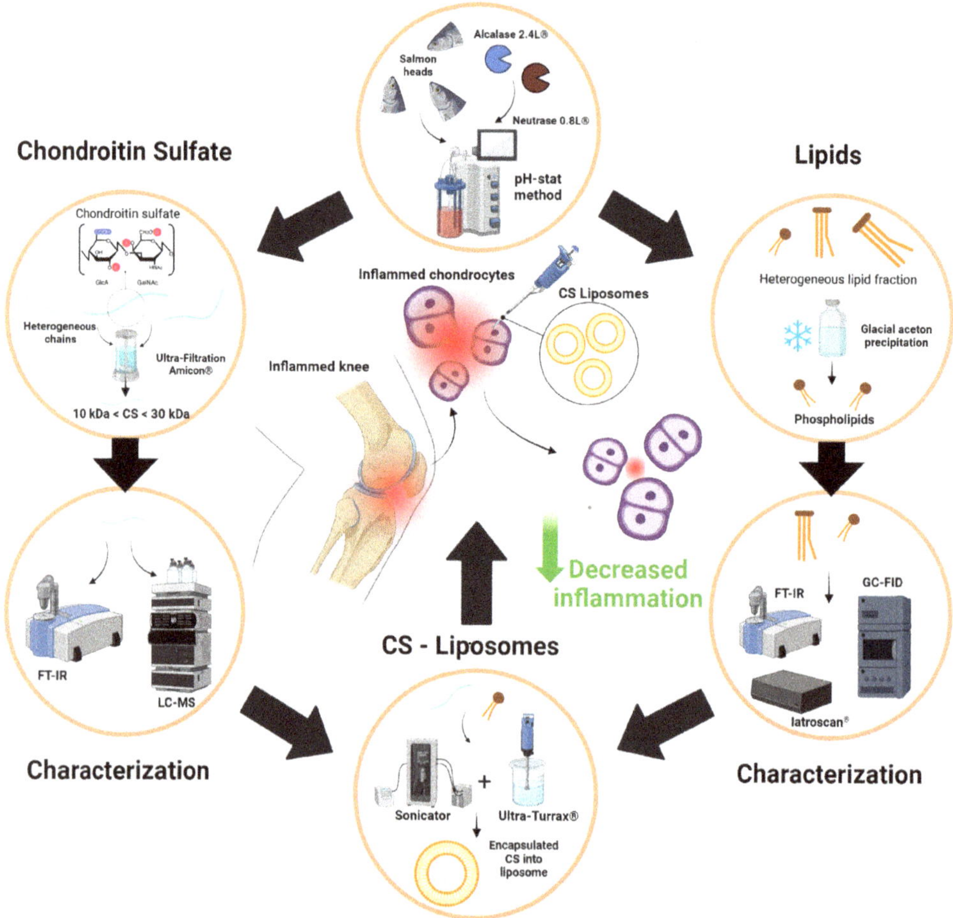

Figure 6. Recapitulative graphical abstract of study design and objectives.

4. Conclusions

As a result of these findings, it is possible to formulate liposomes loaded with chondroitin sulfate, capable of reducing inflammation in joint cells, using a single co-product from salmon (*Salmo salar*). The various characterization techniques used confirmed that chondroitin sulfate and polar lipids were successfully extracted, separated, and concentrated. These biomolecules were used to form liposomes, which, through a synergistic effect between the polar lipids and the chondroitin sulfate, were able to reduce the expression of inflammation markers in human chondrocytes. Moreover, the CS fraction showed different actions on inflammation with a good effect of 10–30 kDa for reducing pathway inflammation markers and the fraction > 30 kDa for the stimulation of aggrecan gene expression and reducing gene expression and the concentration of MMP enzymes. The formulation of such products fully meets contemporary demands with a dual benefit: offering a solution to growing conditions such as osteoarthritis and using food by-products as part of an anti-waste approach. The next steps following this study would be to more precisely characterize the extracted chondroitin sulfate in terms of length and composition. It could also be relevant to scale up production, increase the extraction yields of the different molecules through experimental designs, or test this anti-inflammatory effect on other types of cells.

Author Contributions: Conceptualization, L.P., M.G., C.J.-F.K. and M.L.; methodology, L.P., M.G., C.P., A.B., É.V., C.J.-F.K. and M.L.; validation, C.P., A.B., C.J.-F.K. and M.L.; formal analysis, L.P., M.G. and C.P.; investigation: L.P. and M.G.; resources, M.L. and A.B.; data curation, L.P. and M.G.; writing—original draft preparation, L.P.; writing—review and editing, C.J.-F.K., M.L. and A.B.; supervision, C.J.-F.K. and M.L. All authors have read and agreed to the published version of the manuscript.

Funding: This research received no external funding.

Institutional Review Board Statement: The study was conducted in accordance with the Declaration of Helsinki and approved by the Ethics Committee of the Nancy University Hospital (CHU) (agreement #UF 9607-CPRC 2005; 6 December 2005).

Data Availability Statement: The original contributions presented in the study are included in the article, further inquiries can be directed to the corresponding author.

Conflicts of Interest: The authors declare no conflicts of interest.

Appendix A

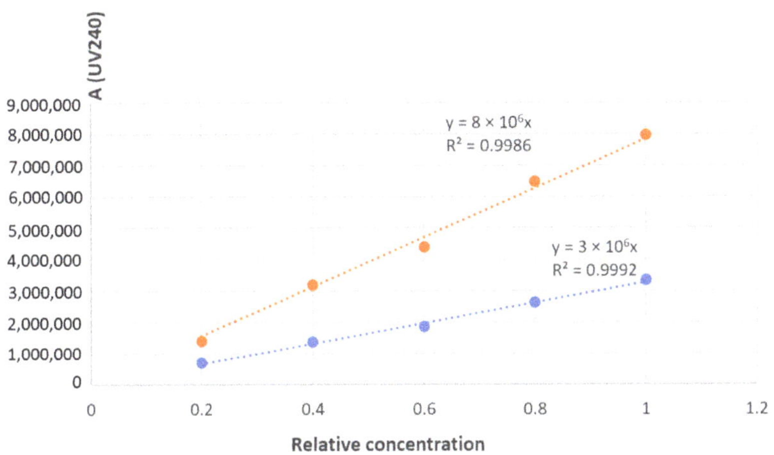

Figure A1. Calibration range of 4S and 6S isomers.

References

1. FAO. *The State of World Fisheries and Aquaculture 2024*; FAO: Rome, Italy, 2024; ISBN 978-92-5-138763-4.
2. Vázquez, J.; Rodríguez-Amado, I.; Montemayor, M.; Fraguas, J.; González, M.; Murado, M. Chondroitin Sulfate, Hyaluronic Acid and Chitin/Chitosan Production Using Marine Waste Sources: Characteristics, Applications and Eco-Friendly Processes: A Review. *Mar. Drugs* **2013**, *11*, 747–774. [CrossRef] [PubMed]
3. AFSSA. Report #2006-SA-0359, Maison-Alfort, Paris. 1 March 2010. Available online: https://www.anses.fr/fr/system/files/NUT2006sa0359.pdf (accessed on 6 September 2024).
4. Hasan, M. Nanovectorisation de la Curcumine Sous Forme Liposomale: Interactions Biomolécule/Membrane, Transferts et Cytotoxicité Dans des Systèmes In Vitro. Ph.D. Thesis, Université de Lorraine, Metz, France, 2015.
5. Mudiyanselage, J.J. Department of Food and Human Nutritional Sciences. Ph.D. Thesis, University of Manitoba Winnipeg, Winnipeg, MB, Canada, 2007.
6. Chaves, M.A.; Ferreira, L.S.; Baldino, L.; Pinho, S.C.; Reverchon, E. Current Applications of Liposomes for the Delivery of Vitamins: A Systematic Review. *Nanomaterials* **2023**, *13*, 1557. [CrossRef] [PubMed]
7. Shionoya, K.; Suzuki, T.; Takada, M.; Sato, K.; Onishi, S.; Dohmae, N.; Nishino, K.; Wada, T.; Linhardt, R.J.; Toida, T.; et al. Comprehensive Analysis of Chondroitin Sulfate and Aggrecan in the Head Cartilage of Bony Fishes: Identification of Proteoglycans in the Head Cartilage of Sturgeon. *Int. J. Biol. Macromol.* **2022**, *208*, 333–342. [CrossRef] [PubMed]
8. Ricard-Blum, S.; Vivès, R.R.; Schaefer, L.; Götte, M.; Merline, R.; Passi, A.; Heldin, P.; Magalhães, A.; Reis, C.A.; Skandalis, S.S.; et al. A Biological Guide to Glycosaminoglycans: Current Perspectives and Pending Questions. *FEBS J.* **2024**, *291*, 3331–3366. [CrossRef] [PubMed]
9. Zhang, W.; Xu, R.; Jin, X.; Wang, Y.; Hu, L.; Zhang, T.; Du, G.; Kang, Z. Enzymatic Production of Chondroitin Oligosaccharides and Its Sulfate Derivatives. *Front. Bioeng. Biotechnol.* **2022**, *10*, 951740. [CrossRef]

10. Bougatef, H.; Volpi, N.; Ben Amor, I.; Capitani, F.; Maccari, F.; Gargouri, J.; Sila, A.; Bougatef, A. Chondroitin Sulfate from Heads of Corb: Recovery, Structural Analysis and Assessment of Anticoagulant Activity. *Carbohydr. Res.* **2024**, *541*, 109163. [CrossRef]
11. Shi, C.; Deng, Y.; An, X.; Chen, Y.; Lv, X.; Liu, Q. Extraction, Physicochemical Properties, and In Vitro Antioxidant Activities of Chondroitin Sulfate from Bovine Nose Cartilage. *Int. J. Food Sci.* **2024**, *2024*, 6328378. [CrossRef]
12. Unver, T.; Erenler, A.S.; Bingul, M.; Boga, M. Comparative Analysis of Antioxidant, Anticholinesterase, and Antibacterial Activity of Microbial Chondroitin Sulfate and Commercial Chondroitin Sulfate. *Chem. Biodivers.* **2023**, *20*, e202300924. [CrossRef]
13. Tian, X.; Zhan, L.; Long, X.; Lin, J.; Zhang, Y.; Luan, J.; Peng, X.; Zhao, G. Multifunctional Natamycin Modified Chondroitin Sulfate Eye Drops with Anti-Inflammatory, Antifungal and Tissue Repair Functions Possess Therapeutic Effects on Fungal Keratitis in Mice. *Int. J. Biol. Macromol.* **2024**, *279*, 135290. [CrossRef]
14. Brito, R.; Costa, D.; Dias, C.; Cruz, P.; Barros, P. Chondroitin Sulfate Supplements for Osteoarthritis: A Critical Review. *Cureus* **2023**, *15*, e40192. [CrossRef]
15. Loeser, R.F.; Goldring, S.R.; Scanzello, C.R.; Goldring, M.B. Osteoarthritis: A Disease of the Joint as an Organ. *Arthritis Rheum.* **2012**, *64*, 1697. [CrossRef] [PubMed]
16. Senni, K.; Gueniche, F.; Changotade, S.; Septier, D.; Sinquin, C.; Ratiskol, J.; Lutomski, D.; Godeau, G.; Guezennec, J.; Colliec-Jouault, S. Unusual Glycosaminoglycans from a Deep Sea Hydrothermal Bacterium Improve Fibrillar Collagen Structuring and Fibroblast Activities in Engineered Connective Tissues. *Mar. Drugs* **2013**, *11*, 1351–1369. [CrossRef] [PubMed]
17. Chou, C.-H.; Jain, V.; Gibson, J.; Attarian, D.E.; Haraden, C.A.; Yohn, C.B.; Laberge, R.-M.; Gregory, S.; Kraus, V.B. Synovial Cell Cross-Talk with Cartilage Plays a Major Role in the Pathogenesis of Osteoarthritis. *Sci. Rep.* **2020**, *10*, 10868. [CrossRef] [PubMed]
18. Terkawi, M.A.; Ebata, T.; Yokota, S.; Takahashi, D.; Endo, T.; Matsumae, G.; Shimizu, T.; Kadoya, K.; Iwasaki, N. Low-Grade Inflammation in the Pathogenesis of Osteoarthritis: Cellular and Molecular Mechanisms and Strategies for Future Therapeutic Intervention. *Biomedicines* **2022**, *10*, 1109. [CrossRef]
19. Pelletier, J.-P.; DiBattista, J.A.; Roughley, P.; McCollum, R.; Martel-Pelletier, J. Cytokines and Inflammation in Cartilage Degradation. *Rheum. Dis. Clin. N. Am.* **1993**, *19*, 545–568. [CrossRef]
20. Kim, H.-A.; Yeo, Y.; Jung, H.A.; Jung, Y.O.; Park, S.J.; Kim, S.J. Phase 2 Enzyme Inducer Sulphoraphane Blocks Prostaglandin and Nitric Oxide Synthesis in Human Articular Chondrocytes and Inhibits Cartilage Matrix Degradation. *Rheumatology* **2012**, *51*, 1006–1016. [CrossRef]
21. Zhang, Y.-Y.; Yao, Y.-D.; Luo, J.-F.; Liu, Z.-Q.; Huang, Y.-M.; Wu, F.-C.; Sun, Q.-H.; Liu, J.-X.; Zhou, H. Microsomal Prostaglandin E2 Synthase-1 and Its Inhibitors: Molecular Mechanisms and Therapeutic Significance. *Pharmacol. Res.* **2022**, *175*, 105977. [CrossRef]
22. Shang, X.B.; Wang, Y.J.; Cai, D.C.; Ma, S.; Wang, Z.; Zhu, Y.K.; Guo, H.H.; Wang, C.; Ma, X.; Hu, Z.Y.; et al. An Inducible Nitric Oxide Synthase Dimerization Inhibitor Prevents the Progression of Osteoarthritis. *Front. Pharmacol.* **2022**, *13*, 861183. [CrossRef]
23. Restaino, O.F.; Schiraldi, C. Chondroitin Sulfate: Are the Purity and the Structural Features Well Assessed? A Review on the Analytical Challenges. *Carbohydr. Polym.* **2022**, *292*, 119690. [CrossRef]
24. Ronca, F.; Palmieri, L.; Panicucci, P.; Ronca, G. Anti-Inflammatory Activity of Chondroitin Sulfate. *Osteoarthr. Cartil.* **1998**, *6*, 14–21. [CrossRef]
25. Iovu, M.; Dumais, G.; Du Souich, P. Anti-Inflammatory Activity of Chondroitin Sulfate. *Osteoarthr. Cartil.* **2008**, *16*, S14–S18. [CrossRef] [PubMed]
26. Zhang, W.; Xu, R.; Chen, J.; Xiong, H.; Wang, Y.; Pang, B.; Du, G.; Kang, Z. Advances and Challenges in Biotechnological Production of Chondroitin Sulfate and Its Oligosaccharides. *Int. J. Biol. Macromol.* **2023**, *253*, 126551. [CrossRef] [PubMed]
27. Fraser, P.E.; Darabie, A.A.; McLaurin, J. Amyloid-β Interactions with Chondroitin Sulfate-Derived Monosaccharides and Disaccharides. *J. Biol. Chem.* **2001**, *276*, 6412–6419. [CrossRef] [PubMed]
28. Alkhalil, A.; Achur, R.N.; Valiyaveettil, M.; Ockenhouse, C.F.; Gowda, D.C. Structural Requirements for the Adherence ofPlasmodium Falciparum-Infected Erythrocytes to Chondroitin Sulfate Proteoglycans of Human Placenta. *J. Biol. Chem.* **2000**, *275*, 40357–40364. [CrossRef]
29. Zhang, W.; Zhang, P.; Wang, H.; Xu, R.; Xie, Z.; Wang, Y.; Du, G.; Kang, Z. Enhancing the Expression of Chondroitin 4-O-Sulfotransferase for One-Pot Enzymatic Synthesis of Chondroitin Sulfate A. *Carbohydr. Polym.* **2024**, *337*, 122158. [CrossRef]
30. Pudełko, A.; Wisowski, G.; Olczyk, K.; Koźma, E.M. The Dual Role of the Glycosaminoglycan Chondroitin-6-sulfate in the Development, Progression and Metastasis of Cancer. *FEBS J.* **2019**, *286*, 1815–1837. [CrossRef]
31. Sakai, T.; Kyogashima, M.; Kariya, Y.; Urano, T.; Takada, Y.; Takada, A. Importance of GlcUAb1-3GalNAc(4S,6S) in Chondroitin Sulfate E for t-PA- and u-PA-Mediated Glu-Plasminogen Activation. *Thromb. Res.* **2000**, *100*, 557–565. [CrossRef]
32. Bergefall, K.; Trybala, E.; Johansson, M.; Uyama, T.; Naito, S.; Yamada, S.; Kitagawa, H.; Sugahara, K.; Bergström, T. Chondroitin Sulfate Characterized by the E-Disaccharide Unit Is a Potent Inhibitor of Herpes Simplex Virus Infectivity and Provides the Virus Binding Sites on gro2C Cells. *J. Biol. Chem.* **2005**, *280*, 32193–32199. [CrossRef]
33. Li, J.; Elkhoury, K.; Barbieux, C.; Linder, M.; Grandemange, S.; Tamayol, A.; Francius, G.; Arab-Tehrany, E. Effects of Bioactive Marine-Derived Liposomes on Two Human Breast Cancer Cell Lines. *Mar. Drugs* **2020**, *18*, 211. [CrossRef]
34. Velot, É.; Elkhoury, K.; Kahn, C.; Kempf, H.; Linder, M.; Arab-Tehrany, E.; Bianchi, A. Efficient TGF-B1 Delivery to Articular Chondrocytes In Vitro Using Agro-Based Liposomes. *Int. J. Mol. Sci.* **2022**, *23*, 2864. [CrossRef]
35. Velot, É.; Ducrocq, F.; Girardeau, L.; Hehn, A.; Piutti, S.; Kahn, C.; Linder, M.; Bianchi, A.; Arab-Tehrany, E. Hop Extract Anti-Inflammatory Effect on Human Chondrocytes Is Potentiated When Encapsulated in Rapeseed Lecithin Nanoliposomes. *Int. J. Mol. Sci.* **2022**, *23*, 12423. [CrossRef] [PubMed]

36. Bianchi, A.; Velot, É.; Kempf, H.; Elkhoury, K.; Sanchez-Gonzalez, L.; Linder, M.; Kahn, C.; Arab-Tehrany, E. Nanoliposomes from Agro-Resources as Promising Delivery Systems for Chondrocytes. *Int. J. Mol. Sci.* **2020**, *21*, 3436. [CrossRef] [PubMed]
37. Henna Lu, F.S.; Nielsen, N.S.; Timm-Heinrich, M.; Jacobsen, C. Oxidative Stability of Marine Phospholipids in the Liposomal Form and Their Applications. *Lipids* **2011**, *46*, 3–23. [CrossRef] [PubMed]
38. Guedes, M.; Vieira, S.F.; Reis, R.L.; Ferreira, H.; Neves, N.M. Fishroesomes as Carriers with Antioxidant and Anti-Inflammatory Bioactivities. *Biomed. Pharmacother.* **2021**, *140*, 111680. [CrossRef]
39. Virk, R.; Cook, K.; Cavazos, A.; Wassall, S.R.; Gowdy, K.M.; Shaikh, S.R. How Membrane Phospholipids Containing Long-Chain Polyunsaturated Fatty Acids and Their Oxidation Products Orchestrate Lipid Raft Dynamics to Control Inflammation. *J. Nutr.* **2024**, *154*, 2862–2870. [CrossRef]
40. Yang, K.-R.; Tsai, M.-F.; Shieh, C.-J.; Arakawa, O.; Dong, C.-D.; Huang, C.-Y.; Kuo, C.-H. Ultrasonic-Assisted Extraction and Structural Characterization of Chondroitin Sulfate Derived from Jumbo Squid Cartilage. *Foods* **2021**, *10*, 2363. [CrossRef]
41. Dong, F.; Quan, X.; Wang, Q.; Liu, Z.; Cui, T.; Wang, W.; Tang, D.; Zhang, R.; Zhang, C.; Wang, H.; et al. Purification, Structural Characterization, and Anticoagulant Activity Evaluation of Chondroitin Sulfate from Codfish (*Gadus macrocephalus*) Bones. *Int. J. Biol. Macromol.* **2022**, *210*, 759–767. [CrossRef]
42. Cavalcanti, O.A.; Pineda, E.A.G.; Hechenleitner, A.A.W. Synthesis and Characterization of Phosphated Crosslinked Chondroitin Sulfate: Potential Ingredient for Specific Drug Delivery. *Acta Farm. Bonaer.* **2005**, *24*, 234.
43. Garnjanagoonchorn, W.; Wongekalak, L.; Engkagul, A. Determination of Chondroitin Sulfate from Different Sources of Cartilage. *Chem. Eng. Process. Process Intensif.* **2007**, *46*, 465–471. [CrossRef]
44. Wan, P.; Zhao, Z.; Wang, Q.-Z.; Chen, D.-W. Use of NMR, FTIR and GC–MS to Monitor the Oxidation Products of Phospholipids in Bighead Carp Head during Cooking Process. *J. Food Compos. Anal.* **2024**, *127*, 105984. [CrossRef]
45. Osago, H.; Shibata, T.; Hara, N.; Kuwata, S.; Kono, M.; Uchio, Y.; Tsuchiya, M. Quantitative Analysis of Glycosaminoglycans, Chondroitin/Dermatan Sulfate, Hyaluronic Acid, Heparan Sulfate, and Keratan Sulfate by Liquid Chromatography–Electrospray Ionization–Tandem Mass Spectrometry. *Anal. Biochem.* **2014**, *467*, 62–74. [CrossRef] [PubMed]
46. Uchisawa, H.; Okuzaki, B.; Ichita, J.; Matsue, H. Binding between Calcium Ions and Chondroitin Sulfate Chains of Salmon Nasal Cartilage Glycosaminoglycan. *Int. Congr. Ser.* **2001**, *1223*, 205–220. [CrossRef]
47. López-Senra, E.; Casal-Beiroa, P.; López-Álvarez, M.; Serra, J.; González, P.; Valcarcel, J.; Vázquez, J.A.; Burguera, E.F.; Blanco, F.J.; Magalhães, J. Impact of Prevalence Ratios of Chondroitin Sulfate (CS)-4 and -6 Isomers Derived from Marine Sources in Cell Proliferation and Chondrogenic Differentiation Processes. *Mar. Drugs* **2020**, *18*, 94. [CrossRef] [PubMed]
48. Maherani, B.; Arab-Tehrany, E.; Kheirolomoom, A.; Geny, D.; Linder, M. Calcein Release Behavior from Liposomal Bilayer; Influence of Physicochemical/Mechanical/Structural Properties of Lipids. *Biochimie* **2013**, *95*, 2018–2033. [CrossRef]
49. Molversmyr, E.; Devle, H.M.; Naess-Andresen, C.F.; Ekeberg, D. Identification and Quantification of Lipids in Wild and Farmed Atlantic Salmon (*Salmo salar*), and Salmon Feed by GC-MS. *Food Sci. Nutr.* **2022**, *10*, 3117–3127. [CrossRef]
50. Gbogouri, G.A.; Linder, M.; Fanni, J.; Parmentier, M. Analysis of Lipids Extracted from Salmon (*Salmo salar*) Heads by Commercial Proteolytic Enzymes. *Eur. J. Lipid Sci. Technol.* **2006**, *108*, 766–775. [CrossRef]
51. Hanachi, A.; Bianchi, A.; Kahn, C.J.F.; Velot, E.; Arab-Tehrany, E.; Cakir-Kiefer, C.; Linder, M. Encapsulation of Salmon Peptides in Marine Liposomes: Physico-Chemical Properties, Antiradical Activities and Biocompatibility Assays. *Mar. Drugs* **2022**, *20*, 249. [CrossRef]
52. Zhang, Z.; Ma, L.; Luo, J. Chondroitin Sulfate-Modified Liposomes for Targeted Co-Delivery of Doxorubicin and Retinoic Acid to Suppress Breast Cancer Lung Metastasis. *Pharmaceutics* **2021**, *13*, 406. [CrossRef]
53. Bozzuto, G.; Molinari, A. Liposomes as Nanomedical Devices. *Int. J. Nanomed.* **2015**, *10*, 975–999. [CrossRef]
54. Nguyen, M.; Battistoni, C.M.; Babiak, P.M.; Liu, J.C.; Panitch, A. Chondroitin Sulfate/Hyaluronic Acid-Blended Hydrogels Suppress Chondrocyte Inflammation under Pro-Inflammatory Conditions. *ACS Biomater. Sci. Eng.* **2024**, *10*, 3242–3254. [CrossRef]
55. Bianchi, A.; Moulin, D.; Sebillaud, S.; Koufany, M.; Galteau, M.-M.; Netter, P.; Terlain, B.; Jouzeau, J.-Y. Contrasting Effects of Peroxisome-Proliferator-Activated Receptor (PPAR)γ Agonists on Membrane-Associated Prostaglandin E2 Synthase-1 in IL-1β-Stimulated Rat Chondrocytes: Evidence for PPARγ-Independent Inhibition by 15-Deoxy-Δ12,14prostaglandin J2. *Arthritis Res. Ther.* **2005**, *7*, R1325. [CrossRef] [PubMed]
56. Francis, K.; Zheng, H.; Suskind, D.; Nuding, M.E.; Morton, G.; Schwartz, M.; Alonge, K.; Scarlett, J. Mo2041 Characterizing the Intestinal Chondroitin Sulfate Glycosaminoglycan Sulfation Signatute in Inflammatory Bowel Disease. *Gastroenterology* **2024**, *166*, S-1208. [CrossRef]
57. Li, X.; Zhou, Y.; Chen, X.; Wang, H.; Yang, S.; Yang, J.; Song, Y.; Zhao, Z.; Zhang, H.; Wu, L. Semi-Synthetic Chondroitin Sulfate CS-Semi5 Upregulates miR-122-5p, Conferring a Therapeutic Effect on Osteoarthritis via the P38/MMP13 Pathway. *Acta Pharm. Sin. B* **2024**, *14*, 3528–3542. [CrossRef] [PubMed]
58. Linder, M.; Matouba, E.; Fanni, J.; Parmentier, M. Enrichment of Salmon Oil with N-3 PUFA by Lipolysis, Filtration and Enzymatic Re-Esterification. *Eur. J. Lipid. Sci.* **2002**, *104*, 455–462. [CrossRef]
59. Folch, J.; Lees, M.; Stanley, G.H.S. A Simple Method for The Isolation and Purification of Total Lipides from Animal Tissues. *J. Biol. Chem.* **1957**, *226*, 497–509. [CrossRef]
60. Zhu, Y.; Zheng, X.; Zeng, Q.; Zhong, R.; Guo, Y.; Shi, F.; Liang, P. The Inhibitory Effect of Large Yellow Croaker Roe Phospholipid as a Potential Antioxidant on Fish Oil Oxidation Stability. *Food Biosci.* **2023**, *56*, 103291. [CrossRef]

61. Chihaoui, M.; Lazreg, H.; M'hamed, A.C.; Bouchemal, N.; Chahed, L.; Messaoudi, I.; Majdoub, H.; Laschet, J.; Boisson-Vidal, C.; Mansour, M.B.; et al. Comparative Analysis of Physicochemical Characteristics of Chondroitin Sulfate from Avian Cartilage: Antioxidant, Anti-Inflammatory and Anti-Nociceptive Properties. *Chem. Afr.* **2024**, *7*, 1269–1282. [CrossRef]
62. Takeda-Okuda, N.; Yeon, S.-J.; Matsumi, Y.; Matsuura, Y.; Hosaka, Y.Z.; Tamura, J. Quantitative, Compositional, and Immunohistochemical Analyses of Chondroitin Sulfate, Dermatan Sulfate, and Hyaluronan in Internal Organs of Deer (*Cervus nippon centralis* and *C. n. yesoensis*) and Cattle (*Bos taurus*). *Int. J. Biol. Macromol.* **2024**, *261*, 129680. [CrossRef]
63. Morrison, W.R.; Smith, L.M. Preparation of Fatty Acid Methyl Esters and Dimethylacetals from Lipids with Boron Fluoride-Methanol. *J. Lipid Res.* **1964**, *5*, 600–608. [CrossRef]
64. Kapoor, M.; Martel-Pelletier, J.; Lajeunesse, D.; Pelletier, J.-P.; Fahmi, H. Role of Proinflammatory Cytokines in the Pathophysiology of Osteoarthritis. *Nat. Rev. Rheumatol.* **2011**, *7*, 33–42. [CrossRef]
65. Amin, A.R.; Dave, M.; Attur, M.; Abramson, S.B. COX-2, NO, and Cartilage Damage and Repair. *Curr. Rheumatol. Rep.* **2000**, *2*, 447–453. [CrossRef]
66. Abramson, S.B.; Attur, M.; Amin, A.R.; Clancy, R. Nitric Oxide and Inflammatory Mediators in the Perpetuation of Osteoarthritis. *Curr. Rheumatol. Rep.* **2001**, *3*, 535–541. [CrossRef]

marine drugs

Review

Recent Advances in Anti-Inflammatory Compounds from Marine Microorganisms

Guihua Yang [1,†], Miaoping Lin [1,†], Kumaravel Kaliaperumal [2], Yaqi Lu [1], Xin Qi [1], Xiaodong Jiang [1], Xinya Xu [1], Chenghai Gao [1], Yonghong Liu [1] and Xiaowei Luo [1,*]

[1] Guangxi Key Laboratory of Marine Drugs, Institute of Marine Drugs, Guangxi University of Chinese Medicine, Nanning 530200, China
[2] Unit of Biomaterials Research, Department of Orthodontics, Saveetha Dental College and Hospitals, Saveetha Institute of Medical and Technical Sciences (SIMATS), Saveetha University, Chennai 600077, India
* Correspondence: luoxiaowei1991@126.com
† These authors contributed equally to this work.

Abstract: Marine microbial secondary metabolites with diversified structures have been found as promising sources of anti-inflammatory lead compounds. This review summarizes the sources, chemical structures, and pharmacological properties of anti-inflammatory natural products reported from marine microorganisms in the past three years (2021–2023). Approximately 252 anti-inflammatory compounds, including 129 new ones, were predominantly obtained from marine fungi and they are structurally divided into polyketides (51.2%), terpenoids (21.0%), alkaloids (18.7%), amides or peptides (4.8%), and steroids (4.3%). This review will shed light on the development of marine microbial secondary metabolites as potential anti-inflammatory lead compounds with promising clinical applications in human health.

Keywords: marine microorganisms; secondary metabolites; chemical structures; anti-inflammatory compounds; structure–activity relationship

1. Introduction

Inflammation is a defense reaction caused when the organism is subjected to certain stimuli, such as trauma and infection, which is characterized by malfunction, heat, redness, swelling, and discomfort. Both the natural defense system and inflammatory response have certain advantages for the body. Nevertheless, an excessive inflammatory response tends to damage the tissues of the organism, leading to the development or rapid deterioration of disease [1,2]. If untreated, this may lead to autoimmune or autoimmune inflammatory diseases, neurodegenerative diseases, or even cancer. A series of studies have indicated that inflammation alters the brain's neurotransmitter systems, which in turn modifies motivation-related behaviors and eventually results in a loss of pleasure [3–5]. Inflammation is a key barrier to the treatment of depression and other related mental diseases. It is a typical symptom of mood and anxiety disorders in psychiatric and medical conditions. Currently, the commonly used anti-inflammatory drugs in clinical practice are steroidal and non-steroidal compounds, such as indomethacin, aspirin, prednisolone, dexamethasone, and hydrocortisone [6–8]. Suppressing various related factors shows anti-inflammatory effects, but long-term use can produce various side effects, such as edema and gastrointestinal ulcers [9]. Hence, there is an urgent need to search for structurally new and highly effective anti-inflammatory drugs with low toxicity.

Marine microorganisms are exposed to special living environments of high pressure, dark conditions, high salinity, and a low concentration of oxygen [10]. For better adaptation to this special environment, marine microorganisms have evolved unique metabolic pathways and can produce diverse bioactive metabolites [11]. Marine microorganisms, especially marine fungi, have elicited increasing interest from the marine natural product research community [12–16]. Moreover, a series of structurally diverse secondary metabolites with anti-inflammatory activity have been obtained from marine microorganisms, including peptides, polyketides, phenols, lactones, alkaloids, steroids, and others [17–19]. Among them, cacospongionolide B and petrosaspongiolide M are two representative examples of anti-inflammatory compounds in experimental models of acute or chronic inflammation [20]. It is anticipated that marine microbial natural products would play a promising role in the search for anti-inflammatory lead compounds [21].

In the previous literature, Xu et al. reviewed 133 marine fungi-derived anti-inflammatory compounds in the period from 2000 to 2018, including alkaloids, terpenoids, polyketides, peptides, and others [22]. Souza Cássio, R.M. et al. summarized 41 marine alkaloids with anti-inflammatory activity and gave future perspectives for their investigation and bioprospecting [23]. Since marine microorganisms have been continuously evidenced as rich sources of anti-inflammatory compounds in recent years, this review summarizes the sources, chemical structures, and pharmacological properties of anti-inflammatory natural products recently reported from marine microorganisms during 2021–2023. A total of 252 compounds with anti-inflammatory activity were obtained from marine microorganisms during 2021–2023, including 129 new ones (51.2%). They were mainly isolated from marine fungi (82.9%), along with marine bacteria or marine actinomycetes (17.1%). The structural types of these reviewed compounds are mainly divided into polyketides (51.2%), terpenoids (21.0%), alkaloids (18.7%), amides or peptides (4.8%) and steroids (4.3%), while 8.5% of them are halogenated compounds.

2. Marine Microbial Anti-Inflammatory Compounds

2.1. Polyketides

In total, 129 polyketides with anti-inflammatory activity were obtained from marine microorganisms during 2021–2023.

Four rare chromone derivatives, epiremisporines D (**1**), E (**2**), G (**3**), and H (**4**), were isolated from marine-derived *Penicillium citrinum*, together with two known compounds, epiremisporine B (**5**) and penicitrinone A (**6**) (Figure 1). They significantly decreased *N*-Formyl-Met-Leu-Phe (fMLP)-induced superoxide anion generation by human neutrophils, with IC_{50} values of 6.4 ± 0.4, 8.3 ± 0.3, 31.7 ± 2.5, 33.5 ± 0.4, 3.6 ± 0.6, and 2.7 ± 0.1 μM, respectively [24,25].

Two known compounds, epitetrahydrotrichodimer ether (**7**) and tetrahydrotrichodimerol (**8**), were isolated and identified from the rhizosphere soil of *Hibiscus tiliaceus* Linn.-derived fungus *Penicillium* sp. DM 815. They inhibited the Gram-negative bacteria lipopolysaccharide (LPS)-induced upregulation of the inducible nitric oxide (NO) synthase (iNOS) at a concentration of 10 μM [26].

A new polyketide, 4-carboxy-5-((1*Z*,3*E*)-1,3-heptadien1-yl)-1,3-benzenediol (**9**), was obtained from the hydrothermal vent-derived fungus *Penicillium* sp. TW58-16. It markedly reduced the amount of NO released in RAW 264.7 cells upon exposure to LPS, which was consistent with a decrease in the production of inducible NO synthase (iNOS) at a concentration of 20 μM [27].

The chemical investigation of the fungus *Fusarium decemcellulare* SYSU-MS 6716 derived from a solid medium yielded two new polypropionate derivatives, decempyrones C (**10**) and J (**11**). Both demonstrated strong anti-inflammatory efficacy with IC_{50} values of 22.4 ± 1.8 and 21.7 ± 1.1 μM, respectively, by preventing LPS-induced NO generation in RAW 264.7 cells. Primary structure-activity relationships (SAR) analysis revealed that the alkyl side chain and pyrone functional groups are mainly responsible for the anti-inflammatory properties [28].

Two new compounds, heterocornols T (**12**) and X (**13**), were produced by the sponge-derived fungus *Pestalotiopsis heterocornis* XWS03F09 based on the one strain many compounds (OSMAC) approach. Both could reduce the amount of NO produced in response to

LPS, which further significantly and dose-dependently reduced the expression of the iNOS protein in LPS-induced RAW 264.7 cells with 33 μM [29].

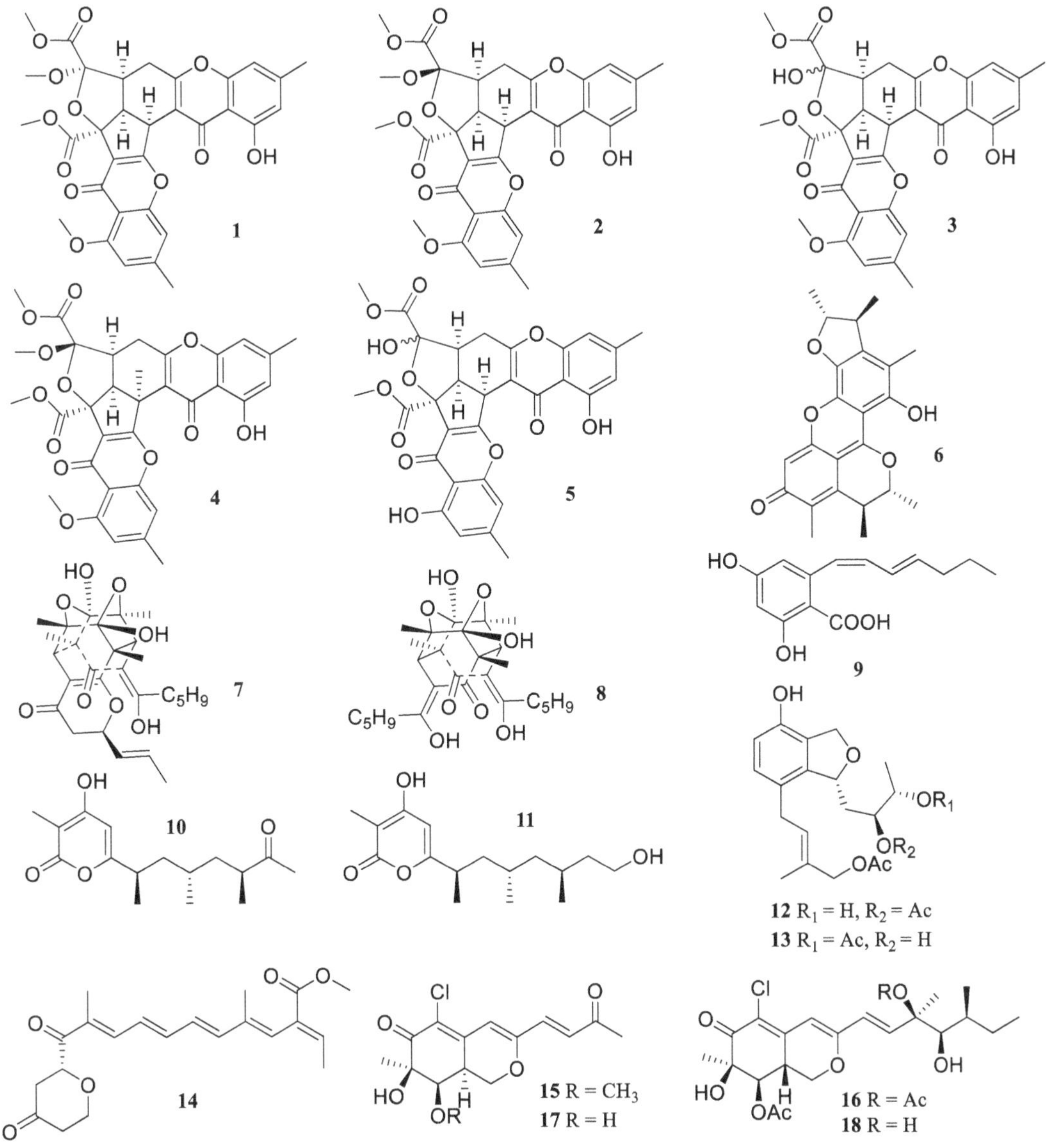

Figure 1. Chemical structures of polyketides (**1–18**).

A chemical investigation of the seawater-derived fungus *Fusarium solani* 7227 yielded one new fusarin derivative, fusarin K (**14**). It exhibited strong anti-inflammatory activity (IC_{50} = 21.9 ± 9.8 μM) by preventing the generation of NO in RAW 264.7 cells that had been stimulated by LPS. The preliminary SAR study showed that the substituent group in polyunsaturated chain is primarily responsible for the anti-inflammatory properties [30].

The chemical study of the sponge-derived fungus *Penicillium sclerotiorum* E23Y-1A resulted in the isolation of two new azaphilones, penicilazaphilones F (**15**) and G (**16**), as well as two known analogs, hypocrellone A (**17**) and penicillazaphilone D (**18**). They reduced the LPS-induced NO generation in BV2 cells with IC_{50} values of 31.7 ± 1.5, 34.5 ± 1.4, 25.3 ± 2.2, and 34.8 ± 1.9 μM, respectively [31].

One new compound, saccharothrixin G (**19**) (Figure 2), was obtained from the deep-sea sediment-derived fungus *Saccharothrix* sp. D09, which revealed inhibition on the production of NO with an IC_{50} value of 28 μM [32].

Two known metabolites, (+)-terrein (**20**) and butyrolactone I (**21**), were isolated and identified from a mangrove plant *Acanthus ilicifolius*-derived fungus, *Aspergillus flavipes* (MTCC 5220), which was collected from Goa, India. Both presented inhibitory activities of interleukine-6 (IL-6) and tumor necrosis factor-*α* (TNF-*α*) with IC_{50} values of 8.5 ± 0.7, 15.8 ± 0.2, 12.0 ± 0.9, and 43.3 ± 0.8 μM, respectively, whereas **21** demonstrated low toxicity to host cells in LPS-stimulated THP-1 cells [33]. Moreover, compound **21** showed noteworthy activity by blocking the release of neutrophil elastase with an IC_{50} value of 2.3 ± 0.3 μM, which was isolated from the annelid *Spirorbis* sp.-derived fungus *Aspergillus terreus* MT 273950 [34].

The chemical study of the alga-derived fungus *Penicillium sclerotiorum* AI-27 yielded one new azaphilone, 8a-*epi*-hypocrellone A (**22**), as well as two known azaphilones, hypocrellone A (**23**) and isochromophilone IV (**24**). They inhibited the TNF-*α*-induced nuclear factor-*κ*B (NF-*κ*B) phosphorylation but without changing the NF-*κ*B activity at a concentration of 20 μM [35]. Two known azaphilone derivatives, compounds **24** and WB (**25**), were produced by co-culturing the mangrove endophytic fungus *P. sclerotiorum* THSH-4 with *P. sclerotiorum* ZJHJJ-18 in PDB medium. When compared to the positive control, indomethacin (IC_{50} = 35.3 μM), both showed a stronger suppression of LPS-induced NO release from RAW 264.7 with IC_{50} values of 17.6 and 4.7 μM, respectively, without clearly deleterious effects within 50 μM [36].

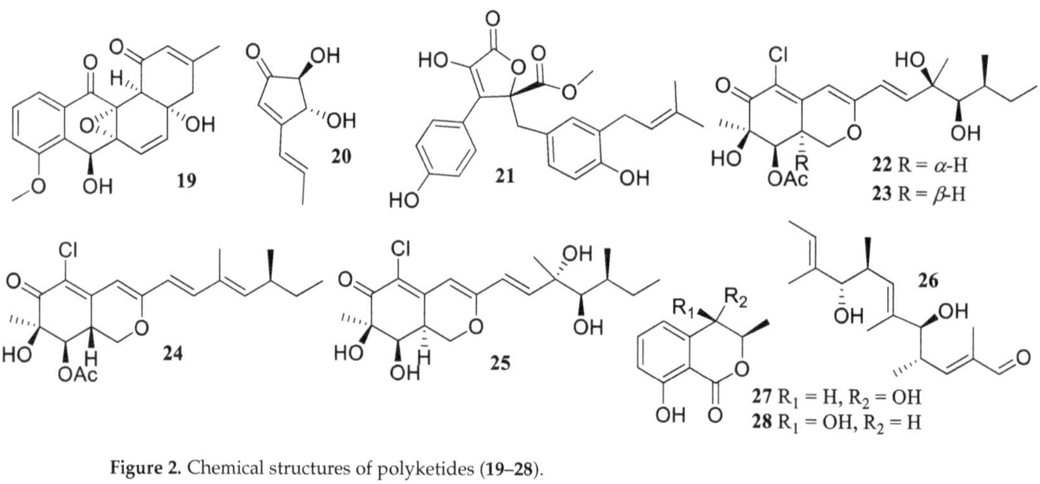

Figure 2. Chemical structures of polyketides (**19–28**).

Three known metabolites, 5,9-dihydroxy-2,4,6,8,10-pentamethyldodeca-2,6,10-trienal (**26**), (3*R*, 4*S*)-(−)-4-hydroxymellein (**27**), and (3*R*, 4*R*)-(−)-4-hydroxymellein (**28**), were isolated from the alga *Hypnea pannosa*-derived fungus *Aspergillus ochraceopetaliformis* SCSIO 41020. They illustrated a dose-dependent inhibitory effect against the excessive generation of NO and pro-inflammatory cytokines in LPS-treated RAW 264.7 macrophages without cytotoxicity at a concentration of 10 μM. Moreover, compound **28** inhibited the release of pro-inflammatory cytokines (IL-6, MCP-1, and TNF-*α*) when LPS was applied in both in vitro and in vivo settings [37].

Six known xanthone dimeric analogs were obtained from the ascidian *Styela plicata*-derived fungus *Diaporthe* sp. SYSU-MS 4722, which were 12-deacetylphomoxanthone A

(**29**), phomoxanthones A (**30**) and B (**31**), dicerandrols B (**32**) and C (**33**), and deacetylphomoxanthone B (**34**) (Figure 3). They indicated anti-inflammatory activity with IC_{50} values ranging from 6.3 to 8.0 μM, which suppressed toward NO generation in LPS-induced RAW 264.7 [38].

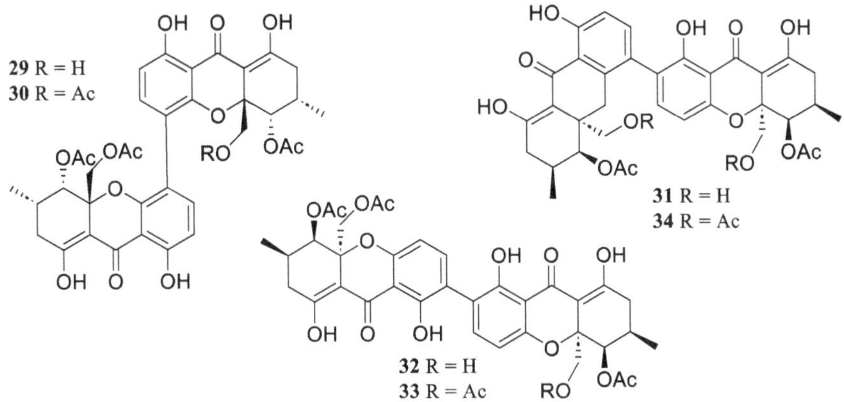

Figure 3. Chemical structures of polyketides (**29–34**).

The fungus *Talaromyces helicus* SCSIO 41311, which is derived from cold seeps in the South China Sea, was shown to contain two distinct compounds, trypacidin (**35**) and fumiquinone B (**36**) (Figure 4). They displayed NO inhibitions with IC_{50} values of 38.6 and 15.5 μM, respectively. Interestingly, compound **36** showed a greater inhibitory effect of NO compared to the positive control, eicosapentaenoic acid (IC_{50} = 50.0 μM) [39].

The chemical investigation of marine sediment-derived actinomyces *Streptomyces* sp. 13G036 yielded six known butenolides, (4*S*)-4,10-dihydroxy-10-methyl-11-oxo-dodec-2-en-1,4-olide (**37**), (4*S*)-4,10-dihydroxy-10-methyl-undec-2-en-1,4-olide (**38**), (4*S*)-4,10-dihydroxy-10-methyl-dodec-2-en-1, 4-olide (**39**), (4*S*,10*R*,11*S*)-4,11-dihydroxy-10-methyl-dodec-2-en-1,4-olide (**40**), (4*S*)-4-hydroxy-10-methyl-11-oxo-dodec-2-en-1,4-olide (**41**), and (4*S*,10*S*,11*S*)-4,10,11-trihydroxy-10-methyl-dodec-2-en-1,4-olide (**42**). They showed anti-inflammatory properties by preventing the generation of NO, TNF-α, and IL-6 in LPS-stimulated macrophages at a concentration of 10 μM [40].

One new compound, aspulvinone V (**43**), together with two known compounds, (+)-terrein (**20**) and butyrolactone I (**21**), were isolated and identified from a marine green alga *Ulva lactuca* L.-derived fungus, *Aspergillus terreus* Thom (Trichocomaceae) strain NTU 243, that was collected from Taiwan's northeast coast. By quantifying the quantity of NO generation in LPS-induced BV2 cells, all isolates were evaluated for their anti-inflammatory action. At a dosage of 10 μM, the isolates showed inhibition rates of 45.0%, 49.2%, and 34.5%, respectively [41].

Saadamysin (**44**) was characterized from the coral-associated *Aspergillus flavus* GXIMD 02503, which demonstrated moderate inhibitory actions of NF-κB activation with an IC_{50} value of 10.7 ± 1.3 μM [42]. The chemical investigation of the sponge-derived fungus *Pestalotiopsis* sp. SWMU-WZ04-2 yielded two new compounds, pestaloketides A (**45**) and B (**46**). Both reduced the activity of NO generation produced by LPS with IC_{50} values of 23.6 and 14.5 μM, respectively, without observed cytotoxicity [43].

Two known compounds, isorhodoptilometrin (**47**) and 5-hydroxy-7-(2′-hydroxypropyl)-2-methyl-chromone (**48**), were discovered from the sponge-derived fungus *Penicillium oxalicum* CLC-MF 05. These compounds inhibited the overproduction of NO and prostaglandin E2 (PGE_2), as well as the overexpression of iNOS and cyclooxygenase-2 (COX-2) in both LPS-stimulated BV2 and rat primary microglia [44].

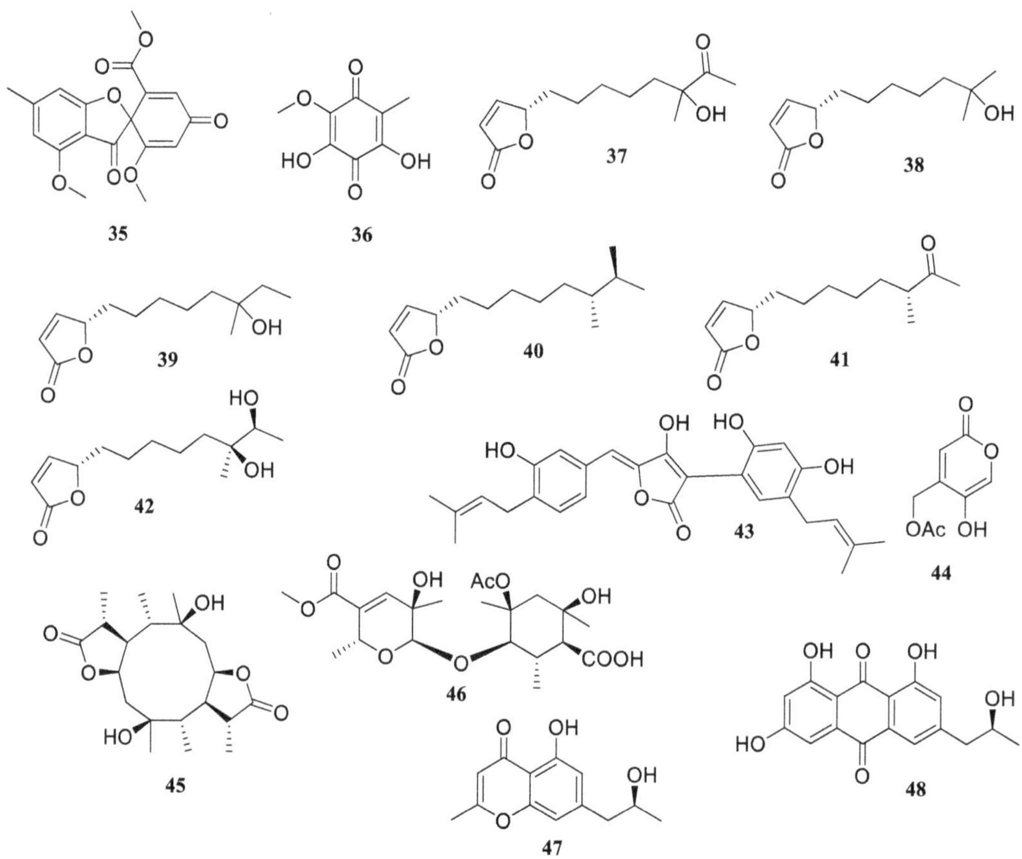

Figure 4. Chemical structures of polyketides (**35**–**48**).

The soft coral-associated fungus *Aspergillus* sp. SCSIO 41036 was the source of one known compound, penicillixanthone A (**49**) (Figure 5). It exhibited an inhibitory effect against NO induced by LPS in RAW 264.7 cells at a dosage of 10 μM [45]. The chemical investigation of *Stratomyces specialis* 208DD-067, an actinomycete obtained from sediment, yielded four new streptoglycerides E–H (**50**–**53**) with a unique 6/5/5/-membered ring structure. They demonstrated strong anti-inflammatory efficacy with IC_{50} values of 10.9, 5.9, 4.7, and 3.5 μM, respectively, in suppressing LPS-induced NO generation in RAW 264.7 cells [46].

A chemical investigation of the mangrove endophytic fungus *Daldinia eschscholtzii* KBJYZ-1 yielded two new polyketides, eschscholin B (**54**) and daldilene A (**55**). They exhibited noteworthy anti-inflammatory properties, with IC_{50} values of 19.3 and 12.9 μM, respectively. Furthermore, compound **54** reduced the expression of COX-2 and iNOS in RAW 264.7 cells that had been exposed to LPS. Further molecular biology study revealed the potential mechanism of compound **54**'s anti-inflammatory function by inactivating the MAPK and NF-κB signaling pathways [47].

The chemical investigation of marine ascidian-derived fungus *Amphichorda felina* SYSU-MS 7908 resulted in the isolation of two new α-pyrone derivatives, amphichopyrones A (**56**) and B (**57**). Both displayed potent anti-inflammatory activity by inhibiting the production of NO in RAW 264.7 cells with IC_{50} values 18.1 ± 4.8 and 7.2 ± 0.9 μM, respectively [48].

Two known polyketides, nectriapyrone (**58**) and monodictyphenone (**59**), were also obtained from marine ascidian-derived *Diaporthe* sp. SYSU-MS 4722. Both indicated anti-inflammatory efficacy by preventing LPS-induced NO production with IC_{50} values of 35.4 and 40.8 μM, respectively (IC_{50} = 35.8 μM for the positive control, indomethacin) [49].

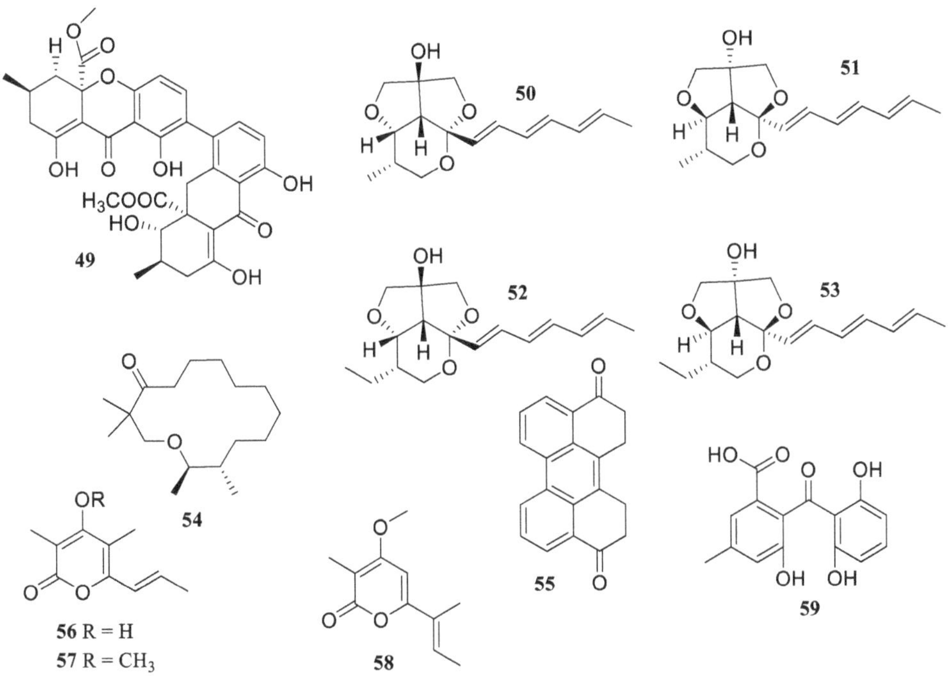

Figure 5. Chemical structures of polyketides (**49–59**).

The chemical investigation of the Beibu Gulf coral-derived fungus *Aspergillus unguis* GXIMD 02505 yielded a new depsidone derivative, aspergillusidone H (**60**), and six known biosynthetically related chlorinated polyketides: aspergillus ethers J (**61**) and F (**62**), nornidulin (**63**), aspergillusidone B (**64**), guisinol (**65**), and 1-(2,6-dihydroxy-4-methoxy-3,5-dimethylphenyl)-2-methylbutan-1-one (**66**) (Figure 6). They demonstrated suppression of LPS-induced NF-κB in RAW 264.7 macrophages at a concentration of 20 μM. Furthermore, the two potent inhibitors (**62** and **65**) dose-dependently reduced the receptor activator of NF-κB ligand (RANKL)-induced osteoclast differentiation in bone marrow macrophage cells (BMMs) without obvious cytotoxicity [50].

The chemical examination of the marine-derived fungal species *Eutypella scoparia* yielded two known compounds, 4,8-dihydroxy-6-methoxy-4,5-dimethyl-3-methyleneisochroman-1-one (**67**) and banksialactone A (**68**). Both illustrated anti-inflammatory properties by inhibiting LPS-induced NO generation in RAW 264.7 macrophages, with inhibition rates of 49.0% and 54.9% at 50.0 μg/mL, respectively [51].

A new indanone derivative, streptinone (**69**), was isolated and identified from a marine sediment-derived *Streptomyces massiliensis* 213DD-128, which suppressed the production of NO, PGE_2, and pro-inflammatory cytokines, such as TNF-α, IL-6, and interleukin-1 beta (IL-1β), by inhibiting the TLR-mediated NF-κB signaling pathway at a concentration of over 5 μM [52].

Secondary metabolites of a deep-sea sediment sample-derived fungus, *Phomopsis lithocarpus* FS 508, were investigated, including three known compounds, lithocarol F (**70**), isoprenylisobenzo-furan A (**71**), and anhydromevalonolactone (**72**). They showed significant anti-inflammatory activities on LPS-induced NO production in RAW 264.7 macrophages, with IC_{50} values of 22.8, 27.2, and 24.1 μM, respectively, all of which were superior to the positive control, indometacin (IC_{50} = 32.9 μM) [53].

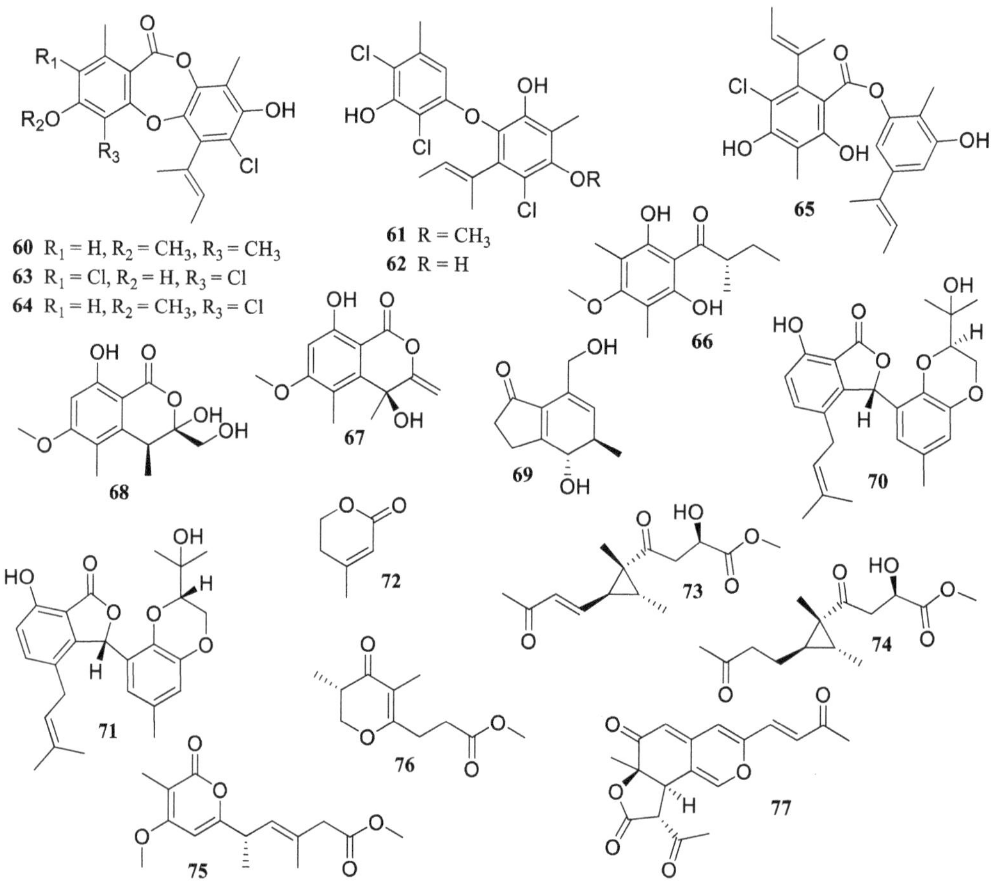

Figure 6. Chemical structures of polyketides (**60**–**77**).

The chemical investigation of *Stragonospora* sp. SYSU-MS 7888, a fungus originating from sponges in the South China Sea, provided two new cyclopropane derivatives, stagonospones A (**73**) and B (**74**), and two new α-pyrone derivatives, stapyrones E (**75**) and G (**76**). They displayed considerable anti-inflammatory efficacy by suppressing LPS-induced NO generation with IC_{50} values of 3.6 ± 1.0, 9.4 ± 1.8, 21.9 ± 3.5, and 22.8 ± 3.9 μM, respectively, surpassing that of the positive control, indomethacin (IC_{50} = 26.5 ± 1.1 μM). The double bond at C-3 in the family of cyclopropane diones may increase cytotoxicity and thereby boost anti-inflammatory efficacy. Meanwhile, the anti-inflammatory properties of pyrones were dependent on the side chain length and ketone position [54].

One new azaphilone, penicilazaphilone N (**77**), was produced by the sponge-derived fungus *Penicillium sclerotiorum* E23Y-1A. It presented moderate anti-inflammatory efficacy by preventing LPS-induced NO production with an IC_{50} value of 22.6 ± 3.0 μM [55].

One new propenylphenol derivate, chlomophenol A (**78**), together with six known compounds, 7-chloro-3,4-dihydro-6,8-dihydroxy-3-methylisocoumarine (**79**), α-acetylorcinol (**80**), (*S*)-5,7-dichloro-6-methoxy-2-methyl-2,3-dihydrobenzofuran-4-carboxylic acid (**81**), 5-chloro-6-hydroxymellein (**82**), 3-methyl-6-hydroxy-8-methoxy-3,4-dihydroisocoumarin

(**83**), and kojic acid (**84**) (Figure 7), were obtained from a mangrove-endophytic fungus *Amorosia* sp. SCSIO 41026. They showed inhibitory effects on the overproduction of NO and pro-inflammatory cytokines in LPS-induced RAW 264.7 macrophages without cytotoxicity at a concentration of 10 μM [56].

Two new chlorinated orsellinic aldehyde derivatives, orsaldechlorins A (**85**) and B (**86**), as well as seven known analogs, ethyl orsellinate (**87**), 5-chloroorsellinic acid (**88**), orcinol (**89**), *O*-methylorcinol (**90**), aryl bromide (**91**), ethyl 4-hydroxyphenylacetate (**92**), and nectriatone C (**93**), were identified from the Beibu Gulf coral-derived fungus *Acremonium sclerotigenum* GXIMD 02501. They displayed suppression of NF-κB activation triggered by LPS in RAW 264.7 cells at the dosage of 20 μM. Additionally, the two new potent inhibitors (**85** and **86**) inhibited RANKL-induced osteoclast differentiation in BMMs without cytotoxicity [57].

The chemical investigation of the mangrove-derived fungus *Diaporthe* sp. XW12–1 resulted in the isolation of two new chromone compounds, diaporspchromanones B (**94**) and C (**95**). Both demonstrated anti-inflammatory activity by inhibiting LPS-induced NO production with IC_{50} values of 19.1 ± 3.6 and 9.6 ± 0.2 μM, respectively, which were stronger than that of the positive control, indomethacin (IC_{50} = 70.3 ± 1.0 μM) [58].

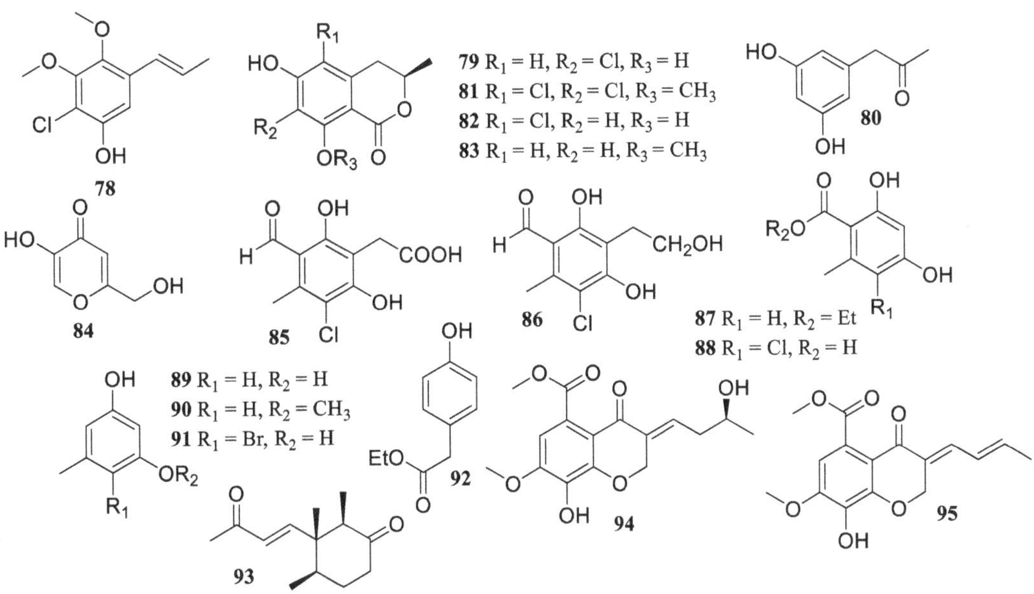

Figure 7. Chemical structures of polyketides (**78**–**95**).

The fungus *Streptomyces* sp. DS-27 was originated from the rhizosphere of marine cordgrass *Spartina alterniflora*. The chemical investigation of its cultures produced two new compounds, streptothiomycin E (**96**) and *S*-methyl (4*R*,5*S*)-2,3-dimethyl-4-hydroxy-4-isopropyl-1-oxocyclopent-3-ene-5-carbothioate (**97**) (Figure 8). Both showed potential anti-inflammatory effects by reducing NO concentration levels in a dose-dependent manner (ranging from 2.5 to 40 μM) [59].

The sediment-derived *Streptomyces* sp. ZSN 77 was found to contain four new compounds, suncheonosides E (**98**), F (**99**), J (**100**), and *S*-methyl 4-hydroxy-6-isopropyl-2-methoxy-3,5-dimethylbenzothioate (**101**), along with one known compound, *S*-methyl 2,4-dihydroxy-6-isopropyl-3,5-dimethylbenzothioate (**102**). They exhibited in vivo anti-inflammatory activity through the suppression of NO generation. Compound pretreatment resulted in a dose-dependent (ranging from 2.5 to 10 μM) significant reduction in the concentration of NO [60].

Neofusicoccum parvum Y2NBKZG 1016, a fungus derived from the fruits of mangrove plant *Sonneratia glauca*, produced a new compound, (4*S*,5*S*,6*S*,7*R*)-4-(3-chloro-1,2-dihydroxybutyl)-butyrolactone (**103**). It presented a minimal anti-inflammatory effect at doses ≥6.3 μM, attaining a maximum inhibition rate of 28.9% without causing cytotoxicity against RAW 264.7 cells [61].

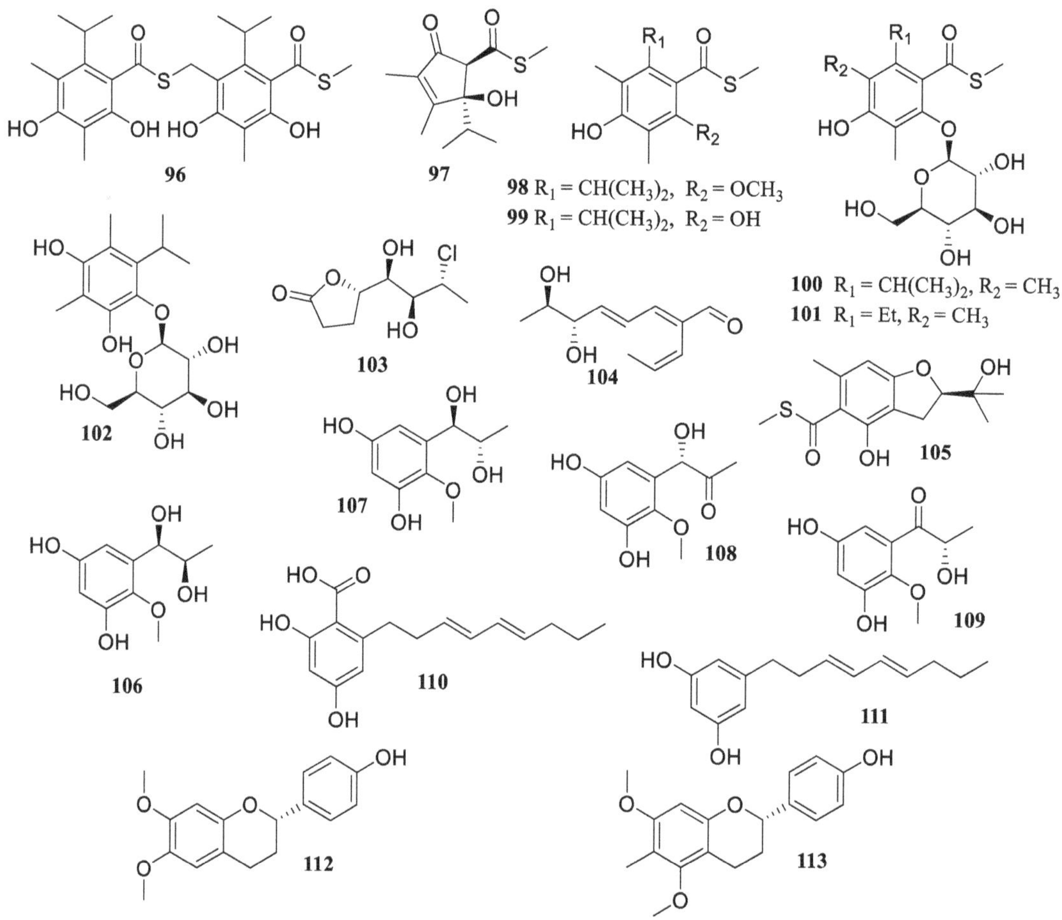

Figure 8. Chemical structures of polyketides (**96–113**).

The chemical examination of the seaweed *Caulerpa* sp.-derived fungus *Talaromyces cyanescens* yielded one new compound, talacyanol B (**104**), and one known polyene molecule, eurothiocin A (**105**). Both reduced the generation of NO and the expression of COX-2 and iNOS in BV2 cells that were triggered by LPS at concentrations of 50, 100, and 200 μM, respectively [62].

Four new phenolic compounds, asperpropanols A–D (**106–109**), and two known congeners, 2,4-dihydroxy-6-((3*E*,5*E*)-nona-3,5-dien-1-yl)-benzoic acid (**110**) and 5-[(3*E*,5*E*)-3,5-nonadienyl]-1,3-benzenediol (**111**), were discovered from the deep-sea sediment-derived fungus *Aspergillus puniceus* SRRC 2155. They showed anti-inflammatory effect on LPS-induced RAW 264.7 cells by reducing the generation of NO, TNF-α, and IL-6 at a dosage of 20 μM [63].

The chemical investigation of the mangrove soil-derived *Isoptericola chiayiensis* BCRC 16888 yielded two new flavonoids, chiayiflavans D (**112**) and E (**113**). Both exhibited stronger NO inhibitory activity than that of the positive control, quercetin (IC_{50} = 37.0 μM), with IC_{50} values of 17.1 and 9.4 μM, respectively [64].

One new α-pyrone derivatives, diaporpyrone A (**114**), was isolated from cultures of the mangrove endophytic fungus *Diaporthe* sp. QYM 12 (Figure 9). It inhibited the production of NO in LPS-induced RAW 264.7 cells with an IC_{50} value of 12.5 μM [65]. The chemical examination of the Antarctic fungi *Pleosporales* sp. SF-7343 revealed one known fungal metabolite, alternariol (**115**). It inhibited the secretion of interleukin-8 and -6 in TNF-α/interferon-γ-treated HaCaT cells at concentrations of 2.5 to 10.0 μM [66].

Three new compounds, guhypoxylonols A (**116**), C (**117**), and D (**118**), were isolated from the mangrove endophytic fungus *Aspergillus* sp. GXNU-Y45, together with one previously reported metabolite, hypoxylonol B (**119**). They presented inhibitory activity against the production of NO, with IC_{50} values of 14.4 ± 0.1, 18.0 ± 0.1, 16.7 ± 0.2, and 21.1 ± 0.1 μM, respectively [67].

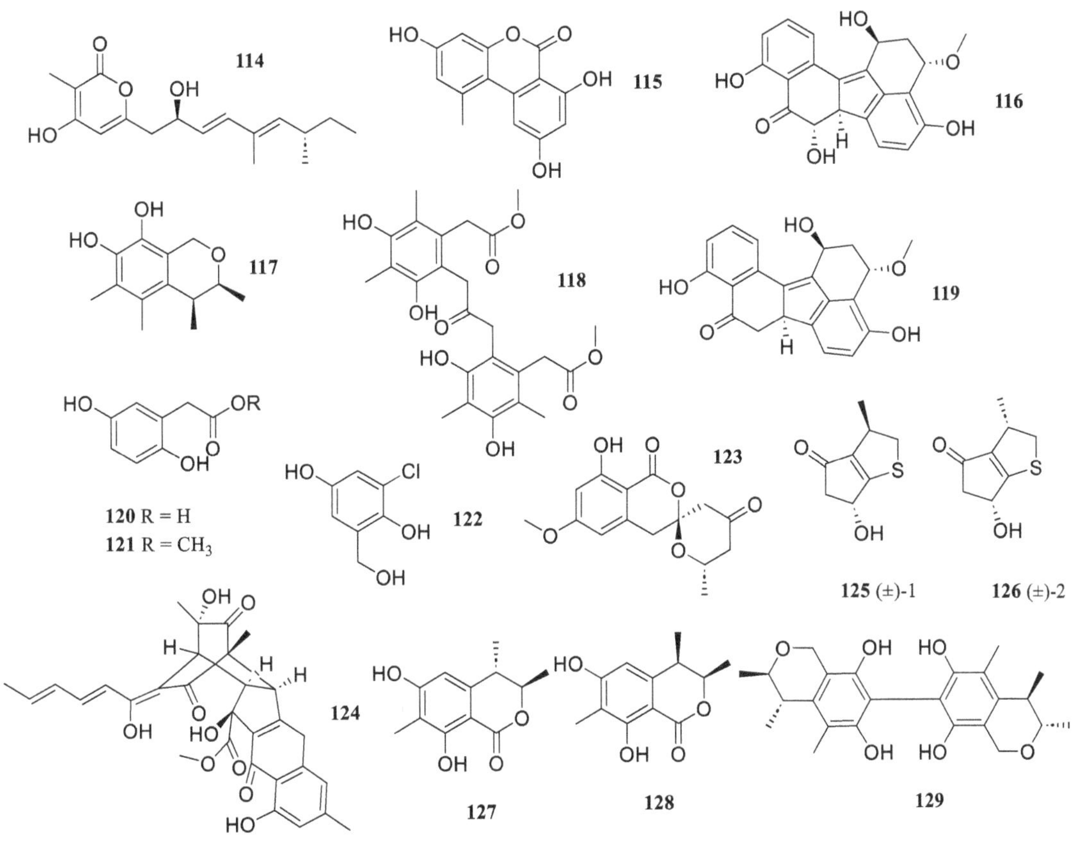

Figure 9. Chemical structures of polyketides (**114–129**).

The chemical investigation of the marine sponge-derived fungal strain *Aspergillus* sp. IMBC-FP2.05 resulted in the isolation of three compounds, namely, homogentisic acid (**120**), methyl (2,5-dihydroxyphenyl) acetate (**121**), and 3-chloro-2,5-dihydroxybenzyl alcohol (**122**). They demonstrated the most inhibitory effects against NO overproduction, with IC_{50} values of 28.2, 14.2, and 41.8 μM, respectively, which was comparable with that of the positive control, N^G-Monomethyl-L-arginine (L-NMMA) (IC_{50} = 44.5 μM) [68].

One new unique isocoumarin, penicillol B (**123**), was isolated from the mangrove endophytic fungus *Penicillium* sp. BJR-P2. It inhibited LPS-induced NO production in RAW 264.7 cells, with an IC_{50} value of 12.0 μM, which was more potent than that of the positive control, indomethacin (IC_{50} = 35.8 ± 5.7 μM). A docking study revealed that it was perfectly docking into the active site of murine inducible NO oxygenase (iNOS) by forming multiple typical hydrogen bonds [69].

Guided by MS/MS-based molecular networking, bisorbicillchaetone B (**124**), a new hybrid sorbicillinoid, was isolated from cultures of the sediment-derived fungus *Penicillium* sp. SCSIO 06868. It exhibited inhibitory effect on NO production in LPS-activated RAW 264.7 cells with an IC_{50} value of 38.4 ± 3.3 μM, without cytotoxicity observed [70].

Ochrathinols A (**125**) and B (**126**), two new sulfur-containing racemates, were isolated from an Antarctic soil-derived fungus, *Aspergillus ochraceopetaliformis* SCSIO 05702. They were obtained as unprecedented sulfur natural products featuring a novel 3-methylhexahydro-2H-cyclopenta [*b*]thiophene core, which suppressed the release of LPS-induced IL-1*β*, IL-6, and TNF-*α* inflammatory cytokines at a concentration of 10.0 μM and alleviated the unbalanced NAD^+/NADH ratio caused by LPS in RAW 264.7 macrophages [71].

Three known compounds, (3*R**,4*S**)-6,8-dihydroxy-3,4,7-trimethylisocoumarin (**127**), sclerotinin C (**128**), and asperbiphenyl (**129**), were isolated from the sediment-derived *Penicillium citrinum* W 17. They exhibited significant inhibitory effects on LPS-stimulated NO production in murine brain microglial BV2 cells in a dose-dependent manner under concentrations of 2.5, 5.0, and 10.0 μM, respectively [72].

2.2. Terpenoids

In total, 53 terpenoids with anti-inflammatory activity were obtained from marine microorganisms during 2021–2023, comprising 29 sesquiterpenes, 4 diterpene, 15 triterpenoids, and 5 meroterpenoids.

2.2.1. Sesquiterpenes

The chemical investigation of the deep-sea sediment-derived fungus *Spiromastix* sp. MCCC 3A00308 yielded three new sesquiterpenes, spiromaterpenes D–F (**130–132**) (Figure 10). The NO production on LPS-induced microglia cells BV2 was significantly inhibited by them, with IC_{50} values of 26 ± 2, 9 ± 1, and 20 ± 1 μM, respectively. The preliminary SAR analyses demonstrated that compound **131** with a 2,11-diol significantly increased the inhibitory effect [73].

A known sesquiterpene, decumbenone A (**133**), was obtained from the Indian Ocean 30 m deep water-derived fungus *Aspergillus austroafricanus* Y32-2, which was found to exhibit a dose-dependent anti-inflammatory activity at concentrations of 30 to 120 μg/mL, by using a zebrafish inflammation model caused by copper sulfate [74].

Five new sesquiterpenes, paraconulones B–E (**134–137**) and G (**138**), along with a known sesquiterpene, 4-*epi*-microsphaeropsisin (**139**), were isolated and identified from coastal sediment-derived from *Paraconiothyrium sporulosum* DL-16. They showed inhibitory effects on LPS-induced NO production in BV2 cells with IC_{50} values of 6.9 ± 2.6, 7.7 ± 2.0, 2.8 ± 0.5, 8.1 ± 2.9, 8.1 ± 3.5, and 4.6 ± 3.5 μM, respectively, which were comparable to the positive control, curcumin (IC_{50} = 8.6 ± 1.6 μM) [75].

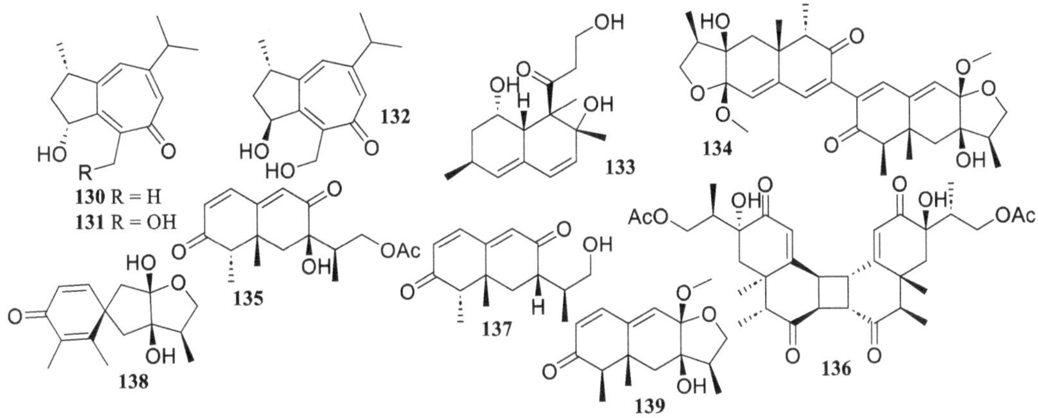

Figure 10. Chemical structures of sesquiterpenoids (**130–139**).

The chemical examination of the deep-sea sediment-derived fungus *Eutypella* sp. MCCC 3A00281 resulted in the isolation of eight sesquiterpenes, including six new ones, eutypeterpenes B (**140**) and C (**141**), eutypeterpene M (**142**), eutypeterpene N (**143**), and eutypeterpenes P (**144**) and Q (**145**), and two known ones, eudesma-3-en-11,15-diol (**146**) and eudesma-4-en-11,15-diol (**147**) (Figure 11). They illustrated inhibitory effects on LPS-induced NO production in RAW 264.7 macrophages with IC_{50} values of 13.4 ± 0.8, 16.8 ± 1.0, 11.8 ± 1.0, 8.6 ± 1.0, 14.3 ± 1.1, 11.5 ± 1.2, 18.3 ± 1.0, and 17.1 ± 1.0 μM, respectively. In addition, compounds **140–145** demonstrated stronger activity than that of quercetin (IC_{50} = 17 ± 1.5 μM) [76].

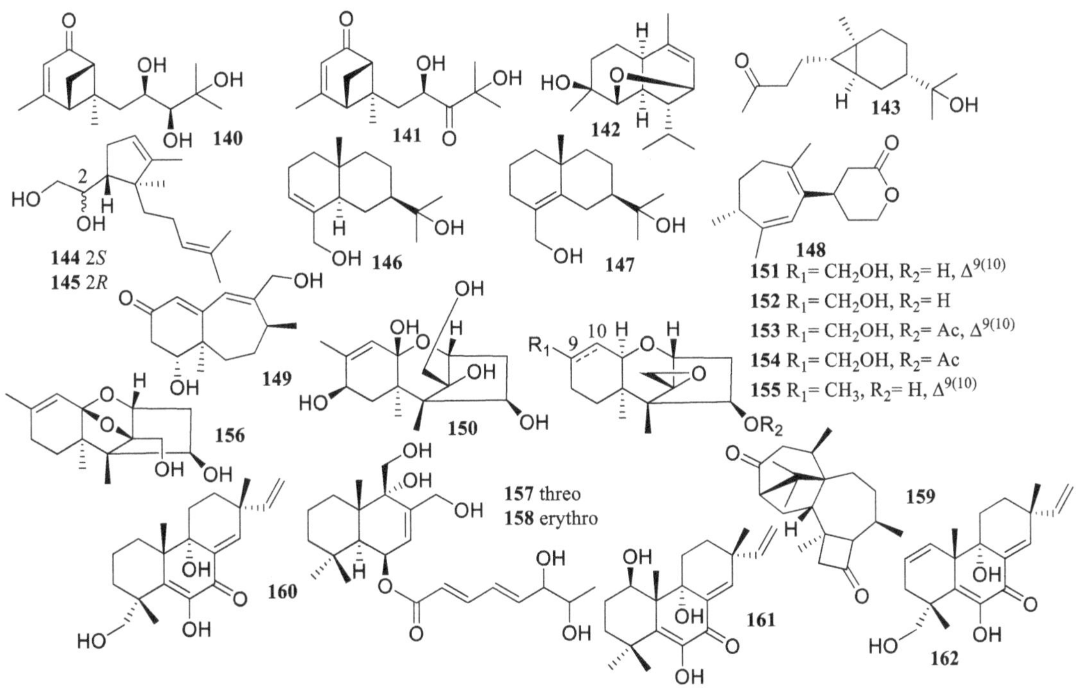

Figure 11. Chemical structures of sesquiterpenoids and diterpene (**140–162**).

Two new sesquiterpenoids, nigerin (**148**) and ochracene J (**149**), were obtained from the South China Sea sponge *Dysidea* sp. symbiotic fungus *Aspergillus niger*. Both exhibited strong inhibitory effects on the generation of NO in LPS-stimulated RAW 264.7 macrophages with IC_{50} values of 8.5 and 4.6 μM, respectively [77].

Seven trichothecenes, including three new compounds, (2*R*,4*R*,5*S*,5a*R*,7*R*,9a*S*,10*S*)-10-(hydroxymethyl)-5,5a,8-trimethyl-3,4,5,5a,6,7-hexahydro-2,5-methanobenzo[*b*]oxepine-4,7,9a,10(2*H*)-tetraol (**150**), (2*S*,2′*R*,4′*R*,5′*S*,5a′*R*,9a′*R*)-8′-(hydroxymethyl)-5′,5a′-dimethyl-2′,3′,4′,5′,5a′,6′,7′,9a′-octahydrospiro[oxirane-2,10′-[2,5] methanobenzo[*b*]oxepin]-4′-ol (**151**), and (2*S*,2′*R*,4′*R*,5′*S*,5a′*R*,9a′*R*)-8′-(hydroxymethyl)-5′,5a′-dimethyldecahydrospiro[oxirane-2,10′-[2,5]methanobenzo[*b*]oxepin]-4′-ol (**152**), and four known ones, trichoderminol (**153**), trichodermarins A (**154**) and E (**155**), and trichodermol (**156**), were isolated from marine alga *Mastophora rosea*-derived fungus *Trichoderma brevicompactum* NTU 439. Compounds **150–154** and **156** displayed minimal inhibitory effects against BV2 cells without cytotoxicity at a dosage of 10 μM. Additionally, compound **159** showed a substantial inhibitory effect on the generation of NO caused by LPS with an IC_{50} value of 5.2 ± 0.4 μM [78].

Meanwhile, two new drimane sesquiterpenes, ustusolates H (**157**) and I (**158**), were isolated from a seagrass-derived fungus, *Aspergillus insuetus* SYSU 6925. Both exhibited a potent inhibition of NO production in RAW 264.7 cells with IC_{50} values of 21.5 ± 1.1, and 32.6 ± 1.2 μM, respectively [79].

2.2.2. Diterpene

A known compound, hazianol J (**159**), was obtained from the deep-sea sediment-derived fungus *Trichoderma* sp. SCSIOW 21, which showed anti-inflammatory activity at 100 μM with a NO inhibition rate of 81.8% [80].

The chemical examination of the fermentation broth of *Eutypella* sp. D-1, using the OSMAC strategy of adding ethanol as a promoter in the culture medium, resulted in the isolation of one new compound, libertellenone Z (**160**), and two known compounds, libertellenones A (**161**) and C (**162**). They exhibited strong NO inhibition rates of 60.9%, 89.4%, and 84.2% at 10.0 μM, respectively, while the latter two were superior to the effect of the positive drug dexamethasone with rates of 72.0% at 10.0 μM [81].

2.2.3. Triterpenoids

Three new compounds, peniscmeroterpenoids A (**163**), D (**164**), and L (**165**), were isolated from the marine-derived fungus *Penicillium sclerotiorum* GZU-XW03-2 (Figure 12), which inhibited the production of NO in RAW 264.7 cells with IC_{50} values of 26.6 ± 1.2, 8.8 ± 1.2, and 48.0 ± 2.5 μM, respectively. Moreover, compound **164** further significantly suppressed the production of pro-inflammatory mediators, tumor necrosis COX-2, IL-1*β*, and IL-6 and the protein expression of the enzyme iNOS [82,83].

Moreover, soyasapogenols B1–B11(**166–176**) were identified from marine actinomycete *Nonomuraea* sp. MYH 522. These compounds presented anti-inflammatory effects in DMXAA-stimulated RAW 264.7 cells by suppressing the STING/TBK1/NF-*κ*B pathway at a concentration of 20 μM [84].

The chemical investigation of the alga-derived fungus *Turbinaria decurrens* yielded one new compound, decurrencyclic B (**177**). It showed superior attenuation properties against COX-2 and 5-lipoxygenase with IC_{50} values of 14.0 and 3.0 μM, respectively [85].

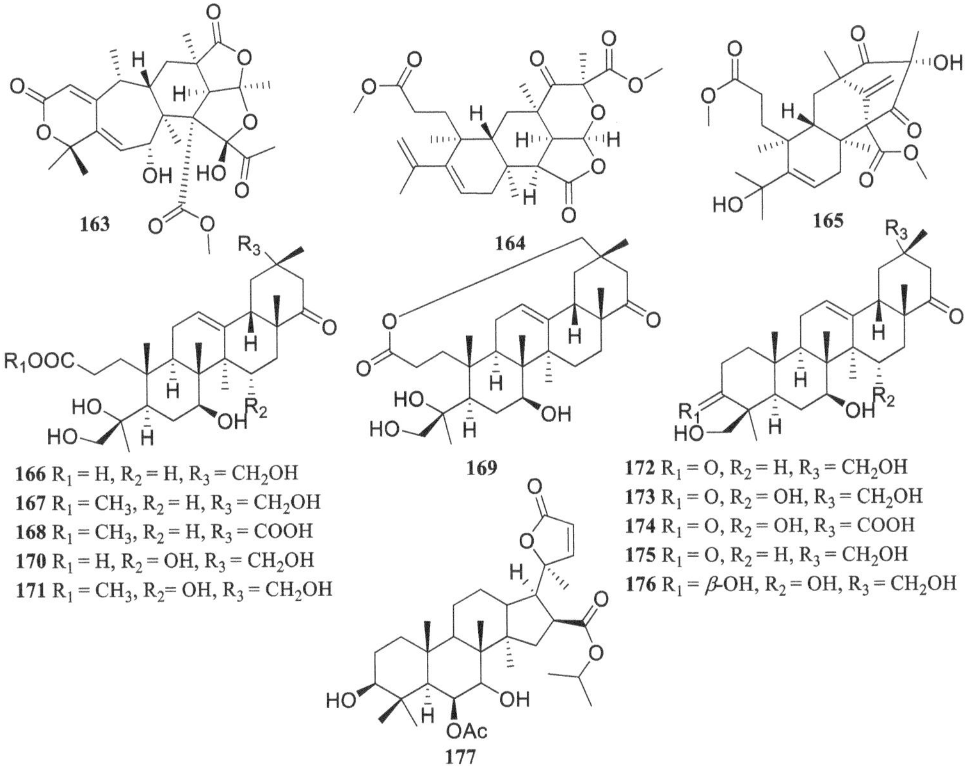

Figure 12. Chemical structures of triterpenoids (**163–177**).

2.2.4. Meroterpenoids

The chemical investigation of marine-derived fungus *Aspergillus terreus* GZU-31-1 yielded five new congeners, aspermeroterpenes D–H (**178–182**) (Figure 13). These compounds prevented RAW 264.7 cells from producing NO in response to LPS. They demonstrated notable anti-inflammatory activity with IC_{50} values of 6.7 ± 0.8, 29.6 ± 3.9, 22.2 ± 0.9, 25.9 ± 3.1, and 26.5 ± 1.0 μM, respectively [86].

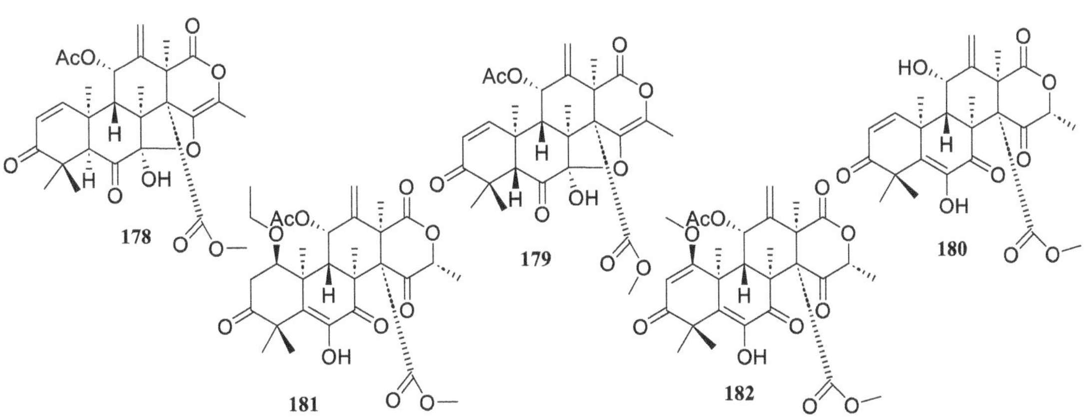

Figure 13. Chemical structures of meroterpenoids (**178–182**).

2.3. *Alkaloids*

In total, 47 alkaloids with anti-inflammatory activity were obtained from marine microorganisms during 2021–2023.

Two new compounds, aspechinulins B (**183**) and C (**184**), together with four known compounds, isoechinulins A (**185**) and B (**186**), neoechinulin B (**187**), and cryptoechinuline G (**188**) (Figure 14), were isolated from the sediment-derived fungus *Aspergillus* sp. FS 445. They illustrated inhibitory effects against NO production with IC_{50} values ranging from 20 to 90 μM [87].

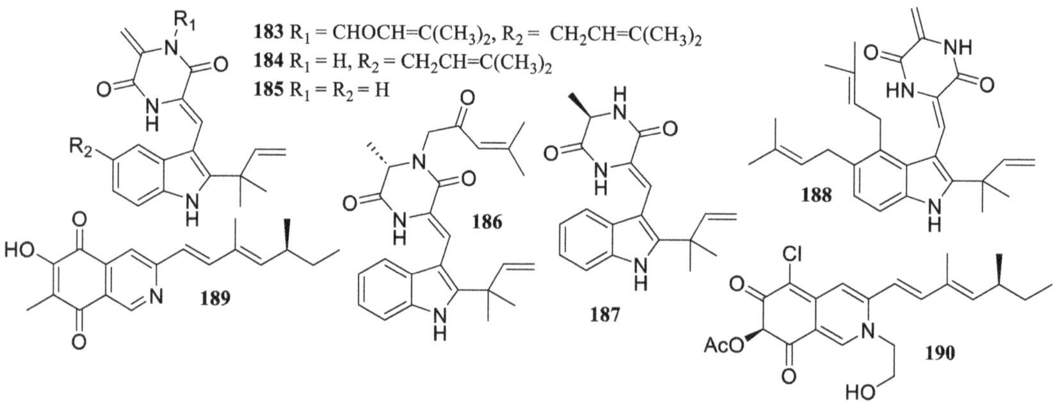

Figure 14. Chemical structures of alkaloids (**183–190**).

The chemical examination of co-cultures of *Penicillium sclerotiorum* THSH–4 and *Penicillium sclerotiorum* ZJHJJ–18 produced one new azaphilone, peniazaphilone A (**189**), and one known azaphilone, isochromophilone VI (**190**). Both revealed a strong suppression of LPS-induced NO release from RAW 264.7 without cytotoxicity with IC_{50} values of 7.1 and 17.0 μM, respectively [36].

Eight known compounds, fumigaclavine C (**191**), isotryptoquivaline F (**192**), fumiquinazoline F (**193**), 12,13-dihydroxyfumitremorgin C (**194**), cyclotryprostatin B (**195**), azaspirofuran A (**196**), 14-norpseurotin A (**197**), and 11-*O*-methylpseurotin A (**198**) (Figure 15), were isolated from the fungus *Talaromyces helicus* SCSIO 41311. They showed moderate NO inhibitory activity with IC_{50} values of 23.5, 26.5, 21.4, 25.0, 29.6, 9.7, 32.4, and 32.2 μM, respectively [39].

In addition to a new oxygenated tricyclic cyclopiazonic acid, asperorydine Q (**199**), the chemical study of the fungus *Aspergillus flavus* GXIMD 02503 produced five known compounds, asperorydines O (**200**) and J (**201**), speradine H (**202**), cyclopiamide A (**203**), and pyrazinemethanol (**204**). They presented suppression of LPS-induced NF-κB activation with IC_{50} values of 14.1 ± 1.5, 21.8 ± 1.9, 8.6 ± 1.3, 17.4 ± 1.7, 11.3 ± 2.0, and 6.5 ± 1.4 μM, respectively [42].

The chemical investigation of a sponge-derived fungus, *Aspergillus tamarii* MCCF 102, resulted in the isolation of two new dipyrrolobenzoquinones, terreusinones B (**205**) and C (**206**), along with one known analog, terreusinone (**207**) (Figure 16). They showed anti-inflammatory activity by inhibiting NO production in a dose-dependent manner (IC_{50} < 1 μM) without any cytotoxicity [88].

Furthermore, a strain of *Cystobasidium laryngis* obtained from deep-sea sediments of the Indian Ocean Ridge produced phenazostatin J (**208**), a new diphenazine derivative. It displayed significant anti-neuroinflammatory activity with an IC_{50} value of 0.3 μM, without cytotoxicity at a concentration of over 1.0 μM [89].

Five new compounds, lecanicilliumins A (**209**), B (**210**), E (**211**), F (**212**), and G (**213**), were obtained from the sediment-derived fungus *Lecanicillium fusisporum* GXIMD 00542. They demonstrated moderate anti-inflammatory activity by reducing LPS-induced NF-κB activation in RAW 264.7 cells with inhibition rates of 50% at 18.5 ± 1.2, 25.8 ± 1.3, 23.1 ± 1.3, 24.7 ± 1.2, and 26.5 ± 1.1 μM, respectively [90].

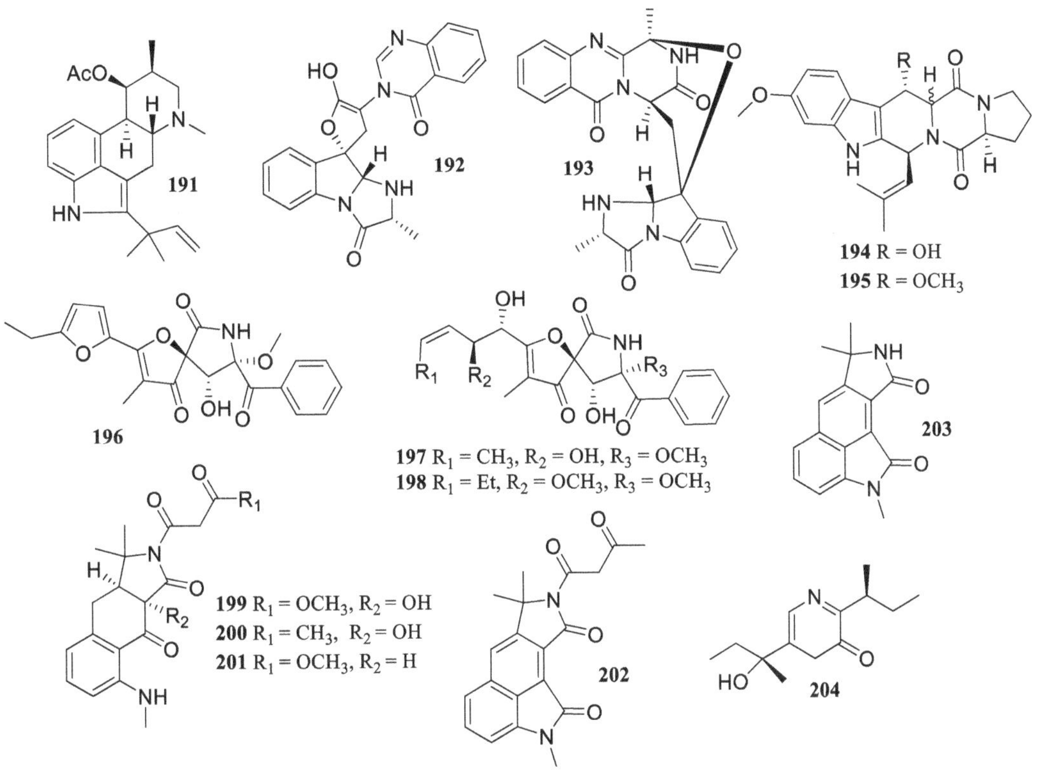

Figure 15. Chemical structures of alkaloids (**191–204**).

The chemical examination of marine sponge *Phakellia fusca*-associated fungus *Actinoalloteichus cyanogriseus* LHW 52806 produced one new β-carboline compound, marinacarboline glucuronide (**214**), as well as two known compounds, marinacarboline L (**215**) and cyanogramide (**216**). They showed anti-inflammatory properties by significantly lowering IL-6 expressions in vitro at 20 μM [91].

Two known compounds, benzomalvin E (**217**) and methylviridicatin (**218**) (Figure 17), were produced by the seawater-derived fungus *Metarhizium* sp. P2100. Both indicated anti-inflammatory activity against LPS-induced NO generation, with IC_{50} values of 37.1 μM and 37.5 μM, respectively [92].

A new compound, sclerotiamide J (**219**), was identified from the coral-derived fungus *Aspergillus sclerotiorum* LZDX-33-4. It prevented NLRP3 inflammasome-induced pyroptosis through the mitigation of mitochondrial damage, and greatly decreased its activation at a concentration of 10 μM [93].

The chemical investigation of the gorgonian coral-associated *Aspergillus candidus* CHNSCLM-0393 provided a pyrrolinone-fused 6/7/5 benzoazepine compound, (+)-asperazepanone B (**220**). It demonstrated strong anti-inflammatory activity by blocking the expression of TNF-α and IL-6 induced by LPS at a concentration of 0.1 μM [94].

Three compounds, cyclopenol (**221**), cyclopenin (**222**), and viridicatol (**223**), were isolated from the fungus *Aspergillus austroafricanus* Y32-2. They showed anti-inflammatory action in an inflammation-induced zebrafish model (ranging from 30 to 120 μg/mL) [75].

A chemical investigation of the fungus *Aspergillus* sp. YJ191021 yielded one new prenylated indole diketopiperazine, asperthrin A (**224**). It revealed strong anti-inflammatory activity with an IC_{50} value of 1.5 ± 0.2 μM in the human monocyte cell line (THP-1) generated by *Propionibacterium acnes* [95].

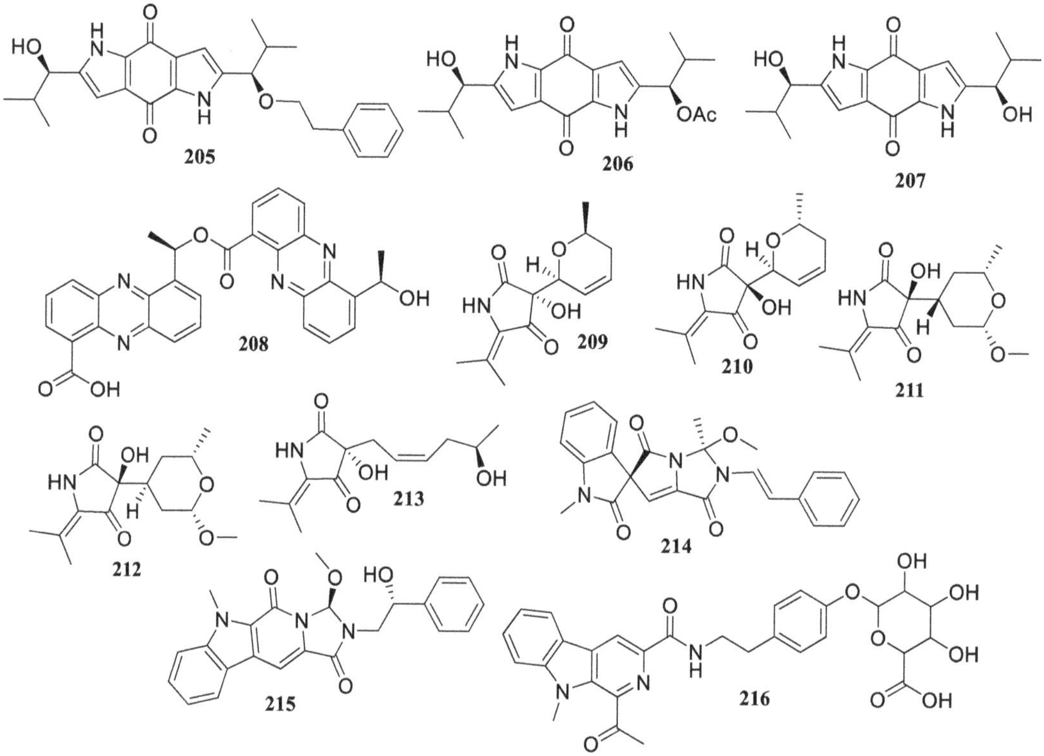

Figure 16. Chemical structures of alkaloids (**205–216**).

A known metabolite, oxaline (**225**), was obtained from cultures of *Penicillium oxalicum* CLC MF 05. It was found to suppress the overproduction of NO and PGE_2, as well as the overexpression of iNOS and COX-2, in both LPS-stimulated BV2 and rat primary microglia with IC_{50} values between 8.8 ± 0.4 and 9.0 ± 0.5 μM [44].

Two compounds, *epi*-aszonalenin A (**226**) and aszonalenin (**227**), were obtained from the coral-derived fungus *Aspergillus terreus* C23-3. Both inhibited the phosphorylation of the MAPK and PI3K/AKT pathways, VEGF protein production, and LOX-1, triggered by ox-LDL at concentrations of 1–10 μM. Moreover, compound **227** inhibited the inflammatory factors (TNF-α, IL-1β, and IL-6) triggered by ox-LDL [96].

A known compound, cyclo (N^8-(α, α-dimethylallyl)-L-Trp-L-Trp) (**228**), was isolated from the hydrothermal vent sediment-derived fungus *Penicillium* sp. LSH-3-1. It decreased the LPS-induced production of pro-inflammatory mediators, including NO, IL-6, and TNF-α at concentrations of 20 to 50 μM [97].

The chemical investigation of the deep-sea sediment-derived fungus *Penicillium chrysogenum* strain S003 yielded one known compound, meleag (**229**). It reduced the levels of IL-6 and IFN-γ, downregulated the expressions of the TLR4, TNF-α, and NF-κB genes, and controlled the Nrf-2/HO-1 cascade [98].

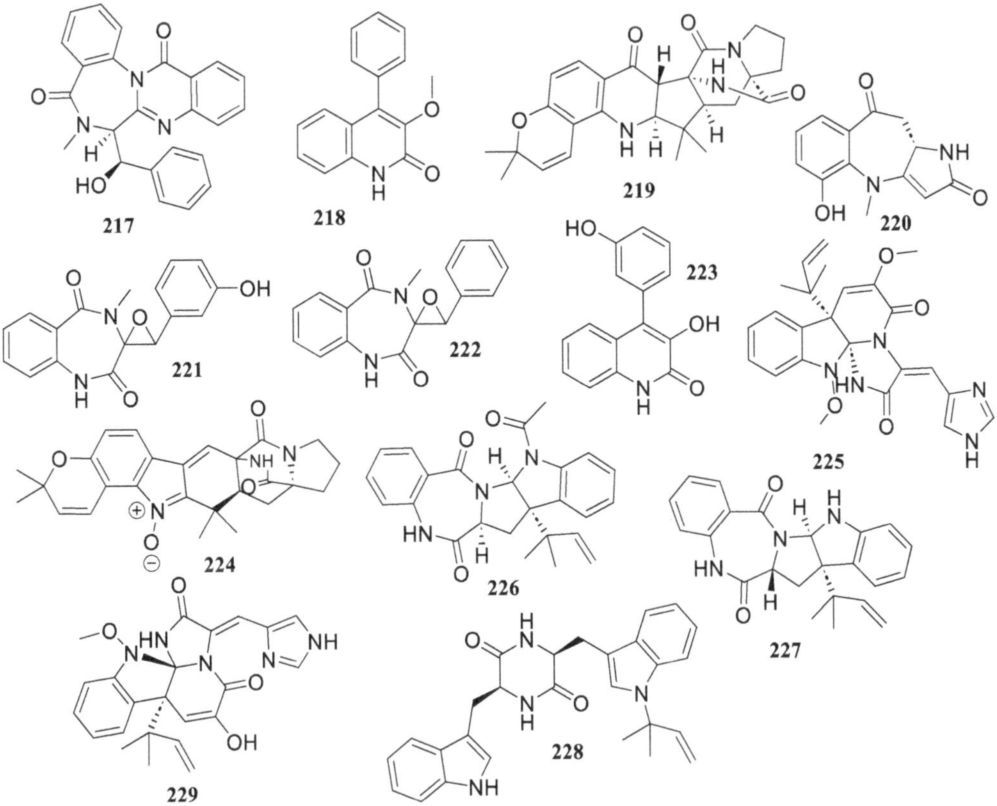

Figure 17. Chemical structures of alkaloids (**217–229**).

2.4. Amides or Peptides

In total, 12 amides or peptides with anti-inflammatory activity were obtained from marine microorganisms during 2021–2023.

Five known compounds, 3,5,7,9-undecatetraenoate (**230**), methyl (2*E*,3*E*,5*E*,7*E*,9*E*)-11-((3a*S*,6*S*,6a*R*)-3a,6-dihydroxy-5-oxohexahydro-2*H*-furo [3,2-b] pyrrol-6-yl)-2-ethylidene-11-hydroxy-4,10-dimethylundeca-3,5,7,9-tetraenoate (**231**), 4*Z*-lucilactaene (**232**), 8*Z*-lucilactaene (**233**), and lucilactaene (**234**) (Figure 18), were isolated from the fungus *Fusarium solani* 7227. They presented strong anti-inflammatory activity by preventing the formation of NO in RAW 264.7 cells stimulated by LPS, with IC_{50} values of 32.2 $\pm$ 5.7, 17.8 $\pm$ 4.9, 7.6 $\pm$ 2.0, 3.6 $\pm$ 2.2, and 8.4 $\pm$ 2.2 μM, respectively. Moreover, the polyunsaturated chain's substitution group increased the anti-inflammatory properties [30].

A new compound, variotin B (**235**), was identified from the ethyl acetate extract of the shrimp-derived fungus *Aspergillus unguis* IV17-109. It indicated anti-inflammatory efficacy by blocking NO generation as well as the expression of iNOS and IL-6 with an IC_{50} value of 20.0 μM [99].

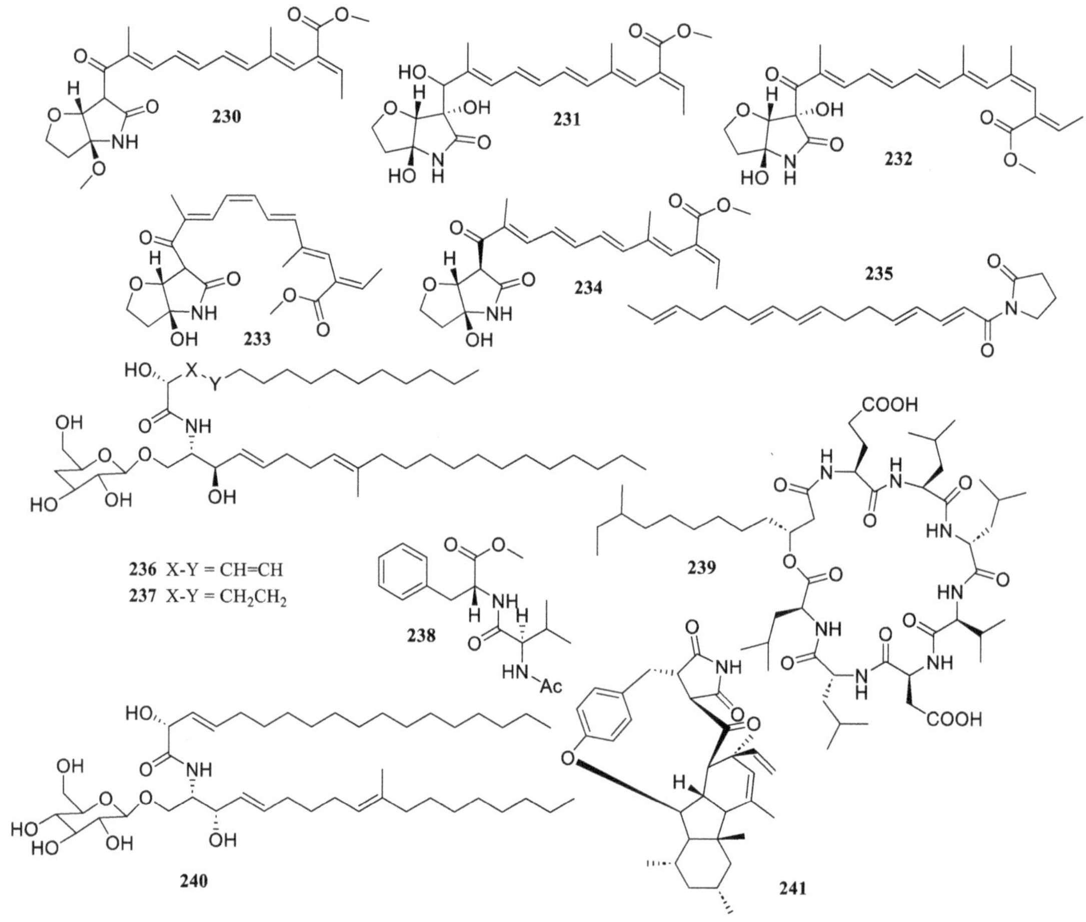

Figure 18. Chemical structures of amides and peptides (230–241).

Two new cerebroside metabolites, hortacerebrosides A (**236**) and B (**237**), were discovered from the sponge-derived fungus *Hortaea werneckii* HN-YPG-2-5. Both showed a notable suppressive impact on the amount of NO generated by RAW 264.7 macrophages activated by LPS, with IC_{50} values of 5 and 7 μM, respectively [100].

One known compound, methyl acetyl-D-valyl-D-phenylalaninate (**238**), was isolated from the fungus *Penicillium* sp. LSH-3-1, which reduced the production of pro-inflammatory mediators, such as NO, IL-6, and TNF-α, at concentrations of 20 to 50 μM, when exposed to LPS [97].

Anteiso-C13-surfactin (IA-1) (**239**) was identified from the marine sediment-derived fungus *Bacillus amyloliquefaciens* strain IA-LB. It ameliorated the inflammatory damage to lung tissue by decreasing neutrophil infiltration, reducing elastase release and oxidative stress in endotoxemic mice at a concentration of 5 μM [101].

The chemical investigation of the sediment-derived fungus *Penicillium islandicum* yielded one known compound, flavuside B (**240**), which significantly reduced LDH release from LPS-induced HaCaT cells to the baseline NO level [102]. One known compound, GKK1032 B (**241**), was isolated from the deep-sea-derived *Penicillium citrinum* W17. It exhibited significant inhibitory effects on LPS-stimulated NO production in murine brain microglial BV2 cells in a dose–response manner with an IC_{50} value of 4.7 μM [72].

2.5. Steroids

In total, 11 steroids with anti-inflammatory activity were obtained from marine microorganisms during 2021–2023.

The fungus *Simplicillium lanosoniveum* SCSIO 41212 produced four new steroids derivatives, arthriniumsteroids A–D (**242–245**), and two known compounds, penicildione B (**246**) and ganodermaside D (**247**) (Figure 19). They displayed poor inhibitory abilities at a dosage of 40 μg/mL, with inhibitory rates ranging from 21.4% to 44.6% [103].

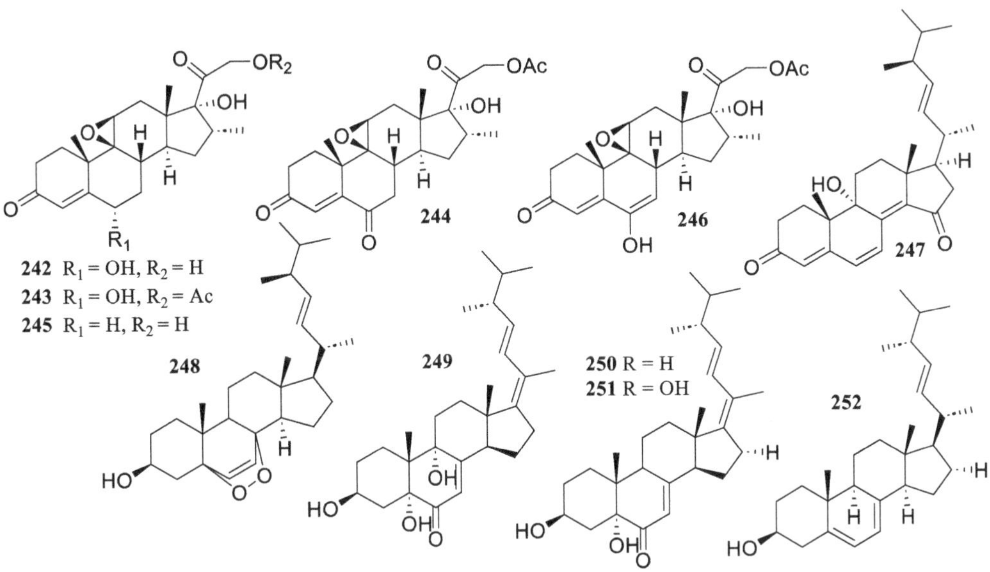

Figure 19. Chemical structures of steroids (**242–252**).

The chemical investigation of the seagrass *Enhalus acoroides*-associated fungus *Penicillium levitum* N33.2 yielded one known compound, ergosterol peroxide (**248**). It indicated an inhibitory effect on macrophages' generation of NO, with an inhibition rate of 81.4 ± 1.4% at 25 mg/mL [104].

Three new ergostane-type sterols, aspersterols B–D (**249–251**), were isolated and identified from the shrimp-derived fungus *Aspergillus unguis* IV17-109. They inhibited LPS-induced NO generation with IC_{50} values of 19.5 ± 1.2, 11.6 ± 1.6, and 14.5 ± 1.5 μM, respectively [105].

One known compound, (22*E*, 24*R*)-ergosta-5,7,22-trien-3*β*-ol (**252**), was obtained from the fungus *Amorosia* sp. SCSIO 41026. It showed inhibitory effects on the overproduction of NO and pro-inflammatory cytokines in LPS-challenged RAW 264.7 macrophages without cytotoxicity at a concentration of 10 μM [56].

3. Conclusions

This review summarizes the sources, chemical structures, and pharmacological properties of anti-inflammatory natural products reported from marine microorganisms in the past three years. A total of 252 natural products with anti-inflammatory activity were recently identified from marine microorganisms, while 51.2% of them were new compounds (Table S1). In addition, 82.9% of them were derived from marine fungi, while 17.1% of them were obtained from marine bacteria or marine actinomycetes (Figure 20). The reviewed marine microorganisms are derived from sediments (31.3%), algae (18.3%), sponges (11.5%), mangroves (9.1%), seawater (7.9%), corals (6.0%), and others (15.9%) (Figure 21). Moreover, the summarized compounds are structurally divided into polyketides (51.2%), terpenoids

(21.0%), alkaloids (18.7%), amides or peptides (4.8%), and steroids (4.3%) (Figure 22). Related anti-inflammatory factors include NO, iNOS, NF-κB, and PGE_2. It is worth noting that the chemical structures of compounds **245–252** with significant anti-inflammatory activity show a high similarity to those of steroidal anti-inflammatory drugs like prednisone.

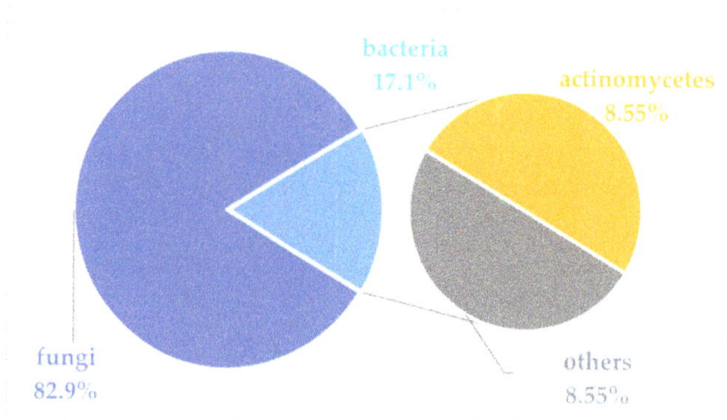

Figure 20. The sources of marine microbial anti-inflammatory natural products (2021–2023).

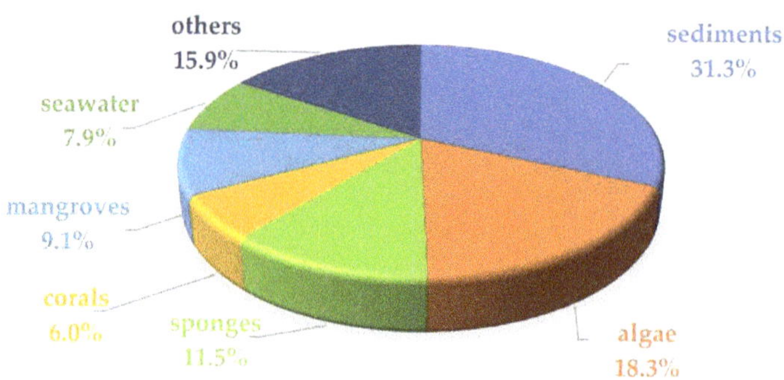

Figure 21. The habitat distribution of anti-inflammatory natural product-producing marine microorganisms.

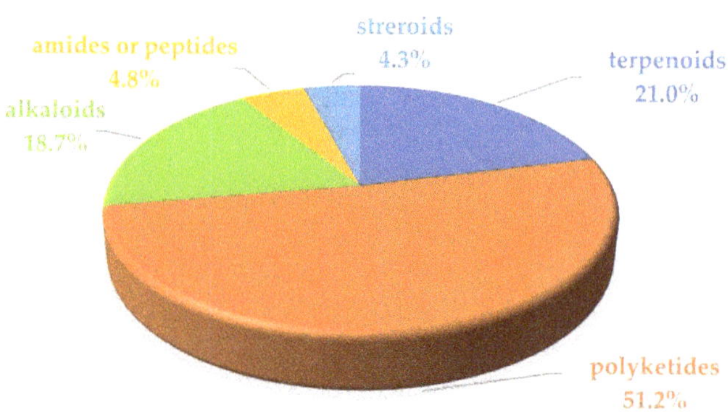

Figure 22. Structural types of marine microbial anti-inflammatory natural products (2021–2023).

Marine microbial natural products are promising sources of anti-inflammatory lead compounds, especially those derived from marine fungi. New effective strategies for dereplication and prioritization to search for minor metabolites should be envisaged for the discovery of new natural compounds from marine microbial sources. Continuously optimizing the fermentation, strengthening the development of extraction and isolation, high-throughput screening, synthetic drug processes, and computer-assisted drug research technologies in the future will promote the mass production as well as the development of anti-inflammatory natural products into clinical agents. Through bioactivity-oriented approaches, diverse natural products with potent anti-inflammatory activity will be found and further structurally modified to improve their drug-forming properties, in order to develop them into anti-inflammatory candidate drugs.

Marine microbial natural products present promising applications in anti-inflammatory drug therapy. However, developing potential anti-inflammatory compounds into clinical agents still faces great challenges owing to their toxicity and selectivity. This review primarily elucidated the pharmacological mechanism of recently reported marine microbial anti-inflammatory natural products, which have attracted great interest and attention in marine microbial anti-inflammatory natural product research, and shed light on their value in the development of clinical anti-inflammatory drugs.

Supplementary Materials: The following supporting information can be downloaded at: https://www.mdpi.com/article/10.3390/md22090424/s1, Table S1: Recently reported marine microbial natural products with anti-inflammatory activity (January 2021 through December 2023).

Author Contributions: Conceptualization, X.L. and Y.L. (Yonghong Liu); data analysis, G.Y., M.L., K.K., Y.L. (Yaqi Lu) and X.Q.; writing—original draft preparation, G.Y. and M.L.; writing—review and editing, X.L., K.K., X.J. and X.X.; funding acquisition X.L. and C.G.; G.Y. and M.L. contributed equally to this work. All authors have read and agreed to the published version of the manuscript.

Funding: This work was supported by Guangxi Natural Science Foundation (2024GXNSFFA010004), the Guangxi Key Research and Development Program (AB24010109), the National Natural Science Foundation of China (82260692, U20A20101), the High-Level Talent Training Project Foundation of Guangxi University of Chinese Medicine (No. 202407, 2022C038), and the Innovation Project of Guangxi Graduate Education (YCSW2024432).

Conflicts of Interest: The authors declare no conflicts of interest.

Abbreviations

IC_{50}	Half maximal inhibitory concentration
NF-κB	Nuclear factor kappa-B
LPS	Lipopolysaccharide
NO	Nitric oxide
IL-6	Interleukine-6
TNF-α	TNF-α

References

1. Almughrbi, A.H.; Crovella, S. Molecular analysis of inflammatory diseases. *Exp. Dermatol.* **2022**, *31*, 9–16. [CrossRef] [PubMed]
2. Deng, L.Y.; He, S.S.; Guo, N.Q.; Tian, W.; Zhang, W.Z.; Luo, L.X. Molecular mechanisms of ferroptosis and relevance to inflammation. *Inflamm. Res.* **2022**, *72*, 281–299. [CrossRef] [PubMed]
3. Lucido, M.J.; Bekhbat, M.; Goldsmith, D.R.; Treadway, M.T.; Haroon, E.; Felger, J.C.; Miller, A.H.; Dantzer, R. Aiding and abetting anhedonia: Impact of inflammation on the brain and pharmacological implications. *Pharmacol. Rev.* **2021**, *73*, 1084–1117. [CrossRef] [PubMed]
4. Coll, R.C.; Schroder, K.; Pelegrín, P. NLRP3 and pyroptosis blockers for treating inflammatory diseases. *Trends Pharmacol. Sci.* **2022**, *43*, 653–668. [CrossRef]
5. Fu, Y.; Xiang, Y.; Li, H.L.; Chen, A.Q.; Dong, Z. Inflammation in kidney repair: Mechanism and therapeutic potential. *Pharmacol. Ther.* **2022**, *237*, 108240. [CrossRef]
6. Squillace, S.; Salvemini, D. Toll-like receptor-mediated neuroinflammation: Relevance for cognitive dysfunctions. *Trends Pharmacol. Sci.* **2022**, *43*, 726–739. [CrossRef]

7. Nicolaes, G.A.F.; Soehnlein, O. Targeting extranuclear histones to alleviate acute and chronic inflammation. *Trends Pharmacol. Sci.* **2024**, *45*, 651–662. [CrossRef]
8. Cryer, B. Nonsteroidal anti-inflammatory drug gastrointestinal toxicity. *Curr. Opin. Gastroen.* **2001**, *17*, 503–512. [CrossRef]
9. Gao, F.; Dai, Z.Q.; Zhang, T.; Gu, Y.H.; Cai, D.S.; Lu, M.J.; Zhang, Z.J.; Zeng, Q.; Shang, B.X.; Xu, B.; et al. Synthesis and biological evaluation of novel sinomenine derivatives as anti-inflammatory and analgesic agent. *RSC Adv.* **2022**, *12*, 30001–30007. [CrossRef]
10. Barzkar, N.; Sukhikh, S.; Babich, O. Study of marine microorganism metabolites: New resources for bioactive natural products. *Front. Microbiol.* **2024**, *14*, 1285902. [CrossRef]
11. Wang, Y.N.; Meng, L.H.; Wang, B.G. Progress in research on bioactive secondary metabolites from deep-sea derived microorganisms. *Mar. Drugs* **2020**, *18*, 614. [CrossRef] [PubMed]
12. Li, C.Q.; Ma, Q.Y.; Gao, X.Z.; Wang, X.; Zhang, B.L. Research progress in anti-inflammatory bioactive substances derived from marine microorganisms, sponges, algae, and corals. *Mar. Drugs* **2021**, *19*, 572. [CrossRef] [PubMed]
13. Ding, Y.; An, F.; Zhu, X.; Yu, H.Y.; Hao, L.L.; Lu, Y.H. Curdepsidones B-G, six depsidones with anti-inflammatory activities from the marine-derived fungus *Curvularia* sp. IFB-Z10. *Mar. Drugs* **2019**, *17*, 266. [CrossRef] [PubMed]
14. Li, H.Y.; Huang, H.M.; Hou, L.K.; Ju, J.H.; Li, W.L. Discovery of antimycin-type depsipeptides from a wbl gene mutant strain of deepsea-derived *Streptomyces somaliensis* SCSIO ZH66 and their effects on pro-inflammatory cytokine production. *Front. Microbiol.* **2017**, *8*, 678. [CrossRef]
15. Carroll, A.R.; Copp, B.R.; Davis, R.A.; Keyzers, R.A.; Prinsep, M.R. Marine natural products. *Nat. Prod. Rep.* **2020**, *37*, 175–223. [CrossRef]
16. Carroll, A.R.; Copp, B.R.; Davis, R.A.; Keyzers, R.A.; Prinsep, M.R. Marine natural products. *Nat. Prod. Rep.* **2021**, *38*, 362–413. [CrossRef]
17. Carroll, A.R.; Copp, B.R.; Davis, R.A.; Keyzers, R.A.; Prinsep, M.R. Marine natural products. *Nat. Prod. Rep.* **2022**, *39*, 1122–1171. [CrossRef]
18. Carroll, A.R.; Copp, B.R.; Davis, R.A.; Keyzers, R.A.; Prinsep, M.R. Marine natural products. *Nat. Prod. Rep.* **2023**, *40*, 275–325. [CrossRef]
19. Carroll, A.R.; Copp, B.R.; Grkovic, T.; Keyzers, R.A.; Prinsep, M.R. Marine natural products. *Nat. Prod. Rep.* **2024**, *41*, 162–207. [CrossRef]
20. Alcaraz, M.J.; Paya, M. Marine sponge metabolites for the control of inflammatory diseases. *Curr. Opin. Investig. Drugs* **2006**, *7*, 974–979.
21. Cheung, R.C.F.; Ng, T.B.; Wong, J.H.; Chen, Y.; Chan, W.Y. Marine natural products with anti-inflammatory activity. *Appl. Microbiol. Biotechnol.* **2015**, *100*, 1645–1666. [CrossRef] [PubMed]
22. Xu, J.Z.; Yi, M.Q.; Ding, L.J.; He, S. A review of anti-inflammatory compounds from marine fungi, 2000–2018. *Mar. Drugs* **2019**, *17*, 636. [CrossRef] [PubMed]
23. Souza, C.R.M.; Bezerra, W.P.; Souto, J.T. Marine alkaloids with anti-inflammatory activity: Current knowledge and future perspectives. *Mar. Drugs* **2020**, *18*, 147. [CrossRef] [PubMed]
24. Chu, Y.C.; Chang, C.H.; Liao, H.R.; Cheng, M.J.; Wu, M.D.; Fu, S.L.; Chen, J.J. Rare chromone derivatives from the marine-derived *Penicillium citrinum* with anti-cancer and anti-inflammatory activities. *Mar. Drugs* **2021**, *19*, 25. [CrossRef]
25. Chu, Y.C.; Chang, C.H.; Liao, H.R.; Fu, S.L.; Chen, J.J. Anti-cancer and anti-inflammatory activities of three new chromone derivatives from the marine-derived *Penicillium citrinum*. *Mar. Drugs* **2021**, *19*, 408. [CrossRef] [PubMed]
26. Ding, W.J.; Wang, F.F.; Li, Q.W.; Xue, Y.X.; Dong, Z.T.; Tian, D.M.; Chen, M.; Zhang, Y.W.; Hong, K.; Tang, J.S. Isolation and characterization of anti-inflammatory sorbicillinoids from the mangrove-derived fungus *Penicillium* sp. DM 815. *Chem. Biodivers.* **2021**, *18*, e2100229.
27. Gou, X.S.; Tian, D.M.; Wei, J.H.; Ma, Y.H.; Zhang, Y.X.; Chen, M.; Ding, W.J.; Wu, B.; Tang, J.S. New drimane sesquiterpenes and polyketides from marine-derived fungus *Penicillium* sp. TW58-16 and their anti-inflammatory and α-glucosidase inhibitory effects. *Mar. Drugs* **2021**, *19*, 416. [CrossRef]
28. Guo, H.; Wu, Q.L.; Chen, D.G.; Jiang, M.H.; Chen, B.; Lu, Y.J.; Li, J.; Liu, L.; Chen, S.H. Absolute configuration of polypropionate derivatives: Decempyrones A-J and their MptpA inhibition and anti-inflammatory activities. *Bioorg. Chem.* **2021**, *115*, 105156. [CrossRef]
29. Lei, H.; Bi, X.X.; Lin, X.P.; She, J.L.; Luo, X.W.; Niu, H.; Zhang, D.; Yang, B. Heterocornols from the sponge-derived fungus *Pestalotiopsis heterocornis* with anti-inflammatory activity. *Mar. Drugs* **2021**, *19*, 585. [CrossRef]
30. Luo, G.Y.; Li, Z.; Wu, Q.L.; Chen, S.H.; Li, J.; Liu, L. Fusarins G-L with Inhibition of NO in RAW 264.7 from marine-derived fungus *Fusarium solani* 7227. *Mar. Drugs* **2021**, *19*, 305. [CrossRef]
31. Wang, S.; Zeng, Y.B.; Yin, J.J.; Chang, W.J.; Zhao, X.L.; Mao, Y. Two new azaphilones from the marine-derived fungus *Penicillium sclerotiorum* E23Y-1A. *Phytochem. Lett.* **2021**, *47*, 76–80. [CrossRef]
32. Shen, Q.Y.; Dai, G.Z.; Li, A.Y.; Liu, Y.; Zhong, G.N.; Li, X.J.; Ren, X.M.; Sui, H.Y.; Fu, J.; Jiao, N.Z.; et al. Genome-guided discovery of highly oxygenated aromatic polyketides, saccharothrixins D-M, from the rare marine actinomycete *Saccharothrix* sp. D09. *J. Nat. Prod.* **2021**, *84*, 2875–2884. [CrossRef] [PubMed]
33. Tilvi, S.; Parvatkar, R.; Singh, K.S.; Devi, P. Chemical investigation of marine-derived fungus *Aspergillus flavipes* for potential anti-inflammatory agents. *Chem. Biodivers.* **2021**, *18*, e2000956. [CrossRef] [PubMed]

34. Uras, I.S.; Ebada, S.S.; Korinek, M.; Albohy, A.; Abdulrazik, B.S.; Wang, Y.H.; Chen, B.H.; Horng, J.T.; Lin, W.; Hwang, T.L.; et al. Anti-inflammatory, antiallergic, and COVID-19 main protease (M^{pro}) inhibitory activities of butenolides from a marine-derived fungus *Aspergillus terreus*. *Molecules* **2021**, *26*, 3354. [CrossRef] [PubMed]
35. Wang, H.C.; Ke, T.Y.; Ko, Y.C.; Lin, J.J.; Chang, J.S.; Cheng, Y.B. Anti-inflammatory azaphilones from the edible alga-derived fungus *Penicillium sclerotiorum*. *Mar. Drugs* **2021**, *19*, 529. [CrossRef]
36. Yang, W.C.; Yuan, J.; Tan, Q.; Chen, Y.; Zhu, Y.J.; Jiang, H.M.; Zou, G.; Zang, Z.M.; Wang, B.; She, Z.G. Peniazaphilones A-I, produced by co-culturing of mangrove endophytic fungi, *Penicillium sclerotiorum* THSH-4 and *Penicillium sclerotiorum* ZJHJJ-18. *Chin. J. Chem.* **2021**, *39*, 3404–3412. [CrossRef]
37. Chen, C.M.; Ren, X.; Tao, H.M.; Cai, W.T.; Chen, Y.C.; Luo, X.W.; Guo, P.; Liu, Y.H. Anti-inflammatory polyketides from an alga-derived fungus *Aspergillus ochraceopetaliformis* SCSIO 41020. *Mar. Drugs* **2022**, *20*, 295. [CrossRef]
38. Chen, S.H.; Guo, H.; Jiang, M.H.; Wu, Q.L.; Li, J.; Shen, H.J.; Liu, L. Mono- and dimeric xanthones with anti-glioma and anti-inflammatory activities from the ascidian-derived fungus *Diaporthe* sp. SYSU-MS 4722. *Mar. Drugs* **2022**, *20*, 51. [CrossRef]
39. Cong, M.J.; Zhang, Y.; Feng, X.Y.; Pang, X.Y.; Liu, Y.H.; Zhang, X.Y.; Yang, Z.Y.; Wang, J.F. Anti-inflammatory alkaloids from the cold-seep-derived fungus *Talaromyces helicus* SCSIO 41311. *3 Biotech* **2022**, *12*, 161. [CrossRef]
40. Gao, M.; Lee, S.B.; Lee, J.E.; Kim, G.J.; Moon, J.; Nam, J.W.; Bae, J.S.; Chin, J.; Jeon, Y.H.; Choi, H. Anti-inflammatory butenolides from a marine-derived *Streptomyces* sp. 13G036. *Appl. Sci.* **2022**, *12*, 4510. [CrossRef]
41. Hsiao, G.; Chi, W.C.; Chang, C.H.; Chiang, Y.R.; Fu, Y.J.; Lee, T.H. Bioactive pulvinones from a marine algicolous fungus *Aspergillus terreus* NTU243. *Phytochemistry* **2022**, *200*, 113229. [CrossRef] [PubMed]
42. Wang, J.M.; Li, Z.Z.; Zhang, Y.T.; Chen, C.M.; Chen, W.H.; Gao, C.H.; Liu, Y.H.; Tan, Y.H.; Luo, X.W. A new α-cyclopiazonic acid alkaloid identified from the Weizhou Island coral-derived fungus *Aspergillus flavus* GXIMD 02503. *J. Ocean Univ. China* **2022**, *21*, 1307–1312. [CrossRef]
43. Jiang, P.; Luo, J.F.; Jiang, Y.; Zhang, L.P.; Jiang, L.Y.; Teng, B.R.; Niu, H.; Zhang, D.; Lei, H. Anti-inflammatory polyketide derivatives from the sponge-derived fungus *Pestalotiopsis* sp. SWMU-WZ04-2. *Mar. Drugs* **2022**, *20*, 711. [CrossRef]
44. Kim, D.C.; Tran Hong, Q.; Nguyen Thuy, T.; Kim, K.W.; Kim, Y.C.; Thanh, N.T.; Cuong, N.X.; Nam, H.N.; Oh, H. Anti-neuroinflammatory effect of oxaline, isorhodoptilometrin, and 5-hydroxy-7-(2′-hydroxypropyl)-2-methyl-chromone obtained from the marine fungal strain *Penicillium oxalicum* CLC-MF05. *Arch. Pharm. Res.* **2022**, *45*, 90–104. [CrossRef]
45. Long, J.Y.; Pang, X.Y.; Lin, X.P.; Liao, S.Y.; Zhou, X.F.; Wang, J.F.; Yang, B.; Liu, Y.H. Asperbenzophenone A and versicolamide C, new fungal metabolites from the soft coral derived *Aspergillus* sp. SCSIO 41036. *Chem. Biodivers.* **2022**, *19*, e202100925. [CrossRef]
46. Shin, H.J.; Heo, C.S.; Anh, C.V.; Yoon, Y.D.; Kang, J.S. Streptoglycerides E-H, unsaturated polyketides from the marine-derived *Bacterium Streptomyces* specialis and their anti-inflammatory activity. *Mar. Drugs* **2022**, *20*, 44. [CrossRef] [PubMed]
47. Wang, G.S.; Yin, Z.H.; Wang, S.Y.; Yuan, Y.L.; Chen, Y.; Kang, W.Y. Diversified polyketides with anti-inflammatory activities from mangrove endophytic fungus *Daldinia eschscholtzii* KBJYZ-1. *Front. Microbiol.* **2022**, *13*, 900227. [CrossRef]
48. Yuan, S.W.; Chen, L.T.; Wu, Q.L.; Jiang, M.H.; Guo, H.; Hu, Z.B.; Chen, S.H.; Liu, L.; Gao, Z.Z. Genome mining of α-pyrone natural products from ascidian-derived fungus *Amphichordafelina* SYSU-MS 7908. *Mar. Drugs* **2022**, *20*, 294. [CrossRef]
49. Zhai, G.F.; Chen, S.H.; Shen, H.J.; Guo, H.; Jiang, M.H.; Liu, L. Bioactive monoterpenes and polyketides from the ascidian-derived fungus *Diaporthe* sp. SYSU-MS4722. *Mar. Drugs* **2022**, *20*, 553. [CrossRef]
50. Zhang, Y.T.; Li, Z.Z.; Huang, B.Y.; Liu, K.; Peng, S.; Liu, X.M.; Gao, C.H.; Liu, Y.H.; Tan, Y.H.; Luo, X.W. Anti-osteoclastogenic and antibacterial effects of chlorinated polyketides from the Beibu Gulf coral-derived fungus *Aspergillus unguis* GXIMD 02505. *Mar. Drugs* **2022**, *20*, 178. [CrossRef]
51. Zhang, Y.H.; Du, H.F.; Gao, W.B.; Li, W.; Cao, F.; Wang, C.Y. Anti-inflammatory polyketides from the marine-derived fungus *Eutypella scoparia*. *Mar. Drugs* **2022**, *20*, 486. [CrossRef] [PubMed]
52. Lee, H.S.; Nagahawatta, D.P.; Jeon, Y.J.; Lee, M.A.; Heo, C.S.; Park, S.J.; Shin, H.J. Streptinone, a new indanone derivative from a marine-derived *Streptomyces massiliensis*, inhibits particulate matter-induced inflammation. *Mar. Drugs* **2023**, *21*, 640. [CrossRef] [PubMed]
53. Tan, Z.L.; Chen, Y.C.; Zhang, J.P.; Liu, H.X.; Zhang, W.M.; Yan, H.J. A new secondary metabolite from the marine-derived fungus *Phomopsis lithocarpus* FS 508. *J. Asian Nat. Prod. Res.* **2023**, *26*, 534–540. [CrossRef]
54. Wu, Z.G.; Guo, H.; Wu, Q.L.; Jiang, M.H.; Chen, J.J.; Chen, B.; Li, H.X.; Liu, L.; Chen, S.H. Absolute configuration of cyclopropanes and the structural revision of pyrones from marine-derived fungus *Stagonospora* sp. SYSU-MS 7888. *Bioorg. Chem.* **2023**, *136*, 106542. [CrossRef]
55. Zeng, Y.B.; Wang, Z.; Chang, W.J.; Zhao, W.B.; Wang, H.; Chen, H.Q.; Dai, H.F.; Lv, F. New azaphilones from the marine-derived fungus *Penicillium sclerotiorum* E23Y-1A with their anti-inflammatory and antitumor activities. *Mar. Drugs* **2023**, *21*, 75. [CrossRef]
56. Ren, X.; Chen, C.M.; Ye, Y.X.; Xu, Z.Y.; Zhao, Q.L.; Luo, X.W.; Liu, Y.H.; Guo, P. Anti-inflammatory compounds from the mangrove endophytic fungus *Amorosia* sp. SCSIO 41026. *Front. Microbiol.* **2022**, *13*, 976399. [CrossRef] [PubMed]
57. Lu, H.M.; Tan, Y.H.; Zhang, Y.T.; Li, Z.C.; Chen, J.Y.; Gao, C.H.; Liu, Y.H.; Luo, X.W. Osteoclastogenesis inhibitory phenolic derivatives produced by the Beibu Gulf coral-associated fungus *Acremonium sclerotigenum* GXIMD 02501. *Fitoterapia* **2022**, *159*, 105201. [CrossRef]
58. Xing, D.X.; Song, X.S.; Pan, W.C.; Cui, H.; Zhao, Z.X. New chromone compounds from the marine derived fungus *Diaporthe* sp. XW12-1. *Fitoterapia* **2023**, *164*, 105384. [CrossRef] [PubMed]

59. Yan, F.H.; Fang, J.B.; Ding, W.J.; Tang, X.Y.; Chen, X.M.; Ma, Z.J.; Wang, J.H. Structurally diverse metabolites from the marine-derived *Streptomyces* sp. DS-27 based on two different culture conditions. *Chem. Biodivers.* **2023**, *20*, 1017. [CrossRef]
60. Jiang, M.; Zhang, Y.; Zhang, Y.X.; Ma, Z.J.; Wang, J.H. Suncheonosides E-M and benzothioate derivatives from the marine-derived *Streptomyces* sp. ZSN77. *J. Nat. Prod.* **2022**, *85*, 1771–1778. [CrossRef]
61. Xie, X.T.; Xiao, S.P.; Liao, H.Y.; Jiang, Q.J.; Chen, G.; Wen, L. A new chloro-containing γ-butyrolactone from the mangrove endophytic fungus *Neofusicoccum parvum* Y2NBKZG1016. *Chem. Nat. Compd.* **2023**, *59*, 424–427. [CrossRef]
62. Shin, H.J.; Anh, C.V.; Cho, D.Y.; Choi, D.K.; Kang, J.S.; Trinh, P.T.H.; Choi, B.-K.; Lee, H.-S. New polyenes from the marine-derived fungus *Talaromyces cyanescens* with anti-neuroinflammatory and cytotoxic activities. *Molecules* **2021**, *26*, 836. [CrossRef]
63. He, J.L.; Wu, X.; Huang, S.H.; Wang, J.; Niu, S.W.; Chen, M.X.; Zhang, G.Y.; Cai, S.Y.; Wu, J.N.; Hong, B.H. Phenolic metabolites from a deep-sea-derived fungus *Aspergillus puniceus* A2 and their Nrf2-dependent anti-inflammatory effects. *Mar. Drugs* **2022**, *20*, 575. [CrossRef] [PubMed]
64. Su, Y.S.; Cheng, M.J.; Wu, M.D.; Chai, C.Y.; Kwan, A.L.; Su, S.H.; Kuo, Y.H. Chemical constituents from a mangrove-derived *Actinobacteria Isoptericola chiayiensis* BCRC 16888 and evaluation of their anti-NO activity. *Chem. Biodivers.* **2021**, *18*, e2100211. [CrossRef]
65. Chen, Y.; Zou, G.; Yang, W.C.; Zhao, Y.Y.; Tan, Q.; Chen, L.; Wang, J.M.; Ma, C.Y.; Kang, W.Y.; She, Z.G. Metabolites with anti-inflammatory activity from the mangrove endophytic fungus diaporthe sp. QYM12. *Mar. Drugs* **2021**, *19*, 56. [CrossRef]
66. Dong, L.X.; Kim, H.J.; Cao, T.Q.; Liu, Z.M.; Lee, H.; Ko, W.; Kim, Y.C.; Sohn, J.H.; Kim, T.K.; Yim, J.H.; et al. Anti-inflammatory effects of metabolites from antarctic fungal strain *Pleosporales* sp. SF-7343 in HaCaT human keratinocytes. *Int. J. Mol. Sci.* **2021**, *22*, 9674. [CrossRef]
67. Qin, X.Y.; Huang, J.G.; Zhou, D.X.; Zhang, W.X.; Zhang, Y.J.; Li, J.; Yang, R.Y.; Huang, X.S. Polyketide derivatives, guhypoxylonols A–D from a mangrove endophytic fungus *Aspergillus* sp. GXNU-Y45 that inhibit nitric oxide production. *Mar. Drugs* **2021**, *20*, 5. [CrossRef]
68. Quang, T.H.; Vien, L.T.; Anh, L.N.; Ngan, N.T.T.; Hanh, T.T.H.; Cuong, N.X.; Nam, N.H.; Van Minh, C. Anti-inflammatory metabolites from a marine sponge-associated fungus *Aspergillus* sp. IMBC-FP2.05. *Vietnam. J. Chem.* **2021**, *59*, 52–56. [CrossRef]
69. Chen, C.; Ye, G.T.; Tang, J.; Li, J.L.; Liu, W.B.; Wu, L.; Long, Y.H. New polyketides from mangrove endophytic fungus *Penicillium* sp. BJR-P2 and their anti-inflammatory activity. *Mar. Drugs* **2022**, *20*, 583. [CrossRef]
70. Pang, X.Y.; Wang, P.; Liao, S.R.; Zhou, X.F.; Lin, X.P.; Yang, B.; Tian, X.P.; Wang, J.F.; Liu, Y.H. Three unusual hybrid sorbicillinoids with anti-inflammatory activities from the deep-sea derived fungus *Penicillium* sp. SCSIO 06868. *Phytochemistry* **2022**, *202*, 113311. [CrossRef]
71. Cong, M.J.; Ren, X.; Song, Y.; Pang, X.Y.; Tian, X.P.; Liu, Y.H.; Guo, P.; Wang, J.F. Ochrathinols A and B, two pairs of sulfur-containing racemates from an antarctic fungus *Aspergillus ochraceopetaliformis* SCSIO 05702 inhibit LPS-induced pro-inflammatory cytokines and NO production. *Phytochemistry* **2023**, *208*, 113593. [CrossRef] [PubMed]
72. Zhang, Y.; Xie, C.L.; Wang, Y.; He, X.W.; Xie, M.M.; Li, Y.; Zhang, K.; Zou, Z.B.; Yang, L.H.; Xu, R.; et al. Penidihydrocitrinins A–C: New polyketides from the deep-sea-derived *Penicillium citrinum* W17 and their anti-inflammatory and anti-osteoporotic bioactivities. *Mar. Drugs* **2023**, *21*, 538. [CrossRef] [PubMed]
73. Guo, X.; Meng, Q.Y.; Niu, S.W.; Liu, J.; Guo, X.C.; Sun, Z.L.; Liu, D.; Gu, Y.C.; Huang, J.; Fan, A.L.; et al. Epigenetic manipulation to trigger production of guaiane-type sesquiterpenes from a marine-derived *Spiromastix* sp. fungus with anti-neuroinflammatory effects. *J. Nat. Prod.* **2021**, *84*, 1993–2003. [CrossRef] [PubMed]
74. Li, P.H.; Zhang, M.Q.; Li, H.N.; Wang, R.C.; Hou, H.R.; Li, X.B.; Liu, K.C.; Chen, H. New prenylated indole homodimeric and pteridine alkaloids from the marine-derived fungus *Aspergillus austroafricanus* Y32-2. *Mar. Drugs* **2021**, *19*, 98. [CrossRef] [PubMed]
75. Sun, B.Y.; Wang, D.D.; Ren, J.W.; Wang, C.J.; Yan, P.C.; Gustafson, K.R.; Jiang, W. Paraconulones A-G: Eremophilane sesquiterpenoids from the marine-derived fungus *Paraconiothyrium sporulosum* DL-16. *J. Nat. Prod.* **2023**, *86*, 1360–1369. [CrossRef]
76. Niu, S.W.; Liu, D.; Shao, Z.Z.; Liu, J.R.; Fan, A.L.; Lin, W.H. Chemical epigenetic manipulation triggers the production of sesquiterpenes from the deep-sea derived *Eutypella* fungus. *Phytochemistry* **2021**, *192*, 112978. [CrossRef]
77. Shang, R.Y.; Cui, J.; Li, J.X.; Miao, X.X.; Zhang, L.; Xie, D.D.; Zhang, L.; Lin, H.W.; Jiao, W.H. Nigerin and ochracenes J−L, new sesquiterpenoids from the marine sponge symbiotic fungus *Aspergillus niger*. *Tetrahedron* **2021**, *104*, 132599. [CrossRef]
78. Safwan, S.; Wang, S.W.; Hsiao, G.; Hsiao, S.W.; Hsu, S.J.; Lee, T.H.; Lee, C.K. New trichothecenes isolated from the marine algicolous fungus *Trichoderma brevicompactum*. *Mar. Drugs* **2022**, *20*, 80. [CrossRef]
79. Hu, Z.B.; Chen, J.J.; Liu, Q.Q.; Wu, Q.L.; Chen, S.H.; Wang, J.J.; Li, J.; Liu, L.; Gao, Z.Z. Cyclohexenone derivative and drimane sesquiterpenes from the seagrass-derived fungus *Aspergillus insuetus*. *Chem. Biodivers.* **2023**, *20*, e202300424. [CrossRef]
80. Li, H.X.; Liu, X.Y.; Li, X.F.; Hu, Z.L.; Wang, L.Y. Novel harziane diterpenes from deep-sea sediment fungus *Trichoderma* sp. SCSIOW 21 and their potential anti-inflammatory effects. *Mar. Drugs* **2021**, *19*, 689. [CrossRef]
81. Ning, Y.D.; Zhang, S.; Zheng, T.; Xu, Y.; Li, S.; Zhang, J.P.; Jiao, B.H.; Zhang, Y.; Ma, Z.L.; Lu, X.L. Pimarane-type diterpenes with anti-inflammatory activity from arctic-derived fungus *Eutypella* sp. D-1. *Mar. Drugs* **2023**, *21*, 541. [CrossRef] [PubMed]
82. Zhao, M.; Chen, X.C.; Pan, W.C.; Liu, X.; Tan, S.L.; Cui, H.; Zhao, Z.X. Meroterpenoids from the fungus *Penicillium sclerotiorum* GZU-XW03-2 and their anti-inflammatory activity. *Phytochemistry* **2022**, *202*, 113307. [CrossRef] [PubMed]
83. Liu, X.; Zhao, M.; Chen, J.; Pan, W.C.; Tan, S.L.; Cui, H.; Zhao, Z.X. Seven new meroterpenoids from the fungus *Penicillium sclerotiorum* GZU-XW03-2. *Fitoterapia* **2023**, *165*, 105428. [CrossRef]

84. Yu, H.; Chen, Y.H.; Cheng, Z.; Li, H.J.; Bian, H.H.; Yang, X.; Lv, J.; Liu, W.; Su, L.; Sun, P. Anti-inflammatory oleanane-type triterpenoids produced by *Nonomuraea* sp. MYH 522 through microbial transformation. *J. Agric. Food Chem.* **2023**, *71*, 3777–3789. [CrossRef] [PubMed]
85. Thambi, A.; Chakraborty, K. Anti-inflammatory decurrencyclics A–B, two undescribed nor-dammarane triterpenes from triangular sea bell *Turbinaria decurrens*. *Nat. Prod. Rep.* **2022**, *37*, 713–724. [CrossRef] [PubMed]
86. Tang, Y.Q.; Chen, X.C.; Zhou, Y.W.; Zhao, M.; He, J.X.; Liu, Y.N.; Chen, G.Y.; Zhao, Z.X.; Cui, H. Furanaspermeroterpenes A and B, two unusual meroterpenoids with a unique 6/6/6/5/5 pentacyclic skeleton from the marine-derived fungus *Aspergillus terreus* GZU-31-1. *Bioorg. Chem.* **2021**, *114*, 105111. [CrossRef]
87. Liu, Z.M.; Chen, Y.C.; Li, S.N.; Hu, C.Y.; Liu, H.X.; Zhang, W.M. Indole diketopiperazine alkaloids from the deep-sea-derived fungus *Aspergillus* sp. FS 445. *Nat. Prod. Res.* **2021**, *36*, 5213–5221. [CrossRef]
88. Niveditha, L.; Fu, P.; Leao, T.F.; Li, T.; Wang, T.; Poulin, R.X.; Gaspar, L.R.; Naman, C.B.; Puthiyedathu, T.S. Targeted isolation of two new anti-inflammatory and UV-a protective dipyrroloquinones from the sponge-associated fungus *Aspergillus tamarii* MCCF 102. *Planta Med.* **2022**, *88*, 774–782.
89. Lee, H.S.; Kang, J.S.; Cho, D.Y.; Choi, D.K.; Shin, H.J. Isolation, structure determination, and semisynthesis of diphenazine compounds from a deep-sea-derived strain of the fungus *Cystobasidium laryngis* and their biological activities. *J. Nat. Prod.* **2022**, *85*, 857–865. [CrossRef]
90. Xu, X.Y.; Tan, Y.H.; Gao, C.H.; Liu, K.; Tang, Z.Z.; Lu, C.J.; Li, H.Y.; Zhang, X.Y.; Liu, Y.H. New 3-acyl tetramic acid derivatives from the deep-sea-derived fungus *Lecanicillium fusisporum*. *Mar. Drugs* **2022**, *20*, 255. [CrossRef]
91. Zhang, D.; Xu, J.; Qin, Q.; An, F.L.; Wang, S.P.; Li, L.; Lin, H.W. Marinacarboline glucuronide, a new member of β-carboline alkaloids from sponge-derived actinomycete *Actinoalloteichus cyanogriseus* LHW 52806. *J. Antibiot.* **2022**, *75*, 523–525. [CrossRef] [PubMed]
92. Yao, G.S.; Ma, Z.L.; Zheng, Y.Y.; Lv, L.; Mao, J.Q.; Wang, C.Y. Bioactive alkaloids from the marine-derived fungus *Metarhizium* sp. P2100. *J. Fungi* **2022**, *8*, 1218. [CrossRef] [PubMed]
93. Meng, Q.Y.; Guo, X.; Wu, J.S.; Liu, D.; Gu, Y.C.; Huang, J.; Fan, A.L.; Lin, W.H. Prenylated notoamide-type alkaloids isolated from the fungus *Aspergillus sclerotiorum* and their inhibition of NLRP3 inflammasome activation and antibacterial activities. *Phytochemistry* **2022**, *203*, 113424. [CrossRef]
94. Xu, L.; Guo, F.W.; Zhang, X.Q.; Zhou, T.Y.; Wang, C.J.; Wei, M.Y.; Gu, Y.C.; Wang, C.Y.; Shao, C.L. Discovery, total syntheses and potent anti-inflammatory activity of pyrrolinone-fused benzoazepine alkaloids asperazepanones A and B from *Aspergillus candidus*. *Commun. Chem.* **2022**, *5*, 80. [CrossRef]
95. Yang, J.; Gong, L.Z.; Guo, M.M.; Jiang, Y.; Ding, Y.; Wang, Z.J.; Xin, X.J.; An, F.L. Bioactive indole diketopiperazine alkaloids from the marine endophytic fungus *Aspergillus* sp. YJ191021. *Mar. Drugs* **2021**, *19*, 157. [CrossRef] [PubMed]
96. Liu, Y.; Li, Y.M.; Chen, M.Q.; Liu, Y.Y.; Liang, J.Y.; Zhang, Y.; Qian, Z.J. Mechanism of two alkaloids isolated from coral endophytic fungus for suppressing angiogenesis in atherosclerotic plaque in HUVEC. *Int. Immunopharmacol.* **2022**, *109*, 108931. [CrossRef]
97. Li, S.H.; Ma, Y.H.; Wang, L.X.; Lan, D.H.; Fu, L.L.; Wu, B. Two new alkaloids from the marine-derived fungus *Penicillium* sp. LSH-3-1. *Chem. Biodivers.* **2022**, *19*, e202200310. [CrossRef]
98. Elhady, S.S.; Goda, M.S.; Mehanna, E.T.; Elfaky, M.A.; Koshak, A.E.; Noor, A.O.; Bogari, H.A.; Malatani, R.T.; Abdelhameed, R.F.A.; Wahba, A.S. Meleagrin isolated from the red sea fungus *Penicillium chrysogenum* protects against bleomycin-induced pulmonary fibrosis in mice. *Biomedicines* **2022**, *10*, 1164. [CrossRef] [PubMed]
99. Anh, C.V.; Yoon, Y.D.; Kang, J.S.; Lee, H.S.; Heo, C.S.; Shin, H.J. Nitrogen-containing secondary metabolites from a deep-sea fungus *Aspergillus unguis* and their anti-inflammatory activity. *Mar. Drugs* **2022**, *20*, 217. [CrossRef]
100. Chen, Y.H.; Wu, X.N.; Xu, L.; El-Shazly, M.; Ma, C.W.; Yuan, S.J.; Wang, P.P.; Luo, L.Z. Two new cerebroside metabolites from the marine fungus *Hortaea werneckii*. *Chem. Biodivers.* **2022**, *19*, e202200008. [CrossRef]
101. Yang, S.C.; Wang, Y.H.; Ho, C.M.; Tsai, Y.F.; Sung, P.J.; Lin, T.E.; Hwang, T.L. Targeting formyl peptide receptor 1 with anteiso-C13-surfactin for neutrophil-dominant acute respiratory distress syndrome. *Br. J. Pharmacol.* **2023**, *180*, 2120–2139. [CrossRef] [PubMed]
102. Chingizova, E.A.; Menchinskaya, E.S.; Chingizov, A.R.; Pislyagin, E.A.; Girich, E.V.; Yurchenko, A.N.; Guzhova, I.V.; Mikhailov, V.V.; Aminin, D.L.; Yurchenko, E.A. Marine fungal cerebroside flavuside B protects HaCaT keratinocytes against staphylococcus aureus induced damage. *Mar. Drugs* **2021**, *19*, 553. [CrossRef] [PubMed]
103. Li, J.X.; Tao, H.M.; Lei, X.X.; Zhang, H.; Zhou, X.F.; Liu, Y.H.; Li, Y.Q.; Yang, B. Arthriniumsteroids A-D, four new steroids from the soft coral-derived fungus *Simplicillium lanosoniveum* SCSIO 41212. *Steroids* **2021**, *171*, 108831. [CrossRef] [PubMed]
104. Hoang, C.K.; Le, C.H.; Nguyen, D.T.; Tran, H.T.N.; Luu, C.V.; Le, H.M.; Tran, H.T.H. Steroid components of marine-derived fungal strain *Penicillium levitum* N33.2 and their biological activities. *Mycobiology* **2023**, *51*, 246–255. [CrossRef]
105. Cao, V.A.; Kwon, J.H.; Kang, J.S.; Lee, H.S.; Heo, C.S.; Shin, H.J. Aspersterols A–D, ergostane-type sterols with an unusual unsaturated side chain from the deep-sea-derived fungus *Aspergillus unguis*. *J. Nat. Prod.* **2022**, *85*, 2177–2183. [CrossRef]

marine drugs

MDPI

Review

Antioxidant and Anti-Inflammatory Properties of Four Native Mediterranean Seagrasses: A Review of Bioactive Potential and Ecological Context

Marzia Vasarri [1,*], Lucia De Marchi [2], Carlo Pretti [2,3], Emanuela Barletta [1] and Donatella Degl'Innocenti [1,3]

1. Department of Experimental and Clinical Biomedical Sciences, University of Florence, Viale Morgagni 50, 50134 Florence, Italy; emanuela.barletta@unifi.it (E.B.); donatella.deglinnocenti@unifi.it (D.D.)
2. Department of Veterinary Sciences, University of Pisa, Viale delle Piagge 2, 56124 Pisa, Italy; lucia.demarchi@unipi.it (L.D.M.); carlo.pretti@unipi.it or pretti@cibm.it (C.P.)
3. Interuniversity Center of Marine Biology and Applied Ecology "G. Bacci" (CIBM), Viale N. Sauro 4, 57128 Leghorn, Italy

* Correspondence: marzia.vasarri@unifi.it

Abstract: This review provides current knowledge of the potential benefits of native Mediterranean seagrasses for human health, specifically focusing on their anti-inflammatory and antioxidant properties. The four main species examined—*Posidonia oceanica*, *Cymodocea nodosa*, *Zostera marina*, and *Zostera noltii*—are integral components of marine ecosystems, providing essential habitats and supporting biodiversity. Recent studies highlight their rich bioactive compounds that show significant therapeutic potential against oxidative stress and chronic inflammation, which are prevalent in various health disorders. This overview synthesizes the current literature, emphasizing the mechanisms through which these seagrasses exert their beneficial effects. Furthermore, it addresses the environmental implications of the excessive use and abuse of conventional anti-inflammatory drugs, advocating for a shift towards natural alternatives derived from marine resources. By exploring the bioactivity of these Mediterranean seagrasses, research here collected underscores the importance of integrating marine plants into health and wellness strategies, thereby promoting both human health and ecosystem sustainability. This exploration not only enriches the understanding of their applications on human health but also stimulates further research in this promising field, paving the way for innovative approaches to combat chronic diseases and support environmental conservation.

Keywords: native Mediterranean plants; antioxidant; anti-inflammatory; seagrass; *Posidonia oceanica*; *Cymodocea nodosa*; *Zostera marina*; *Zostera noltii*

1. Introduction

Inflammation is a crucial and complex biological process that plays a fundamental role in the body's defense mechanism. It occurs as a response to injury, infection, or exposure to harmful stimuli, serving to protect the body by eliminating the source of damage, removing dead or damaged cells, and promoting tissue repair [1]. The acute inflammatory response is essential for healing and maintaining health; however, when inflammation becomes persistent or uncontrolled, it can have detrimental effects [2].

Chronic inflammation has been linked to the development and progression of numerous diseases, including cardiovascular disease, diabetes, cancer, and neurodegenerative disorders, among many others. Therefore, regulating the inflammatory process is vital for developing strategies to prevent and treat these chronic conditions, emphasizing the importance of maintaining a balanced immune response for overall health [3].

A key factor intertwined with inflammation is the production of free radicals: unstable molecules that contain unpaired electrons that make them highly reactive. Common free radicals, such as reactive oxygen species (ROS) like superoxide anion, hydroxyl radical, and hydrogen peroxide, are naturally produced within the cells during metabolic processes, especially in the mitochondria during energy production [4].

The body's antioxidant defense system is essential in protecting cells, DNA, and tissues from the damaging effects of these reactive molecules. This system includes endogenous antioxidants, such as enzymes like superoxide dismutase (SOD), catalase (CAT), glutathione peroxidase (GPx), and glutathione reductase (GR), which are produced internally to neutralize ROS. Additionally, exogenous antioxidants obtained from the diet, including vitamin C, vitamin E, polyphenols, flavonoids, and carotenoids, contribute significantly to reducing oxidative stress. Maintaining a robust antioxidant system is essential for overall health and for preventing diseases associated with oxidative damage [4]. However, while low to moderate levels of ROS play essential roles in cell signaling, immune defense, and maintaining homeostasis, excessive ROS production can cause oxidative damage to lipids, proteins, and DNA. This damage impairs cellular function and integrity, potentially leading to various health issues if left unchecked [5,6]. Indeed, oxidative stress arises when there is an imbalance between the production of free radicals and the body's ability to neutralize them with antioxidants. This imbalance results in damage to cellular components and contributes to aging and the development of numerous diseases. During inflammation, immune cells such as macrophages and neutrophils generate large amounts of ROS to destroy pathogens. However, excessive or prolonged ROS production can also harm host tissues, perpetuating inflammation and creating a vicious cycle of oxidative stress.

The relationship between inflammation, free radicals, and oxidative stress is complex and bidirectional, each process influencing the other. Inflammation can increase ROS production, leading to oxidative stress, which in turn can activate further inflammatory pathways in a persistent cycle [7,8]. This interplay is central to many chronic diseases, highlighting the importance of antioxidant defenses and anti-inflammatory strategies. Understanding the roles of inflammation, free radicals, and oxidative stress is crucial for developing therapies aimed at reducing oxidative damage and controlling chronic inflammation. A comprehensive approach that addresses these interconnected processes is essential for preventing and managing a wide array of health conditions linked to inflammation and oxidative damage [4].

1.1. Seagrasses: Marine Flowering Plants, Ecosystem Functions, and Societal Significance

Seagrasses, named for their long green leaves, are often mistaken for algae; however, they are more closely related to land plants [9]. These fascinating marine flowering plants originated from terrestrial ancestors that made their way back to the ocean approximately 70–100 million years ago [10,11]. Seagrasses form dense underwater meadows that are among the most productive ecosystems on Earth, serving as crucial carbon sinks and providing habitat and sustenance for a diverse array of marine life, rivaling the biodiversity found in coral reefs [12–14]. These underwater meadows play a vital role in maintaining the health and sustainability of marine environments, significantly contributing to biodiversity, coastal stability, and water quality [15].

For millennia, seagrass meadows have been intertwined with human culture, representing a natural resource that has sustained humanity throughout history [16,17]. Over the last 180,000 years, these seagrass meadows have provided spiritual, medicinal, and material benefits, serving as a food source for both humans and marine life, and influencing various cultural practices and local economies. Although many traditional customs have been lost or modified, recent rediscoveries and innovations, such as the use of seagrasses in sustainable food production and construction material, demonstrate the ongoing connection between these ecosystems and human communities. The importance of sustainable harvesting practices is highlighted to prevent overexploitation and promote conservation, linking the health of seagrass ecosystems to broader environmental and social well-being. This connection supports the integration of seagrasses into modern economic practices to achieve the Sustainable Development Goals (SDG, also known as the Global Goals), adopted by the United Nations in 2015 to achieve a better and more sustainable future for all by 2030 [16].

Globally, there are about 60 species of marine flowering plants, with only 4 considered native to the Mediterranean Sea [18]. These species belong to four families: *Posidoniaceae*, *Zosteraceae*, *Hydrocharitaceae*, and *Cymodoceaceae*, which are all classified within the order Alismatales and the clade of monocotyledons (Figure 1).

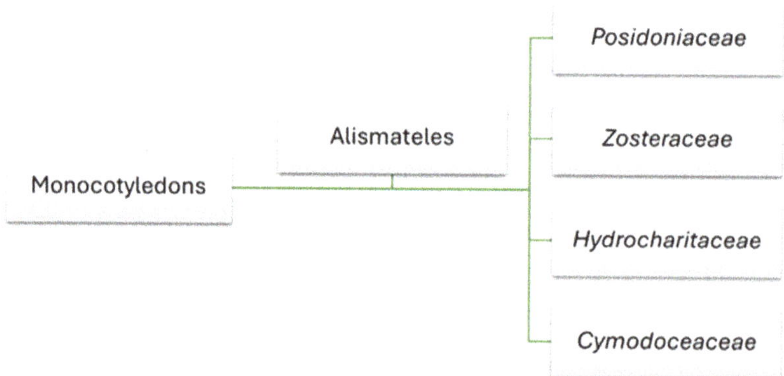

Figure 1. Seagrass family within the order Alismatales in the monocot clade.

The four native species found in Mediterranean waters are *Posidonia oceanica*, *Cymodocea nodosa*, *Zostera marina*, and *Zostera noltii* [19]. Among these, *Posidonia oceanica* and *Cymodocea nodosa* play a fundamental role as structuring species within marine flowering plant communities. These plants not only provide essential habitat for a variety of marine organisms but are also capable of hosting various epiphytic algae, thereby contributing to the biodiversity of marine ecosystems [20,21]. Their presence is crucial for the health of coastal environments, performing vital ecological functions and supporting marine life [12,22].

1.1.1. *Posidonia oceanica*

P. oceanica, commonly known as "Neptune Grass", is an endemic species of the Mediterranean Sea that thrives in clear, shallow waters, up to 25–30 m deep, and occasionally up to 40 m in insular areas [23] (Figure 2A). Recognized as one of the planet's oldest and most remarkable organisms, *P. oceanica* can live for nearly 100,000 years [24]. Its extremely slow growth and remarkable longevity enable the formation of seagrass meadows that can persist for millennia. However, this slow growth also renders it susceptible to environmental stresses, meaning that recovery from any damage can take decades or even centuries [25]. While *P. oceanica* can tolerate some fluctuations in temperature, thriving best between 10–25 °C, prolonged exposure to extreme conditions can adversely affect its health and vitality [26]. This species is found exclusively in Mediterranean waters, where it creates barriers of compact sediments that help stabilize marine ecosystems. Its broad, elongated leaves grow in bundles attached to vertical rhizomes that spread horizontally, making the plant easily identifiable. Flowering occurs infrequently; its propagation primarily occurs through vegetative means via rhizome branching, further increasing the species' vulnerability to human activities and climate change [27].

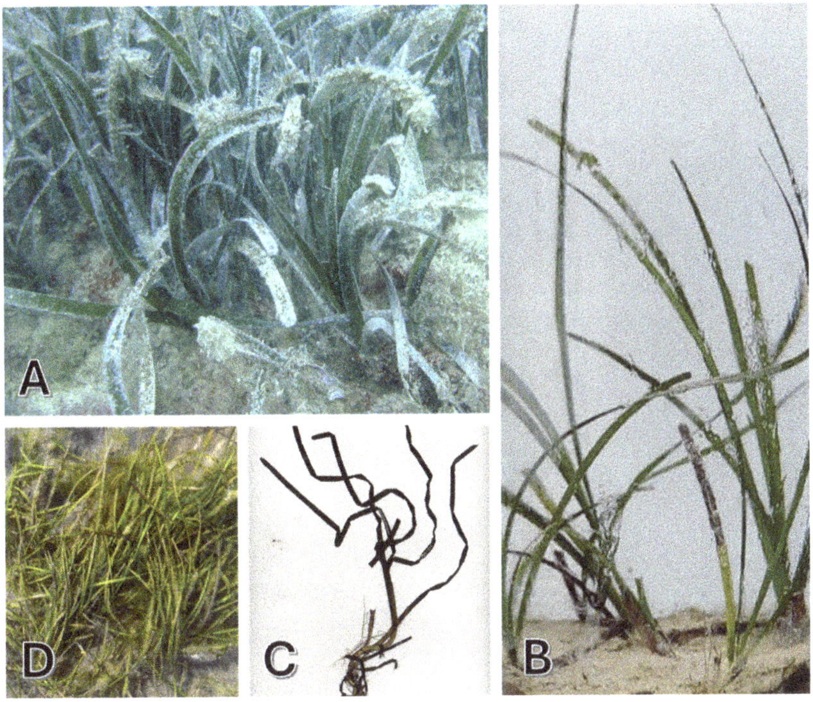

Figure 2. Representative images of the native Mediterranean plants: (**A**) *Posidonia oceanica*, (**B**) *Cymodocea nodosa*, (**C**) *Zostera marina*, and (**D**) *Zostera noltii*.

1.1.2. *Cymodocea nodosa*

C. nodosa, known as "seahorse grass", is a seagrass species that grows in warm waters of the Mediterranean, the Canary Islands, and along the North African coast up to southern Portugal (Figure 2B). It prefers depths between 0–60 m. The leaves are 2–4 mm wide and 10–45 cm long, and the white or pink rhizomes grow vertically and branch horizontally, facilitating the colonization of bare substrates. The flowering, which occurs rarely between May and August, produces seeds that are larger than those of *Z. marina* [19]. Considered a pioneer species, *C. nodosa* is more tolerant of environmental fluctuations compared to *P. oceanica* [28,29] and often precedes the climax communities of *P. oceanica* [30,31]. It thrives best in shallow coastal waters, estuaries, and lagoons [32], preferring muddy or sandy substrates up to 35 m deep. It requires good illumination and tolerates moderate water movement, with an optimal temperature range between 10–32 °C, making it relatively resilient to future climate changes [33,34].

1.1.3. *Zostera marina* and *Zostera noltii*

Z. marina, commonly referred to as "greater eelgrass", a perennial marine plant essential for the coastal ecosystems of the Northern Hemisphere, is found in shallow waters at 10–25 °C (Figure 2C). In the Mediterranean, *Z. marina* grows in small colonies in areas of low salinity. Its stems can reach up to 1.5 m, and the leaves have an average length of

20–35 cm. Reproduction occurs both vegetatively and sexually, but fruiting is rare [19]. In recent years, *Z. marina* has declined in the Mediterranean due to pollution and anthropization. Seagrass meadows of *Z. marina* are vital habitats for many marine species, and their disappearance threatens biodiversity. The conservation of this plant is crucial for the health of coastal marine ecosystems [14,35]. Interestingly, research conducted in 2016 by Olsen et al. reported for the first time the sequencing of the whole genome of the seagrass *Z. marina*, becoming the first angiosperm to be sequenced [36].

Z. noltii, or "dwarf eelgrass", is a Mediterranean marine plant forming dense beds in intertidal muddy sands (Figure 2D). Notable for its tolerance to desiccation, it thrives in areas with significant tidal changes, unlike *Z. marina*. Its leaves, 5 to 25 cm long and 0.5–2 mm wide, are anchored to a horizontal rhizome, providing stability in coastal environments. The plant's hermaphroditic flowers produce seeds likely dispersed by waterfowl, aiding its propagation. *Z. noltii* thrives in shallow waters, tolerating temperatures up to 38 °C, which enhances its adaptability. This resilience makes it vital for marine biodiversity, offering habitat for various organisms and contributing to coastal stability and ecosystem sustainability. In essence, *Z. noltii* is crucial for the health of marine environments and coastal protection [14,37].

1.2. Ecological Functions of Seagrasses and Their Secondary Metabolites

Seagrasses such as *P. oceanica*, *C. nodosa*, *Z. marina*, and *Z. noltii* are known to produce a diverse array of secondary metabolites that serve as vital defense mechanisms during stressful conditions. These compounds help protect the plants from oxidative stress caused by environmental challenges like UV radiation, temperature fluctuations, and water pollution. These secondary metabolites, like polyphenols, flavonoids, and polysaccharides, have been reported to possess a wide range of beneficial properties, including anticancer, antifungal, anti-inflammatory, antimicrobial, antiviral, antidiabetic, antimalarial, antioxidant, anti-aging, and cytotoxic effects. Moreover, these seagrass species are considered effective in the prevention of various human diseases, highlighting their potential as valuable sources for therapeutic applications [38,39].

2. Inflammation and Oxidative Stress: The Power of Marine Plants and Their Potential Environmental Impact

Since ancient times, early societies have used crude extracts of plants to treat infections, inflammation, pain and a variety of other ailments [38]. In recent decades, attention has been paid to marine herbal medicine to develop new therapeutic approaches or for other medical purposes [40]. In fact, studies worldwide have shown that several crude extracts derived from marine plants contain innovative bioactive compounds that can benefit health and can be used in medicine or food [41–43].

Research indicates that marine plants are abundant in micronutrients and secondary metabolites such as polyphenols, flavonoids, and carotenoids, which are essential in the prevention and/or treatment of chronic diseases, and in the promotion of human health [43,44]. Among these bioactive compounds, some are recognized for their therapeutic potential against inflammation and oxidative stress, two important aspects of many chronic diseases that are nowadays a global economic and health challenge [45,46].

Chronic inflammation and oxidative stress are a common factor of a wide range of disorders and diseases. Inflammatory processes not only affect short-term health, but also contribute to an overall decline in long-term health [47,48], negatively affecting health status and increasing susceptibility to various diseases that are not necessarily inflammatory. Chronic inflammation is characterized by a persistent immune response that can damage tissues and organs, while oxidative stress results from an excess of free radicals in the body, leading to cell damage and accelerated ageing [2,49]. Therefore, curbing the inflammatory process and oxidative stress is an important global goal in both medicine and prevention.

Currently, among the various methods to address inflammation, non-steroidal anti-inflammatory drugs (NSAIDs) are among the most widely used. NSAIDs are commonly employed to relieve pain, reduce inflammation, and lower fever [50]. While these drugs are effective for many patients, they are not universally suitable and can lead to a range of side effects [51–53]. Furthermore, the ease of access to NSAIDs, often available over the counter, encourages self-medication and can contribute to their excessive use and abuse [54]. This widespread drug consumption raises significant concerns regarding environmental contamination, as NSAIDs frequently enter aquatic ecosystems through wastewater effluents and household waste, posing risks to both wildlife and human health [55–58].

In light of these challenges, there is a growing interest in exploring natural products as alternative therapies. Indeed, natural substances are often renewable resources and generally exhibit a lower toxicity profile compared to conventional drugs [46]. This shift from chemicals to naturals can help mitigate the side effects associated with conventional treatments. Moreover, many natural compounds and/or phytocomplexes possess multiple mechanisms of action, which may enhance the efficacy of existing treatments.

The exploration of marine-derived therapies presents an opportunity not only to address health concerns but also to reduce environmental pollution, aligning with the principles of a circular economy: utilizing resources from the sea that can ultimately return to the marine environment in a sustainable manner (Figure 3). In this context, the identification and application of natural marine substances with anti-inflammatory and antioxidant properties are becoming increasingly important [46,59–61].

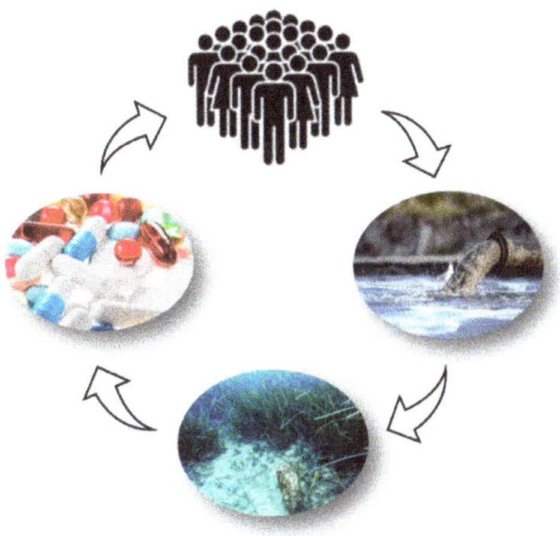

Figure 3. Marine pharmaceuticals: a virtuous cycle for human health and the preservation of marine ecosystems. The effects of pharmaceuticals extend far beyond the human body. All medications are eventually excreted from the body. Active ingredients or mixtures of metabolites are expelled through feces and urine. These substances flow into sewage treatment, which often struggles to eliminate the pharmaceutical residues that inevitably end up in the planet's waters.

By harnessing the potential of these compounds, we can effectively tackle health issues related to chronic inflammation and oxidative stress while simultaneously minimizing the ecological impact of pharmaceutical waste. This approach not only supports individual health but also promotes environmental sustainability, paving the way for a more responsible and holistic healthcare system [16].

As the Mediterranean native plants are poorly known in terms of their bioactivity, this review aims to provide a comprehensive analysis of the scientific evidence on their anti-inflammatory and antioxidant properties. By synthesizing the current literature, we will highlight the mechanisms through which these marine plants exert their beneficial effects, as well as their potential applications for human health. This exploration will not only enhance our understanding of the therapeutic potential of marine plants native to the Mediterranean but will also stimulate further research in this promising and rapidly expanding field. As we continue to explore the health benefits of these extraordinary plants, we may discover new strategies to address chronic diseases and promote general well-being.

3. Exploring the Antioxidant and Anti-Inflammatory Benefits of the Native Mediterranean Seagrasses

3.1. *Posidonia oceanica Bioactivity*

Since ancient times, the marine plant *P. oceanica* has been valued not only for its ecological role but also for its remarkable therapeutic properties. The ancient Egyptians, for example, used it to treat various ailments, demonstrating a long tradition in folk medicine [17]. Historical documentation confirms the use of *P. oceanica* to alleviate inflammation, acne, colitis, and respiratory infections, making it a valuable remedy for multiple pathologies [62,63]. Currently, contemporary research is rediscovering and delving into its potential, highlighting its beneficial properties and contributing to a renewed interest in a plant that has much to offer for human health and well-being.

This paragraph will analyze in detail the antioxidant and anti-inflammatory effects of *P. oceanica*, which could open new avenues in the treatment of various diseases.

For the first time, Gokce et al. (2008) described the antioxidant activity of a hydroalcoholic extract of *P. oceanica* leaves in an alloxane-induced diabetic Wistar albino rat model. The authors showed that oral administration of the extract (150 and 250 mg/kg body weight) led to a decrease in blood glucose and in a reduction in oxidative stress markers in the livers of diabetic rats, accompanied by increased levels of glutathione, GPx, SOD, CAT, nitric oxide (NO), and malondialdehyde (MDA) [63].

In the last decade, extracts of *P. oceanica* have attracted increasing scientific attention for their potential in the field of human health. In this context, *P. oceanica* stands out as a significant source of bioactive compounds, particularly polyphenols. These compounds, including phenolic acids and flavonoids, have been recognized for their ability to neutralize free radicals, reduce oxidative stress, and protect cells from damage caused by external agents [17].

In the research conducted by Messina et al. (2021), HPLC analysis revealed significant differences in the phenolic compound content of *P. oceanica* leaves, depending on their physiological state. Green leaves, rich in chlorophyll and photosynthetically active, show a higher polyphenol content compared to brown leaves and exhibit better antioxidant potential. This suggests that the harvesting and analysis of *P. oceanica* leaves could provide valuable insights for nutritional and therapeutic applications [64]. Additionally, extraction conditions, such as the grinding method and the type of solvent used, have a significant impact on the yield and antioxidant activity of the extracts. For instance, the Gd-E4 extract (obtained from green leaves dried at 60 °C for two days) showed the highest yield, with a polyphenols content of 19.712 ± 0.496 mg gallic acid equivalents (GAE)/g, as well as superior biological activity, evidenced by a DPPH IC_{50} value of 0.090 µg/µL. Particularly, HPLC analysis revealed chicoric acid as the most abundant phenolic compound in Gd-E4 (4991.813 µg/g). These findings underscore the importance of optimizing drying parameters to preserve heat-sensitive phenolic compounds, thereby maximizing extract quality and bioactivity [64]. Furthermore, the authors tested the photoprotective capacity of *P. oceanica* green leaf (Gd-E4) extracts in human skin fibroblasts (HS-68 cells) subjected to UV-induced oxidative stress. The reported results suggest that *P. oceanica* Gd-E4 extracts (0.15–1.5 μg/mL) induce significant protection against oxidative stress and mortality associated with UV exposure. In this context, the potential cosmetic applications of compounds extracted from *P. oceanica* appear promising, especially in the prevention of skin aging [64]. Additionally, the analysis of the ethanolic extract of *P. oceanica* leaves (PEE) by Cornara et al. (2018) highlighted chicoric acid as the main component of the extract (55.8 ± 7 mg/g dry weight in the PEE). Other major PEE compounds identified by HPLC-MS and tandem MS/MS were flavonoids, including procyanidin C2, procyanidin B2, isorhamnetin-3-*O*-glucoside, quercetin-3-*O*-glucoside, quercetin-3-*O*-malonylglucoside, and isorhamnetin-3-*O*-malonylglucoside. These compounds possesses remarkable in vitro antioxidant properties. The PEE showed an IC_{50} value of 32 ± 2 μg/mL in the DPPH radical scavenging assay, corresponding to 6.5 mM (1.14 mg/mL) ascorbic acid equivalents (AAE) [65]. The authors attributed the antioxidant activity of the extract rich in chicoric acid and flavonoids to its ability to stimulate human skin fibroblasts activity (20 μg/mL of PEE), promoting the collagen synthesis essential for maintaining skin elasticity and reducing signs of aging. The extract also demonstrated potential skin whitening effects by inhibiting the in vitro activity of the mushroom enzyme tyrosinase, with an estimated IC_{50} of 14.7 μg/mL of the PEE. Additionally, the PEE at a concentration of 50 μg/mL reduced melanin content in melanoma cells by approximately 50% within 72 h, suggesting a multifunctional approach to address hyperpigmentation problems [65]. The lipolytic effects observed by measuring the glycerol released by adipocytes following the triglyceride degradation indicate that the PEE (10–200 μg/mL) could have applications in the treatment of cellulite, improving skin texture.

By delving deeper into the focus on bioactive compounds in the research by Messina et al. (2021) and Cornara et al. (2018), it is highlighted that phenolic components (primarily chlorogenic acid) are fundamental in the bioactive profile of *Posidonia oceanica* extracts, with significant therapeutic and cosmetic potential, although the authors do not describe a molecular mechanism through which the extracts act on this process.

The antioxidant activity of *P. oceanica* was also reported by Piva et al. (2017), who evaluated a hydroalcoholic leaf extract (PO) rich in polyphenols using the DPPH assay [66]. The *P. oceanica* extract exhibited a total phenolic content of 711 mg GAE/g extract, and demonstrated an antioxidant capacity with an IC_{50} value of 72.42 ± 22.9 mg/L [66]. Additionally, Kevrekidou et al. (2024) investigated the methanolic extract of *P. oceanica* living leaves (LP). The total phenolic content of the LP extract was 222.80 ± 13.99 mg GAE/g dry weight. This study identified chicoric acid as the main polyphenol present in the extract (7.059%). The antioxidant activity was assessed using multiple methods, including the DPPH assay (IC_{50} value of 8.2 ± 0.8 μg/mL), ABTS radical scavenging assay (IC_{50} value of 1.6 ± 0.9 μg/mL), hydroxyl radical scavenging assay (IC_{50} value of 267 μg/mL), superoxide anion radical scavenging assay (IC_{50} 71.0 ± 2.0 μg/mL), and reducing power assay (19.5 ± 0.6 mg/mL) [67].

These data from Piva et al. (2017) and Kevrekidou et al. (2024) collectively confirm that *P. oceanica* possesses substantial antioxidant activity, largely driven by its high polyphenolic content, including chicoric acid. Its efficacy across multiple radical scavenging assays underscores its potential as a natural source of antioxidants.

The role of *P. oceanica* in counteracting oxidative stress and its anti-inflammatory properties was studied in a lipopolysaccharide (LPS)-stimulated murine macrophage model (RAW264.7 cells). The tested hydro-ethanolic extract from *P. oceanica* leaves (POE) contained 3.6 ± 3 mg GAE/mL of total polyphenols. Using UPLC analysis, the authors characterized the extract, revealing a large amount of catechins and smaller quantities of other polyphenols (gallic acid, chlorogenic acid, ferulic acid, epicatechin) [68]. Additionally, the POE exhibited a radical scavenging activity in the DPPH assay and antioxidant activity in the FRAP assay, with values of 11.0 ± 0.7 mg AAE/mL and 0.9 ± 0.2 mg AAE/mL, respectively.

The POE (2.88 μg GAE/mL) was shown to provide non-toxic protection against LPS-induced damage by reducing intracellular ROS levels and cytotoxicity and by modulating inflammatory mediators such as NO, inducible nitric oxide synthase (iNOS), and cyclooxygenase-2 (COX-2) [68]. Furthermore, it was shown that the POE prevented the phosphorylation and activation of NF-κB, a crucial signaling pathway in the inflammatory response, and its upstream pathways, ERK1/2 and Akt [68]. The implications of these findings are significant: they not only contribute to understanding *P. oceanica* as an anti-inflammatory agent but also highlight its potential role in the co-treatment of chronic diseases associated with inflammation. In the work of Micheli et al. (2021), a polyphenol-rich hydroalcoholic extract of *P. oceanica* leaves (POE) showed a radical scavenging activity of 1.2 ± 0.04 mg AAE/mL (tested by a DPPH assay) and an antioxidant activity of 0.24 ± 0.05 mg AAE/mL (tested by a FRAP assay). The authors tested the POE in an in vivo experimental model of acute inflammatory pain in CD-1 mice. The POE demonstrated a dose-dependent effect when orally administered (10–100 mg/kg body weight), reducing inflammatory and oxidative markers, increasing the pain threshold, and decreasing edema formation [69]. The POE (100 mg/kg body weight) has been shown to decrease myeloperoxidase (MPO) activity and levels of inflammatory cytokines, such as IL-1β and TNF-α, in tissues, underscoring its ability to modulate inflammatory responses. This study represents a significant step, as it is the first to provide pharmacological evidence regarding the ability of *P. oceanica* to alleviate inflammatory pain in vivo [69].

Based on these findings, the research conducted by Micheli et al. (2024) examined the effect of POE on C57BL/6 murine model of psoriasis-like skin lesions induced by Imiquimod for 5 days. The antioxidant activity of POE was measured in vitro by DPPH and FRAP assays, with values of 1.1 ± 0.2 mg AAE/mL and 0.13 ± 0.07 mg AAE/mL, respectively. The oral administration of the POE (100 mg/kg body weight) showed promising results, significantly reducing the PASI score (Psoriasis Area Severity Index) and the histological features characteristic of psoriasis, such as hyperkeratosis [70]. The *P. oceanica* extract inhibited the expression of key inflammatory cytokines, such as TNF-α, IL-17A, and IL-23, suggesting that this plant extract not only modulates inflammatory signals but may also prevent the activation of the NF-κB pathway, which is fundamental in the pathogenesis of psoriasis. Furthermore, the reduction of the plasma levels of lipocalin-2, a potential therapeutic target for psoriasis, further highlights the modulatory action of the *P. oceanica* extract [70].

Both the in vitro and in vivo results consistently indicate that the POE exerts antioxidant and anti-inflammatory effects through modulation of key signaling pathways such as NF-κB and upstream kinases. The in vitro data elucidate molecular mechanisms at the cellular level, including ROS scavenging and cytokine suppression, while the in vivo studies demonstrate tangible therapeutic benefits, such as pain reduction and skin lesion improvement.

The potential antioxidant and anti-inflammatory mechanisms of action attributed to *P. oceanica* extracts described in this review are overall schematically reported in Figure 4.

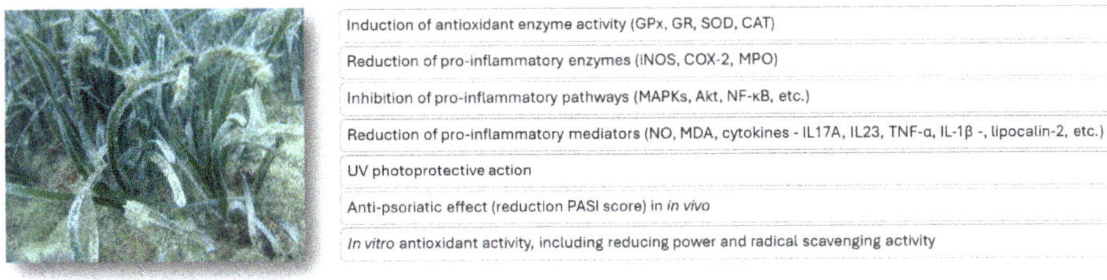

Figure 4. Putative mechanisms of the antioxidant and anti-inflammatory action of extracts from the *P. oceanica* marine plant.

In conclusion, the scientific research summarized in Table 1 underscores the significant antioxidant and anti-inflammatory properties of *P. oceanica*. Traditionally valued for its therapeutic potential, actual scientific studies have confirmed its capacity to neutralize free radicals, reduce oxidative stress, and modulate inflammatory pathways. The bioactive compounds, particularly polyphenols, play a central role in these effects, with extract preparations showing promise in protecting skin cells, mitigating inflammatory responses, and potentially addressing chronic inflammatory conditions. Importantly, *P. oceanica* exhibits no notable toxicity both in vitro and in vivo, highlighting its safety profile for future therapeutic and cosmetic applications. Collectively, these findings position *P. oceanica* as a promising natural marine resource for developing novel strategies to prevent and treat oxidative stress-related and inflammatory diseases, warranting further exploration and clinical validation.

Table 1. Experimental details of scientific research on the antioxidant and anti-inflammatory properties of *P. oceanica*.

Plant Material	Extraction Method	Compound Class	Cellular Model	Animal Model	In Vitro Assay	Ref.
Leaves	Hydro-ethanolic	Polyphenols		Wistar albino rats (150–250 mg/kg b.w.)		[63]
Leaves	Hydro-ethanolic (Gd-E4)	Polyphenols	Human skin HS-68 fibroblasts (0.15–1.5 μg/mL)		DPPH (IC_{50} 0.090 μg/mL)	[64]
Leaves	Hydro-ethanolic (PEE)	Polyphenols			DPPH (IC_{50} 32 ± 2 μg/mL)	[65]
Leaves	Hydro-ethanolic (PO)	Polyphenols			DPPH (IC_{50} 72.42 ± 22.9 mg/L)	[66]
Leaves	Methanolic (LP)	Polyphenols			DPPH (IC_{50} 8.2 ± 0.8 μg/mL); ABTS (IC_{50} 1.6 ± 0.9 μg/mL); hydroxyl radical scavenging (IC_{50} 267 μg/mL); superoxide anion radical scavenging (IC_{50} 71.0 ± 2.0 μg/mL); reducing power (19.5 ± 0.6 mg/mL)	[67]
Leaves	Hydro-ethanolic (POE)	Polyphenols	Murine RAW 264.7 macrophages (2.88 μg GAE/mL)		DPPH (11.0 ± 0.7 mg AAE/mL); FRAP (0.9 ± 0.2 mg AAE/mL)	[68]
Leaves	Hydro-ethanolic (POE)	Polyphenols		CD-1 mice (10–100 mg/kg b.w.)	DPPH (1.2 ± 0.04 mg AAE/mL); FRAP (0.24 ± 0.05 mg AAE/mL)	[69]
Leaves	Hydro-ethanolic (POE)	Polyphenols		C57BL/6 mice (100 mg/kg b.w.)	DPPH (1.1 ± 0.2 mg AAE/mL); FRAP (0.13 ± 0.07 mg AAE/mL)	[70]

3.2. *Cymodocea nodosa* Bioactivity

The marine plant *C. nodosa* has emerged as a subject of interest in the realm of natural health due to its promising antioxidant and anti-inflammatory benefits.

The antioxidant capacity of *C. nodosa* was first prominently documented by Kolsi et al. (2015). This study represented a significant innovation by thoroughly examining the chemical composition, biological properties, and potential nutritional benefits of a polysaccharide extracted from the leaves of the seagrass *C. nodosa* [71]. The authors isolated the sulphated polysaccharide from *C. nodosa* (CNSP) via hot water extraction and analyzed its chemical composition. The polysaccharide fraction was rich in sulphates and carbohydrates, while proteins and lipids were present in moderate and low amounts, respectively. Studies on CNSP in high-fat diet (HFD)-fed rats revealed significant antioxidant activity, evidenced by increased activities of SOD, CAT, and GPx, as well as enhanced reducing power—all of which were strongly dependent on concentration—and protecting the liver and kidneys of rats [71]. In 2017 Kolsi et al. revealed that CNSP exhibits a range of interesting properties, including antioxidant, antimicrobial, and cytotoxic activities, making it a promising candidate for future applications in nutraceuticals and functional foods, as well as in alternative medicine and natural therapies [72]. The results revealed that CNSP had high activity in the total antioxidant assay (59.03 mg AAE/g extract), reducing power (OD = 0.3), DPPH radical scavenging (IC_{50} = 1.22 mg/mL), and ABTS radical scavenging (IC_{50} = 1.14 mg/mL). Notably, CNSP demonstrated significant antioxidant activity in Hela cells subjected to oxidative stress induced by Fe_2SO_4 (100 mM). After oxidative stress induction, it was observed that Hela cells pre-treated with different concentrations of CNSP (0.015, 0.0035 and 0.0015 μg/mL for 72 h) showed a significant reduction in lipid oxidation. These findings open new opportunities for the use of CNSP in preventive and therapeutic strategies, laying the groundwork for future developments in the field of health and wellness [72].

The research underscores CNSP's strong antioxidant capacity both in vitro and in vivo, highlighting its potential as a natural antioxidant agent for health promotion and disease prevention. These results align with the existing literature, as marine polysaccharides extracted from algae and marine organisms are attracting increasing interest for their potential anti-inflammatory and antioxidant properties [73–75].

In a further study by Kolsi et al. (2017), flavonoids and phenolic acid derivatives were characterized from a hydro-ethanolic extract of *C. nodosa* (CNE). Specifically, four flavonoids (catechin, quercetin-3-O-rutinoside, quercetin-3-O-glucoside, and isorhamnetin-3-O-rutinoside) and three phenolic acid derivatives (sinapinic acid, ferulic acid, and cinnamic acid) were characterized from the CNE. The CNE (100–2000 mg/kg body weight) demonstrated the ability to enhance antioxidant defenses by increasing levels of SOD, CAT, and GPx in the pancreas, liver, and kidneys of alloxan-induced diabetic rats. Additionally, it reduced lipid peroxidation (LPO) in these organs. Histological analyses confirmed tissue protection and regeneration [76]. This highlights how these bioactive compounds can bolster antioxidant defenses by increasing antioxidant enzymes in vital organs, thereby reducing oxidative stress and lipid peroxidation. The findings also suggest tissue protection and regenerative effects, which are significant for developing natural interventions for diabetes-related oxidative damage and organ protection.

In a related study, Chaabani et al. (2024) investigated the efficacy of ultrasound-assisted extraction techniques to maximize the recovery of phenolic compounds from *C. nodosa* [77]. The results revealed that, under optimized extraction conditions, both the total phenolic content (113.07 mg GAE/g dry extract) and antioxidant activity (67.02%)—assessed by a DPPH assay—of the extracts obtained were significantly high. In particular, the study identified synaptic acid, myricetin, and quercetin-3-O-rutinoside, well documented for their potent antioxidant and anti-inflammatory properties, as key phenolic compounds. In addition, the authors demonstrated the anti-inflammatory activity of *C. nodosa* extracts by measuring their ability to inhibit the production of NO, a recognized biomarker of inflammation, in RAW264.7 murine macrophage cells stimulated with LPS. A slight inhibition of NO production was observed at a non-cytotoxic dose of 400 μg/mL of *C. nodosa* extracts. The combined antioxidant and anti-inflammatory activity of the tested eco-friendly extracts suggests that they could be used in skincare cream to combat oxidative stress and skin inflammation [77]. This study provides scientific validation for the potential use of *C. nodosa*-derived phenolic-rich extracts as natural, eco-friendly ingredients in skincare products targeting oxidative damage and inflammation, aligning with current trends favoring plant-based and sustainable formulations.

The potential antioxidant and anti-inflammatory mechanisms of action attributed to *C. nodosa* extracts described in this review are overall schematically reported in Figure 5.

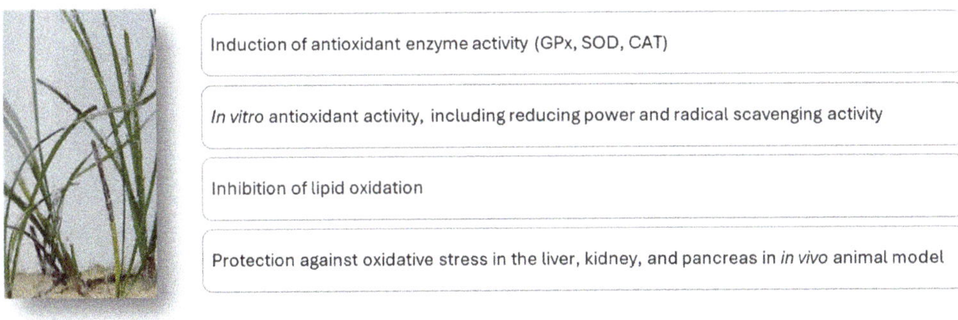

Figure 5. Putative mechanisms of the antioxidant and anti-inflammatory action of extracts from the *C. nodosa* marine plant.

In conclusion, *C. nodosa* has demonstrated significant potential as a natural marine source with antioxidant and anti-inflammatory properties (Table 2). The reviewed studies reveal that its bioactive polysaccharides and phenolic constituents possess robust free radical scavenging, reducing, and anti-inflammatory activities, which could be harnessed in the development of functional foods, nutraceuticals, and topical formulations. Future research should focus on further elucidating its mechanisms of action, optimizing extraction techniques, and evaluating its efficacy and safety in clinical settings.

Table 2. Experimental details of scientific research on the antioxidant and anti-inflammatory properties of *C. nodosa*.

Plant Material	Extraction Method	Compound Class	Cellular Model	Animal Model	In vitro Assay	Ref.
Raw material (CNSP)	Hot water	Polysaccharides		HDF-rats		[71]
Leaves (CNSP)	Water with ethanol precipitation	Polysaccharides	Epithelial cervical Hela cells (0.015–0.0015 μg/mL)		DPPH (IC_{50} = 1.22 mg/mL); ABTS (IC_{50} = 1.14 mg/mL); total antioxidant (59.0 mg AAE/g); reducing power (OD = 0.3)	[72]
Raw material (CNE)	Hydro-ethanolic	Pholyphenols		Male Wistar rats (100–2000 mg/kg b.w.)		[76]
Raw material	Hydro-ethanolic, ultrasound assisted	Polyphenols	Murine RAW 264.7 macrophage (400 μg/mL)		Total antioxidant (113.07 mg GAE/g); DPPH (67.02%)	[77]

3.3. *Zostera marina* and *Zostera noltii* Bioactivity

The marine plant *Z. marina* has garnered significant attention in recent years due to its remarkable therapeutic properties, particularly in the domains of skin health and anti-aging.

A study indicates that hydroalcoholic extracts of *Z. marina* leaves possess substantial antioxidant activity and the ability to inhibit matrix metalloproteinase-1 (MMP-1) [78]. MMPs are the primary enzymes responsible for extracellular matrix breakdown; particularly, MMP-1 is a crucial enzyme in collagen degradation and skin aging processes. Inhibiting MMPs is crucial for maintaining youthful skin [79]. The authors investigated the role of three major compounds isolated from an ethyl acetate-soluble fraction of *Z. marina*, namely apigenin-7-O-β-D-glucoside, chrysoeriol, and luteolin. These compounds demonstrated significant antioxidant activity. Their effectiveness was quantified through SC_{50} values in DPPH assay and in xanthine/xanthine oxidase system, with luteolin showing the strongest activity (0.01 mM). Additionally, luteolin showed the most potent radical scavenging activity, demonstrating a remarkable ability to inhibit MMP-1 expression by up to 44% at 4 μM in a UVA-irradiated human skin fibroblast (Hs68) cell model. This effect is particularly significant, as it is directly related to the preservation of collagen integrity in the skin. In addition, luteolin was also found to suppress the production of IL-6 by 30% at 4 μM, which is a cytokine that promotes MMP-1 expression, in a UVB-irradiated human (HaCaT) keratinocyte cell model. These results further consolidate the role of *Z. marina* extracts as a potential photoprotective agent given its strong antioxidant activity [78]. This study underscores the relevance of *Z. marina* extracts as potent natural agents capable of combating skin aging processes through antioxidant activity and enzyme inhibition, highlighting their potential in skincare formulations aimed at photoprotection and anti-aging.

Free radicals are often the cause of LPO, and they are therefore responsible for the destruction of biological membranes; therefore, the use of antioxidant agents could ensure the protection of tissues against the effect of free radicals. In the work of Khasina et al. (2003), the authors induced LPO in a murine model using white male mice and evaluated the MDA liver levels, as well as the activity of GR and GPx in the liver [80]. LPO activation was induced by lead acetate (20 mg/kg of body weight), tetrachloromethane (300 mg/kg), sodium nitrite (50 mg/kg), or a mixture of polychlorinated biphenyls (SOVOL; 5 mg/kg). All tested substances caused an increase in hepatic MDA levels by an average of 1.8–2.5 times and a decrease in the activity of GR and GPx by 31–54%. The study demonstrated that two weeks after intragastric administration of a low-esterified pectin, named pectin-zosterin, in the form of a 1% gel at a dose of 100 mg/kg—isolated from raw material of *Z. marina*—the pro-oxidant process induced by LPO in mice was suppressed. These results provided the first evidence that pectin-zosterin from *Z. marina* enhances antioxidant mechanisms. However, the mechanism of the in vivo antioxidant effect of pectin-zosterin has not yet been elucidated. The authors hypothesize an antioxidant effect associated with the absorption properties of low-esterified pectins [80].

A comparative study conducted by Kolenchenko et al. (2005) further reinforced the antioxidant activity of the low-esterified pectin extracted from *Z. marina* raw material. This research demonstrated that the pectin exhibited superior reducing activity compared to established antioxidant agents used in medicine, namely Mildronate and Emoxipin. This was assessed through the inhibition of Fe^{2+} ascorbate-induced oxidation of Tween 80 (sorbitan monooleate) to malonic dialdehyde [81]. The study revealed that increasing the pectin concentration tenfold from 0.1% to 1% (0.1% solution: 1.7 ± 0.3%; 0.5% solution: 5.3 ± 0.4%; 1% solution: 10.9 ± 0.6%) significantly enhanced its reducing activity, resulting in an average 4.1-fold increase in reduced iron content after 60 min. In contrast, Emoxipin and Mildronat showed only about a 1.9-fold increase under similar conditions.

When assessing inhibitory effects, solutions of 1%, 0.5%, and 0.1% concentrations of pectin and Emoxipin demonstrated that pectin's inhibiting activity was higher—53.4%, 67.5%, and 80.2%, respectively—compared to Emoxipin's 72.2%, 60.1%, and 76.7%, all relative to Mildronat. Overall, the low-etherified pectin exhibits stronger reducing properties in vitro than the antioxidative drugs Mildronat and Emoxipin. Its capacity to inhibit Fe^{2+}-induced ascorbate oxidation of Tween 80 to malonic dialdehyde was less effective than Mildronat but comparable to Emoxipin, indicating its potential as a potent antioxidant with notable reducing activity.

According to the studies by Khasina et al. (2003) and Kolenchenko et al. (2005), it has been shown that polysaccharides, such as low-esterified pectin, are significant because they can directly scavenge free radicals, inhibit lipid peroxidation, and enhance endogenous antioxidant enzymes. The efficacy demonstrated in these studies suggests potential therapeutic applications for preventing diseases related to oxidative damage, preserving membrane integrity, and maintaining cellular health.

In a study conducted by Choi et al. (2009), a methanol crude extract of *Z. marina*, organic solvent fractions (n-hexane, chloroform, ethyl acetate, n-butanol), and a water fraction were screened for antioxidant activity [82]. The crude extract of *Z. marine* contained total polyphenols of 204.63 μg GAE/mg dry extract and showed a dose-dependent DPPH inhibitory activity (from 0.1 to 20 mg/mL) ranging from 3.12 ± 0.75% to 90.55 ± 2.34% and a dose-response reducing power (from 0.1 to 20 mg/mL) ranging from 0.03 ± 0.00% to 1.28 ± 0.06%. The water fraction was the most abundant (around 60.45%), but it contained the lowest phenolic content (50.25 μg/mg) and exhibited minimal antioxidant activity (<10% DPPH scavenging), indicating limited phenolic presence. Conversely, the ethyl acetate fraction, richest in phenolics (968.50 μg/mg), showed the strongest antioxidant effects, achieving over 95% DPPH scavenging with an IC_{50} of 0.46 mg/mL, which is comparable to standard antioxidants (BHA and ascorbic acid). The n-butanol fraction also demonstrated high scavenging activity (91.27% DPPH). Reducing power assays revealed that the n-butanol fraction (0.1 mg/mL) had the highest electron-donating capacity at lower concentrations, with both the ethyl acetate and n-butanol fractions exhibiting enhanced reducing activity at higher concentrations,' correlating with their phenolic richness. Overall, phenolic compounds are predominantly concentrated in semi-polar and non-polar fractions, such as ethyl acetate and n-butanol, which possess significant antioxidant activities, underscoring *Z. marina*'s potential as a natural source of bioactive antioxidants for functional applications [82]. This research enhances the understanding of the antioxidant potential of *Z. marina* extracts, emphasizing the importance of phenolic compounds concentrated in specific solvent fractions. It supports the exploration of *Z. marina* as a promising natural source for antioxidant agents that can be harnessed in various health and industrial applications to mitigate oxidative stress and associated disorders.

In addition to its antioxidant properties, the marine plant *Z. marina* has been studied for its anti-inflammatory effects. A research conducted in 2015 by Kim et al. showed that an ethanolic extract of *Z. marina*, called ZMEE, significantly reduced NO production and iNOS expression in LPS-induced RAW264.7 murine macrophages in a dose-dependent manner (0.1–100 μg/mL) [83]. Furthermore, ZMEE (0.1–100 μg/mL) was found to significantly inhibit the secretion of pro-inflammatory cytokines, including IL-6, IL-1β, and TNF-α. It also suppressed NF-κB activation and phosphorylation of mitogen-activated protein kinases (MAPKs) such as JNK, ERK, and p38 after treatment [83]. Furthermore, the authors demonstrated that topical administration of ZMEE (20 μL/ear) alleviated the oedema induced by 5% croton oil in the ears of IRC mice. Histological analyses of mouse ear tissues revealed a reduction in dermal thickness and a decrease in infiltrating mast cells. These results suggest an anti-inflammatory potential of *Z. marina* [83]. This information underscores the potential therapeutic applications of *Z. marina* as an anti-inflammatory agent, contributing to the broader understanding of marine plants' pharmacological properties.

The potential antioxidant and anti-inflammatory mechanisms of action attributed to *Z. marina* extracts described in this review are overall schematically reported in Figure 6.

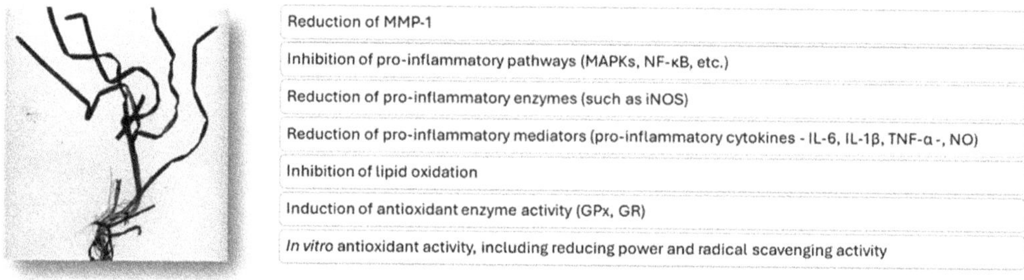

Figure 6. Putative mechanisms of the antioxidant and anti-inflammatory action of extracts from the *Z. marina* marine plant.

Belonging to the Zosteraceae family, *Z. noltii* shares a similar habitat with *Z. marina*, but presents significant differences in terms of bioactive properties and potential therapeutic applications. In a research conducted by Custódio et al. in 2014, a raw material methanol extract of *Z. marina*, collected in southern Portugal, showed a significantly higher total phenolic content (0.14 ± 0.01 mg GAE/g, dry weight) than that of *Z. noltii* (0.09 ± 0.00 mg GAE/g, dry weight). Rosmarinic acid, quantified by HPLC analysis, was found in the extracts for the two species and was the main component in *Z. marina* (0.24 mg/g dry weight), but not in *Z. noltei* (0.09 mg/g dry weight) [84]. This characteristic translates into a greater scavenging capacity for DPPH radicals (IC_{50} values of 0.31 ± 0.01 mg/mL and 1.10 ± 0.15 mg/mL in *Z. marina* and *Z. noltii*, respectively) and an effective copper chelation ability, suggesting potential therapeutic applications against oxidative stress. On the other hand, *Z. noltii* extract has shown lower antioxidant activity, although some capacity for chelation of metal ions has been identified. This difference in antioxidant activity may limit the therapeutic applications of *Z. noltii* compared to *Z. marina*. Overall, while *Z. marina* stands out for its promising antioxidant properties, *Z. noltii* shows significant limitations in these areas.

In conclusion, *Z. marina* exhibits a promising antioxidant and anti-inflammatory activities, which are primarily attributed to its rich content of phenolic compounds, summarized in Table 3. These constituents demonstrate significant radical scavenging capabilities, inhibition of matrix metalloproteinases involved in skin aging, and suppression of pro-inflammatory mediators, supporting its potential as a natural agent for skin health and photoprotection. Furthermore, the *Z. marina* ability to enhance endogenous antioxidant defenses underscores its capacity to mitigate oxidative stress at the tissue level. Comparative studies also highlight the superior antioxidant properties of *Z. marina* over related species like *Z. noltii*, emphasizing its therapeutic potential.

Table 3. Experimental details of scientific research on the antioxidant and anti-inflammatory properties of *Z. marina* and *Z. noltii*.

Plant Material	Extraction Method	Compound Class	Cellular Model	Animal Model	In Vitro Assay	Ref.
Leaves (*Z. marina*)	Hydro-ethanolic	Polyphenols (luteolin)	Human skin Hs68 fibroblasts and human HaCaT keratinocytes (4 μM)		DPPH (0.01 mM); xanthine/xanthine oxidase system (0.01 mM).	[78]

Table 3. *Cont.*

Plant Material	Extraction Method	Compound Class	Cellular Model	Animal Model	In Vitro Assay	Ref.
Raw material (*Z. marina*)	Ammonium oxalate with ethanol precipitation	Polysaccharide (pectin-zosterin)		White male mice (100 mg/kg b.w.)		[80]
Raw material (*Z. marina*)	Ammonium oxalate with ethanol precipitation	Polysaccharide (pectin)			Fe^{2+} ascorbate-induced oxidation (0.1, 0.5, 1%; solution: 1.7 ± 0.3%; 5.3 ± 0.4%; 10.9 ± 0.6%)	[81]
Raw material (*Z. marina*)	Methanol (crude extract)	Polyphenols			DPPH (0.1–20 mg/mL: 3.12 ± 0.75%–90.55 ± 2.34%); IC_{50} = 0.46 mg/mL); FRAP (0.1–20 mg/mL: 0.03 ± 0.00%–1.28 ± 0.06)	[82]
Raw material (*Z. marina*)	Hydro-ethanolic (ZMEE)	Undescribed	Murine RAW264.7 cells macrophages (0.1–100 μg/mL)	IRC mice (20 μL/ear)		[83]
Raw material (*Z. marina*)	Methanol	Polyphenols			DPPH (IC_{50} = 0.31 ± 0.01 mg/mL)	[84]
Raw material (*Z. noltii*)	Methanol	Polyphenols			DPPH (IC_{50} = 1.10 ± 0.15 mg/mL)	[84]

4. Bioactive Compounds from the Native Mediterranean Seagrasses and Their Therapeutic Potential

The ecological functions of seagrasses, such as providing protection against environmental stressors through the production of antioxidant and anti-inflammatory compounds, are directly related to their potential as sources of natural bioactive substances for human health [85]. The same secondary metabolites that help seagrasses defend against abiotic and oxidative stress also exhibit potent antioxidant and anti-inflammatory activities beneficial to human health, as previously discussed.

The work collected in this review clearly shows that native Mediterranean seagrasses are a rich source of secondary metabolites. In particular, it has been shown that the seagrass extracts described here are mainly composed of polyphenols, which have been attributed antioxidant and anti-inflammatory functions.

The main polyphenols identified in these seagrass extracts include chicoric acid, gallic acid, chlorogenic acid, catechin, epicatechin, ferulic acid, synaptic acid, myricetin, quercetin-3-O-rutinoside, quercetin, luteolin, apigenin-7-O-β-D-glucoside, chrysoeriol, quercetin-3-O-rutinoside, quercetin-3-O-glucoside, quercetin-3-O-malonylglucoside, isorhamnetin-3-O-rutinoside, isorhamnetin-3-O-glucoside, isorhamnetin-3-O-malonylglucoside, sinapinic acid, cinnamic acid, rosmarinic acid, procyanidin C2, and procyanidin B2.

It is important to emphasize that the bioactive properties of the seagrasses described have mainly been attributed to polyphenol-rich extracts. In particular, these extracts act as a phytocomplex, and their antioxidant and anti-inflammatory properties cannot be attributed to a single specific compound.

This aspect underlines the importance of considering the phytocomplex rather than the single compound, since the phytocomplex represents the entirety and abundance of the many secondary metabolites of the specific seagrass.

Among secondary metabolites, polysaccharides have also been extracted, such as the sulfated polysaccharide from *C. nodosa* (CNSP) and low-esterified pectin from *Z. marina*. These polysaccharides have demonstrated the ability to neutralize free radicals and reduce oxidative stress. According to the literature, it was observed that the chemical antioxidant activity of polysaccharides in vitro is greatly influenced by factors such as their solubility, sugar ring configuration, molecular weight, presence of charged groups, protein components, and covalently attached phenolic compounds [86].

It should be noted that the studies collected in this review describe the antioxidant and anti-inflammatory activities of seagrass extracts obtained through a wide variety of extraction methods. Variations in extraction protocols can influence the yield, potency, and composition of the bioactive compounds, thereby limiting the ability to draw definitive conclusions. Furthermore, phytochemical analysis was not conducted for all tested and reported extracts, making detailed comparative analysis difficult. This gap hampers the ability to identify specific active compounds responsible for the observed biological activities and restricts detailed mechanistic understanding. Additionally, when phytochemical characterization was performed, it was observed that the chemical composition varies depending on several factors, such as collection site, seasonality, depth, harvesting period, and others. In addition, most of the studies conducted so far are in vitro or preliminary in vivo, and there is therefore a paucity of clinical investigations to substantiate the health claims of compounds derived from seagrasses.

In summary, while the collected studies support the promising role of seagrass secondary metabolites in promoting human health, these limitations highlight the need for more standardized, comprehensive, and mechanistically oriented research to fully elucidate their potential and facilitate clinical translation.

5. Research Methodology

This overview collected 18 research articles found in the literature from 2003 to 2024 on the description of antioxidant and anti-inflammatory properties of native Mediterranean plants. Extensive searches were performed in PubMed, ScienceDirect, Web of Science, and Google Scholar databases using one or a combination of the following terms: "marine plants", "seagrasses", "marine natural compounds", "marine plants with antioxidant properties", "marine plants with anti-inflammatory properties", "*Posidonia oceanica* bioactivity", "*Cymodocea nodosa* bioactivity", "*Zostera marina* bioactivity", and "*Zostera noltii* bioactivity". The marine plant images were provided by the staff of the Interuniversity Center of Marine Biology and Applied Ecology "G. Bacci" (CIBM) of Leghorn (Italy) and by Prof. Valentino Casolo of the University of Udine (Italy). Figures were created by Microsoft PowerPoint per Microsoft 365 MSO (Version 2502 Build 18526.20168).

6. Future Perspectives

With the increasing awareness of the importance of human health and well-being, seagrasses are emerging as a promising resource capable of providing innovative and sustainable solutions to address public health and environmental conservation challenges [85]. Integrating these resources into natural treatments could represent a significant step towards a holistic approach to health that recognizes the deep connection between humans and the marine environment.

Native Mediterranean seagrasses, in particular, offer a unique opportunity to improve human health, promote environmental sustainability, and stimulate innovation. These species, often adapted to specific conditions of the marine ecosystem, can provide bioactive compounds with potential health benefits, such as antioxidant and anti-inflammatory properties. The growing interest in the sustainable use of marine resources can also contribute to the protection of these delicate ecosystems, ensuring the availability of such resources for future generations.

NSAIDs are among the most well-known and widely used medications in both human and veterinary medicine. However, their widespread use has led to their identification as emerging contaminants in the environment. For example, in recent decades, the use of NSAIDs in companion animals has significantly increased, becoming a standard practice. In this context, the veterinary community must look to human studies as a crucial source of information to gain insights into the potential of new natural drugs that are free from side effects. Given the increasing abuse of NSAIDs in both human and veterinary medicine, this collection of scientific data, aligned with the "One Health" approach, highlights the anti-inflammatory potential of seagrasses and aims to serve and guide future research in this area [16].

We hope that the research compiled in this overview can stimulate a greater understanding of the potential of native Mediterranean seagrass and encourage the development of new strategies for the management and conservation of marine biodiversity, promoting a more sustainable and healthier future for all.

Author Contributions: Conceptualization, M.V. and D.D.; writing—original draft preparation, M.V. and D.D.; writing—review and editing, L.D.M., C.P. and E.B.; and funding acquisition, D.D. All authors have read and agreed to the published version of the manuscript.

Funding: This research was funded by the University of Florence (Fondi di Ateneo 2025 to D.D.).

Acknowledgments: Images of *Posidonia oceanica* (Figure 2A) and *Cymodocea nodosa* (Figure 2B) were provided by the CIBM staff (Leighorn, Italy); images of *Zostera marina* (Figure 2C) and *Zostera noltii* (Figure 2D) were provided courtesy of Valentino Casolo of the University of Udine (Italy).

Conflicts of Interest: The authors declare no conflict of interest.

References

1. Calhelha, R.C.; Haddad, H.; Ribeiro, L.; Heleno, S.A.; Carocho, M.; Barros, L. Inflammation: What's There and What's New? *Appl. Sci.* **2023**, *13*, 2312. [CrossRef]
2. Chen, L.; Deng, H.; Cui, H.; Fang, J.; Zuo, Z.; Deng, J.; Li, Y.; Wang, X.; Zhao, L. Inflammatory responses and inflammation-associated diseases in organs. *Oncotarget* **2017**, *9*, 7204–7218. [CrossRef]
3. Megha, K.B.; Joseph, X.; Akhil, V.; Mohanan, P.V. Cascade of immune mechanism and consequences of inflammatory disorders. *Phytomedicine* **2021**, *91*, 153712. [CrossRef] [PubMed]
4. Chaudhary, P.; Janmeda, P.; Docea, A.O.; Yeskaliyeva, B.; Abdull Razis, A.F.; Modu, B.; Calina, D.; Sharifi-Rad, J. Oxidative stress, free radicals and antioxidants: Potential crosstalk in the pathophysiology of human diseases. *Front Chem.* **2023**, *11*, 1158198. [CrossRef]
5. Jena, A.B.; Samal, R.R.; Bhol, N.K.; Duttaroy, A.K. Cellular Red-Ox system in health and disease: The latest update. *Biomed. Pharmacother.* **2023**, *162*, 114606. [CrossRef]
6. de Almeida, A.J.P.O.; de Oliveira, J.C.P.L.; da Silva Pontes, L.V.; de Souza Júnior, J.F.; Gonçalves, T.A.F.; Dantas, S.H.; de Almeida Feitosa, M.S.; Silva, A.O.; de Medeiros, I.A. ROS: Basic Concepts, Sources, Cellular Signaling, and its Implications in Aging Pathways. *Oxid. Med. Cell. Longev.* **2022**, *2022*, 1225578. [CrossRef]
7. Bhol, N.K.; Bhanjadeo, M.M.; Singh, A.K.; Dash, U.C.; Ojha, R.R.; Majhi, S.; Duttaroy, A.K.; Jena, A.B. The interplay between cytokines, inflammation, and antioxidants: Mechanistic insights and therapeutic potentials of various antioxidants and anti-cytokine compounds. *Biomed. Pharmacother.* **2024**, *178*, 117177. [CrossRef]
8. Olaniyan, M.F.; Muhibi, M.A.; Olaniyan, T.B. Oxidative Stress and Inflammatory Response Interplay. *J. Prev. Med.* **2023**, *2*, 94–100. [CrossRef]
9. Trache, D.; Tarchoun, A.F.; De Vita, D.; Kennedy, J.F. *Posidonia oceanica* (L.) Delile: A Mediterranean seagrass with potential applications but regularly and erroneously referred to as an algal species. *Int. J. Biol. Macromol.* **2023**, *230*, 122624. [CrossRef]
10. Wissler, L.; Codoñer, F.M.; Gu, J.; Reusch, T.B.H.; Olsen, J.L.; Procaccini, G.; Bornberg-Bauer, E. Back to the sea twice: Identifying candidate plant genes for molecular evolution to marine life. *BMC Evol. Biol.* **2011**, *11*, 8. [CrossRef]
11. Ma, X.; Vanneste, S.; Chang, J.; Ambrosino, L.; Barry, K.; Bayer, T.; Bobrov, A.A.; Boston, L.; Campbell, J.E.; Chen, H.; et al. Seagrass genomes reveal ancient polyploidy and adaptations to the marine environment. *Nat. Plants* **2024**, *10*, 240–255. [CrossRef]
12. Duarte, C.M. The future of seagrass meadows. *Environ. Conserv.* **2002**, *29*, 192–206. [CrossRef]
13. Fourqurean, J.; Duarte, C.; Kennedy, H.; Marbà, N.; Holmer, M.; Mateo, M.A.; Apostolaki, E.T.; Kendrick, G.A.; Krause-Jensen, D.; McGlathery, K.J.; et al. Seagrass ecosystems as a globally significant carbon stock. *Nat. Geosci.* **2012**, *5*, 505–509. [CrossRef]
14. Orth, R.J.; Carruthers, T.J.B.; Dennison, W.C.; Duarte, C.M.; Fourqurean, J.W.; Heck, K.L.; Hughes, A.R.; Kendrick, G.A.; Kenworthy, W.J.; Olyarnik, S.; et al. A Global Crisis for Seagrass Ecosystems. *Bioscience* **2006**, *56*, 987–996. [CrossRef]
15. Unsworth, R.K.; van Keulen, M.; Coles, R.G. Seagrass meadows in a globally changing environment. *Mar. Pollut. Bull.* **2014**, *83*, 383–386. [CrossRef]

16. Foster, N.R.; Apostolaki, E.T.; DiBenedetto, K.; Duarte, C.M.; Gregory, D.; Inostroza, K.; Krause-Jensen, D.; Jones, B.L.H. Serrano, E.; Zakhama-Sraieb, R.; et al. Societal value of seagrass from historical to contemporary perspectives. *Ambio* **2025** [CrossRef]
17. Vasarri, M.; De Biasi, A.M.; Barletta, E.; Pretti, C.; Degl'Innocenti, D. An Overview of New Insights into the Benefits of the Seagrass *Posidonia oceanica* for Human Health. *Mar. Drugs* **2021**, *19*, 476. [CrossRef]
18. Green, E.P.; Short, F.T. *World Atlas of Seagrasses Prepared by the UNEP World Conservation Monitoring Centre*; University of California Press: Berkeley, CA, USA, 2003; pp. 48–58.
19. Borum, J.; Greve, T. The four European seagrass species. In *European Seagrasses: An Introduction to Monitoring and Management* The M&MS Project; EU: Brussels, Belgium, 2004; pp. 1–7.
20. Balata, D.; Bertocci, I.; Piazzi, L.; Nesti, U. Comparison between epiphyte assemblages of leaves and rhizomes of the seagrass *Posidonia oceanica* subjected to different levels of anthropogenic eutrophication. *Estuar. Coast. Shelf Sci.* **2008**, *79*, 533–540. [CrossRef]
21. Tsioli, S.; Papathanasiou, V.; Rizouli, A.; Kosmidou, M.; Katsaros, C.; Papastergiadou, E.; Küpper, F.C.; Orfanidis, S. Diversity and composition of algal epiphytes on the Mediterranean seagrass *Cymodocea nodosa*: A scale-based study. *Bot. Mar.* **2021**, *64*, 101–118. [CrossRef]
22. Katsaros, C.; Orfanidis, S.; Küpper, F.C. What's new in marine botany of the Eastern Mediterranean? *Bot. Mar.* **2022**, *65*, 221–230. [CrossRef]
23. Panayotidis, P.; Papathanasiou, V.; Gerakaris, V.; Fakiris, E.; Orfanidis, S.; Papatheodorou, G.; Kosmidou, M.; Georgiou, N. Drakopoulou, V.; Loukaidi, V. Seagrass meadows in the Greek Seas: Presence, abundance and spatial distribution. *Bot. Mar.* **2022**, *65*, 289–299. [CrossRef]
24. Guerrero-Meseguer, L.; Sanz-Lázaro, C.; Marín, A. Understanding the sexual recruitment of one of the oldest and largest organisms on Earth, the seagrass *Posidonia oceanica*. *PLoS ONE* **2018**, *13*, e0207345. [CrossRef]
25. Pansini, A.; Bosch-Belmar, M.; Berlino, M.; Sarà, G.; Ceccherelli, G. Collating evidence on the restoration efforts of the seagrass *Posidonia oceanica*: Current knowledge and gaps. *Sci. Total Environ.* **2022**, *851*, 158320. [CrossRef]
26. Stipcich, P.; Marín-Guirao, L.; Pansini, A.; Pinna, F.; Procaccini, G.; Pusceddu, A.; Soru, S.; Ceccherelli, G. Effects of Current and Future Summer Marine Heat Waves on *Posidonia oceanica*: Plant Origin Matters? *Front. Clim.* **2022**, *4*, 844831. [CrossRef]
27. Telesca, L.; Belluscio, A.; Criscoli, A.; Ardizzone, G.; Apostolaki, E.T.; Fraschetti, S.; Gristina, M.; Knittweis, L.; Martin, C.S.; Pergent, G.; et al. Seagrass meadows (*Posidonia oceanica*) distribution and trajectories of change. *Sci. Rep.* **2015**, *5*, 12505. [CrossRef]
28. Infantes, E.; Orfila, A.; Bouma, T.J.; Simarro, G.; Terrados, J. *Posidonia oceanica* and *Cymodocea nodosa* seedling tolerance to wave exposure. *Limnol. Oceanogr.* **2011**, *56*, 2223–2232. [CrossRef]
29. Pergent, G.; Bazairi, H.; Bianchi, C.N.; Boudouresque, C.F.; Buia, M.C.; Calvo, S.; Clabaut, P.; Harmelin-Vivien, M.; Mateo, M.A.; Montefalcone, M.; et al. Climate change and Medditeranean seagrass meadows: A synopsis for environmental managers. *Mediterr. Mar. Sci.* **2014**, *15*, 462–473. [CrossRef]
30. Nadzari, M.; Papathanasiou, V.; Tsioli, S.; Küpper, F.C.; Orfanidis, S. Effects of flooding on the Mediterranean *Cymodocea nodosa* population in relation to environmental degradation. *Bot. Mar.* **2022**, *65*, 301–313. [CrossRef]
31. Cancemi, G.; Buia, M.C.; Mazzella, L. Structure and growth dynamics of *Cymodocea nodosa* meadows. *Sci. Mar.* **2002**, *66*, 365–373. [CrossRef]
32. Cunha, S.H.; Araújo, A. New distribution limits of seagrass beds in West Africa. *J. Biogeogr.* **2009**, *36*, 1613–1622. [CrossRef]
33. Ivajnšič, D.; Orlando-Bonaca, M.; Donša, D.; Grujić, V.J.; Trkov, D.; Mavrič, B.; Lipej, L. Evaluating Seagrass Meadow Dynamics by Integrating Field-Based and Remote Sensing Techniques. *Plants* **2022**, *11*, 1196. [CrossRef]
34. Egea, L.G.; Jiménez-Ramos, R.; Vergara, J.J.; Hernández, I.; Brun, F.G. Interactive effect of temperature, acidification and ammonium enrichment on the seagrass *Cymodocea nodosa*. *Mar. Pollut. Bull.* **2018**, *134*, 14–26. [CrossRef] [PubMed]
35. Boudouresque, C.-F.; Blanfuné, A.; Pergent, G.; Thibaut, T. Restoration of Seagrass Meadows in the Mediterranean Sea: A Critical Review of Effectiveness and Ethical Issues. *Water* **2021**, *13*, 1034. [CrossRef]
36. Olsen, J.L.; Rouzé, P.; Verhelst, B.; Lin, Y.C.; Bayer, T.; Collen, J.; Dattolo, E.; De Paoli, E.; Dittami, S.; Maumus, F.; et al. The genome of the seagrass *Zostera marina* reveals angiosperm adaptation to the sea. *Nature* **2016**, *530*, 331–335. [CrossRef]
37. Short, F.T.; Wyllie-Echeverria, S. Natural and human-induced disturbance of seagrasses. *Environ. Conserv.* **1996**, *23*, 17–27. [CrossRef]
38. Petrovska, B.B. Historical Review of Medicinal Plants usage. *Pharm. Rev.* **2012**, *6*, 1–5. [CrossRef]
39. Stiller, A.; Garrison, K.; Gurdyumov, K.; Kenner, J.; Yasmin, F.; Yates, P.; Song, B.-H. From Fighting Critters to Saving Lives: Polyphenols in Plant Defense and Human Health. *Int. J. Mol. Sci.* **2021**, *22*, 8995. [CrossRef]
40. Buonocore, E.; Grande, U.; Franzese, P.P.; Russo, G.F. Trends and Evolution in the Concept of Marine Ecosystem Services: An Overview. *Water* **2021**, *13*, 2060. [CrossRef]
41. Alves, A.; Sousa, E.; Kijjoa, A.; Pinto, M. Marine-Derived Compounds with Potential Use as Cosmeceuticals and Nutricosmetics. *Molecules* **2020**, *25*, 2536. [CrossRef]

42. Nieto, G.; Martínez-Zamora, L.; Peñalver, R.; Marín-Iniesta, F.; Taboada-Rodríguez, A.; López-Gómez, A.; Martínez-Hernández, G.B. Applications of Plant Bioactive Compounds as Replacers of Synthetic Additives in the Food Industry. *Foods* **2024**, *13*, 47. [CrossRef]
43. Ahmad, M.; Tahir, M.; Hong, Z.; Zia, M.A.; Rafeeq, H.; Ahmad, M.S.; Rehman, S.U.; Sun, J. Plant and marine-derived natural products: Sustainable pathways for future drug discovery and therapeutic development. *Front. Pharmacol.* **2025**, *15*, 1497668. [CrossRef] [PubMed]
44. Pandey, K.B.; Rizvi, S.I. Plant polyphenols as dietary antioxidants in human health and disease. *Oxid. Med. Cell. Longev.* **2009**, *2*, 270–278. [CrossRef]
45. Dash, U.C.; Bhol, N.K.; Swain, S.K.; Samal, R.R.; Nayak, P.K.; Raina, V.; Panda, S.K.; Kerry, R.G.; Duttaroy, A.K.; Jena, A.B. Oxidative stress and inflammation in the pathogenesis of neurological disorders: Mechanisms and implications. *Acta Pharm. Sin. B* **2025**, *15*, 15–34. [CrossRef]
46. Atanasov, A.G.; Zotchev, S.B.; Dirsch, V.M.; International Natural Product Sciences Taskforce; Supuran, C.T. Natural products in drug discovery: Advances and opportunities. *Nat. Rev. Drug Discov.* **2021**, *20*, 200–216. [CrossRef]
47. Furman, D.; Campisi, J.; Verdin, E.; Carrera-Bastos, P.; Targ, S.; Franceschi, C.; Ferrucci, L.; Gilroy, D.W.; Fasano, A.; Miller, G.W.; et al. Chronic inflammation in the etiology of disease across the life span. *Nat. Med.* **2019**, *25*, 1822–1832. [CrossRef]
48. Pizzino, G.; Irrera, N.; Cucinotta, M.; Pallio, G.; Mannino, F.; Arcoraci, V.; Squadrito, F.; Altavilla, D.; Bitto, A. Oxidative Stress: Harms and Benefits for Human Health. *Oxid. Med. Cell. Longev.* **2017**, *2017*, 8416763. [CrossRef]
49. Yang, J.; Luo, J.; Tian, X.; Zhao, Y.; Li, Y.; Wu, X. Progress in Understanding Oxidative Stress, Aging, and Aging-Related Diseases. *Antioxidants* **2024**, *13*, 394. [CrossRef]
50. Gunaydin, C.; Bilge, S.S. Effects of Nonsteroidal Anti-Inflammatory Drugs at the Molecular Level. *Eurasian J. Med.* **2018**, *50*, 116–121. [CrossRef]
51. Stöllberger, C.; Finsterer, J. Side effects of conventional nonsteroidal anti-inflammatory drugs and celecoxib: More similarities than differences. *South. Med. J.* **2004**, *97*, 209. [CrossRef]
52. Davis, A.; Robson, J. The dangers of NSAIDs: Look both ways. *Br. J. Gen. Pract.* **2016**, *66*, 172–173. [CrossRef]
53. Sohail, R.; Mathew, M.; Patel, K.K.; Reddy, S.A.; Haider, Z.; Naria, M.; Habib, A.; Abdin, Z.U.; Razzaq Chaudhry, W.; Akbar, A. Effects of Non-steroidal Anti-inflammatory Drugs (NSAIDs) and Gastroprotective NSAIDs on the Gastrointestinal Tract: A Narrative Review. *Cureus* **2023**, *15*, e37080. [CrossRef] [PubMed]
54. Marcum, Z.A.; Hanlon, J.T. Recognizing the Risks of Chronic Nonsteroidal Anti-Inflammatory Drug Use in Older Adults. *Ann. Long-Term Care* **2010**, *18*, 24–27.
55. Jiang, T.; Wu, W.; Ma, M.; Hu, Y.; Li, R. Occurrence and distribution of emerging contaminants in wastewater treatment plants: A globally review over the past two decades. *Sci. Total Environ.* **2024**, *951*, 175664. [CrossRef]
56. Justi, L.H.Z.; Silva, J.F.; Santana, M.S.; Laureano, H.A.; Pereira, M.E.; Oliveira, C.S.; Guiloski, I.C. Non-steroidal anti-inflammatory drugs and oxidative stress biomarkers in fish: A meta-analytic review. *Toxicol. Rep.* **2025**, *14*, 101910. [CrossRef]
57. Jan-Roblero, J.; Cruz-Maya, J.A. Ibuprofen: Toxicology and Biodegradation of an Emerging Contaminant. *Molecules* **2023**, *28*, 2097. [CrossRef]
58. Menicagli, V.; Ruffini Castiglione, M.; Cioni, E.; Spanò, C.; Balestri, E.; De Leo, M.; Bottega, S.; Sorce, C.; Lardicci, C. Stress responses of the seagrass *Cymodocea nodosa* to environmentally relevant concentrations of pharmaceutical ibuprofen: Ecological implications. *J. Hazard. Mater.* **2024**, *476*, 135188. [CrossRef]
59. Blagov, A.V.; Summerhill, V.I.; Sukhorukov, V.N.; Zhigmitova, E.B.; Postnov, A.Y.; Orekhov, A.N. Potential use of antioxidants for the treatment of chronic inflammatory diseases. *Front. Pharmacol.* **2024**, *15*, 1378335. [CrossRef]
60. Vasarri, M.; Degl'Innocenti, D. Antioxidant and Anti-Inflammatory Agents from the Sea: A Molecular Treasure for New Potential Drugs. *Mar. Drugs* **2022**, *20*, 132. [CrossRef]
61. Gouda, N.A.; Alshammari, S.O.; Abourehab, M.A.S.; Alshammari, Q.A.; Elkamhawy, A. Therapeutic potential of natural products in inflammation: Underlying molecular mechanisms, clinical outcomes, technological advances, and future perspectives. *Inflammopharmacology* **2023**, *31*, 2857–2883. [CrossRef]
62. El-Mokasabi, F.M. Floristic composition and traditional uses of plant species at Wadi Alkuf, Al-Jabal Al-Akhder, Libya. *Am. Eur. J. Agric. Environ. Sci.* **2014**, *14*, 685–697.
63. Gokce, G.; Haznedaroglu, M.Z. Evaluation of antidiabetic, antioxidant and vasoprotective effects of *Posidonia oceanica* extract. *J. Ethnopharmacol.* **2008**, *115*, 122–130. [CrossRef]
64. Messina, C.M.; Arena, R.; Manuguerra, S.; Pericot, Y.; Curcuraci, E.; Kerninon, F.; Renda, G.; Hellio, C.; Santulli, A. Antioxidant Bioactivity of Extracts from Beach Cast Leaves of *Posidonia oceanica* (L.) Delile. *Mar. Drugs* **2021**, *19*, 560. [CrossRef]
65. Cornara, L.; Pastorino, G.; Borghesi, B.; Salis, A.; Clericuzio, M.; Marchetti, C.; Damonte, G.; Burlando, B. *Posidonia oceanica* (L.) Delile Ethanolic Extract Modulates Cell Activities with Skin Health Applications. *Mar. Drugs* **2018**, *16*, 21. [CrossRef] [PubMed]

66. Piva, G.; Fracassetti, D.; Tirelli, A.; Mascheroni, E.; Musatti, A.; Inglese, P.; Piergiovanni, L.; Rollini, M. Evaluation of the antioxidant/antimicrobial performance of *Posidonia oceanica* in comparison with three commercial natural extracts and as a treatment on fresh-cut peaches (Prunus persica Batsch). *Postharvest Biol. Technol.* **2017**, *124*, 54–61. [CrossRef]
67. Kevrekidou, A.; Assimopoulou, A.N.; Trachana, V.; Stagos, D.; Malea, P. Antioxidant Activity, Inhibition of Intestinal Cancer Cell Growth and Polyphenolic Compounds of the Seagrass *Posidonia oceanica*'s Extracts from Living Plants and Beach Casts. *Mar. Drugs* **2024**, *22*, 130. [CrossRef]
68. Vasarri, M.; Leri, M.; Barletta, E.; Ramazzotti, M.; Marzocchini, R.; Degl'Innocenti, D. Anti-inflammatory properties of the marine plant *Posidonia oceanica* (L.) Delile. *J. Ethnopharmacol.* **2020**, *247*, 112252. [CrossRef]
69. Micheli, L.; Vasarri, M.; Barletta, E.; Lucarini, E.; Ghelardini, C.; Degl'Innocenti, D.; Di Cesare Mannelli, L. Efficacy of *Posidonia oceanica* Extract against Inflammatory Pain: In vivo Studies in Mice. *Mar. Drugs* **2021**, *19*, 48. [CrossRef]
70. Micheli, L.; Vasarri, M.; Degl'Innocenti, D.; Di Cesare Mannelli, L.; Ghelardini, C.; Emiliano, A.; Verdelli, A.; Caproni, M.; Barletta, E. *Posidonia oceanica* (L.) Delile Is a Promising Marine Source Able to Alleviate Imiquimod-Induced Psoriatic Skin Inflammation. *Mar. Drugs* **2024**, *22*, 300. [CrossRef]
71. Kolsi, R.B.A.; Ben Gara, A.; Chaaben, R.; El Feki, A.; Paolo Patti, F.; El Feki, L.; Belghith, K. Anti-obesity and lipid lowering effects of *Cymodocea nodosa* sulphated polysaccharide on high cholesterol-fed-rats. *Arch. Physiol. Biochem.* **2015**, *5*, 210–217. [CrossRef]
72. Kolsi, R.B.A.; Gargouri, B.; Sassi, S.; Frikha, D.; Lassoued, S.; Belghith, K. In vitro biological properties and health benefits of a novel sulfated polysaccharide isolated from *Cymodocea nodosa*. *Lipids Health Dis.* **2017**, *16*, 252. [CrossRef] [PubMed]
73. Khursheed, M.; Ghelani, H.; Jan, R.K.; Adrian, T.E. Anti-Inflammatory Effects of Bioactive Compounds from Seaweeds, Bryozoans, Jellyfish, Shellfish and Peanut Worms. *Mar. Drugs* **2023**, *21*, 524. [CrossRef] [PubMed]
74. Reddy, S.M.; Suresh, V.; Pitchiah, S.; Subramanian, B., 4th. Anti-inflammatory Activities of Sulfated Polysaccharides from Ethanol Crude Extract of Spyrida Species Red Seaweed. *Cureus* **2023**, *15*, e50284. [CrossRef]
75. Carrasqueira, J.; Bernardino, S.; Bernardino, R.; Afonso, C. Marine-Derived Polysaccharides and Their Potential Health Benefits in Nutraceutical Applications. *Mar. Drugs* **2025**, *23*, 60. [CrossRef] [PubMed]
76. Kolsi, R.B.A.; Ben Salah, H.; Jardak, N.; Chaaben, R.; El Feki, A.; Rebai, T.; Jamoussi, K.; Allouche, N.; Belghith, H.; Belghith, K. Effects of *Cymodocea nodosa* extract on metabolic disorders and oxidative stress in alloxan-diabetic rats. *Biomed. Pharmacother.* **2017**, *89*, 257–267. [CrossRef]
77. Chaabani, E.; Mgaidi, S.; Ben Abdennebi, A.; Dakhlaoui, S.; Hammami, M.; Selmi, S.; Zariat, M.; Shili, A.; Merah, O.; Bettaieb Rebey, I. Enhancing Antioxidant Activity from Aquatic Plant *Cymodocea nodosa* for Cosmetic Formulation Through Optimized Ultrasound-Assisted Extraction Using Response Surface Methodology. *Cosmetics* **2024**, *11*, 186. [CrossRef]
78. Kim, J.H.; Cho, Y.H.; Park, S.M.; Lee, K.E.; Lee, J.J.; Lee, B.C.; Pyo, H.B.; Song, K.S.; Park, H.D.; Yun, Y.P. Antioxidants and inhibitor of matrix metalloproteinase-1 expression from leaves of *Zostera marina* L. *Arch. Pharmacal Res.* **2004**, *27*, 177–183. [CrossRef]
79. Feng, C.; Chen, X.; Yin, X.; Jiang, Y.; Zhao, C. Matrix Metalloproteinases on Skin Photoaging. *J. Cosmet. Dermatol.* **2024**, *23*, 3847–3862. [CrossRef]
80. Khasina, E.I.; Kolenchenko, E.A.; Sgrebneva, M.N.; Kovalev, V.V.; Khotimchenko, Y.S. Antioxidant Activities of a Low Etherified Pectin from the Seagrass *Zostera marina*. *Russ. J. Mar. Biol.* **2003**, *29*, 259–261. [CrossRef]
81. Kolenchenko, E.A.; Sonina, L.N.; Khotimchenko, Y.S. Comparative in vitro Assessment of Antioxidant Activities of Low-Etherified Pectin from the Eelgrass *Zostera marina* and Antioxidative Medicines. *Russ. J. Mar. Biol.* **2005**, *31*, 331–334. [CrossRef]
82. Choi, H.G.; Lee, J.H.; Park, H.H.; Sayegh, F. Antioxidant and Antimicrobial Activity of *Zostera marina* L. Extract. *Algae* **2009**, *24*, 179–184. [CrossRef]
83. Kim, M.J.; Bae, N.Y.; Kim, K.B.W.R.; Park, J.H.; Park, S.H.; Cho, Y.J.; Ahn, D.H. Anti-inflammatory Effect of *Zostera marina* Ethanolic Extract on LPS-induced RAW264.7 Cells and Mouse Model. *KSBB J.* **2015**, *30*, 182–190. [CrossRef]
84. Custódio, L.; Laukaityte, S.; Engelen, A.H.; Rodrigues, M.J.; Pereira, H.; Vizetto-Duarte, C.; Barreira, L.; Rodríguez, H.; Albericio, F.; Varela, J. A Comparative Evaluation of Biological Activities and Bioactive Compounds of the Seagrasses *Zostera marina* and Zostera Noltei from Southern Portugal. *Nat. Prod. Res.* **2015**, *30*, 724–728. [CrossRef] [PubMed]
85. Ribas-Taberner, M.d.M.; Mir-Rossello, P.M.; Gil, L.; Sureda, A.; Capó, X. Potential Use of Marine Plants as a Source of Bioactive Compounds. *Molecules* **2025**, *30*, 485. [CrossRef]
86. Fernandes, P.A.R.; Coimbra, M.A. The antioxidant activity of polysaccharides: A structure-function relationship overview. *Carbohydr. Polym.* **2023**, *314*, 120965. [CrossRef] [PubMed]

MDPI AG
Grosspeteranlage 5
4052 Basel
Switzerland
Tel.: +41 61 683 77 34

Marine Drugs Editorial Office
E-mail: marinedrugs@mdpi.com
www.mdpi.com/journal/marinedrugs

www.ingramcontent.com/pod-product-compliance
Lightning Source LLC
Chambersburg PA
CBHW040816250926
51850CB00007BA/1182